NEUROLOGICAL INVESTIGATIONS

NEUROLOGICAL INVESTIGATIONS

Edited by

R A C Hughes

Professor of Neurology, UMDS, Guy's Hospital, London

BMJ
Publishing
Group

First published in 1997
by the BMJ Publishing Group, BMA House, Tavistock Square, London WC1H 9JR

British Library Cataloguing in Publication Data

A catalogue record for this book is available from the British Library

ISBN 0-7279-1080-9

Typeset by Thanet Press Limited, Margate, Kent
Printed and bound by Graphy Cems, Navarra, Spain

Contents

Contributors

J F Acheson
Consultant Ophthalmologist
Department of Neuro-Ophthalmology, The National Hospital for Neurology and Neurosurgery, London, UK

C D Binnie
Professor of Clinical Neurophysiology
Department of Clinical Neurophysiology, King's College Hospital, London, UK

A M Bronstein
2nd Hon Consultant Neurologist, Consultant Clinical Scientist
MRC Human Movement and Balance Unit,
The National Hospital for Neurology and Neurosurgery, London, UK

Lisa Cipolotti
Consultant Neuropsychologist
Psychology Department, The National Hospital for Neurology and Neurosurgery, London, UK

M Czosnyka
Senior Research Assistant
MRC Centre for Brain Repair and Academic Neurosurgical Unit, Addenbrooke's Hospital, Cambridge, UK

Clare J Fowler
Consultant in Uro-Neurology
Department of Uro-Neurology, The National Hospital for Neurology and Neurosurgery, London, UK

R A C Hughes
Professor of Neurology
UMDS, Guy's Hospital, London, UK

C Kennard
Professor of Clinical Neurology
Department of Clinical Neurosciences, Charing Cross Hospital, London, UK

CONTRIBUTORS

P J Kirkpatrick
Lecturer and Consultant in Neurosurgery
MRC Cambridge Centre for Brain Repair and Academic
Neurosurgical Unit, Addenbrooke's Hospital, Cambridge, UK

N G Laing
Assistant Professor
Australian Neuromuscular Research Institute, University Department
of Medicine and Pathology and Department of Neurology and Clinical
Neurophysiology, Queen Elizabeth II Medical Centre, Perth, Australia

Christian J Lueck
Consultant Neurologist
Department of Clinical Neurosciences, Western General Hospital,
Edinburgh, UK

J G McLeod
Bushell Professor of Neurology and Bosch Professor of Medicine
The University of Sydney Department of Medicine, Sydney, Australia

F L Mastaglia
Professor of Neurology
Australian Neuromuscular Research Institute, University Department
of Medicine and Pathology and Department of Neurology and Clinical
Neurophysiology, Queen Elizabeth II Medical Centre, Perth, Australia

Ivan Moseley
Consultant Radiologist and Director
Lysholm Department of Radiology, The National Hospital for
Neurology and Neurosurgery, London, and Department of Radiology,
Moorfields Eye Hospital, London, UK

E O'Sullivan
Research Fellow
Department of Clinical Neurosciences, Charing Cross Hospital,
London, UK

J D Pickard
Professor of Neurosurgery
MRC Cambridge Centre for Brain Repair and Academic Neurosurgical
Unit, Addenbrook's Hospital, Cambridge, UK

P F Prior
Consultant Clinical Neurophysiologist
Department of Clinical Neurophysiology, St Bartholomew's Hospital, London, UK

P Rudge
Consultant Neurologist
The National Hospital for Neurology and Neurosurgery, London, UK

M D Sanders
Consultant Ophthalmologist
Department of Neuro-Ophthalmology, The National Hospital for Neurology and Neurosurgery, London, UK

Guy V Sawle
Consultant Neurologist
Division of Clinical Neurology, Queen's Medical Centre, Nottingham, UK

R J Sellar
Consultant Neuroradiologist
Department of Neuroradiology, Western General Hospital, Edinburgh, UK

S Shaunak
Research Fellow
Department of Clinical Neurosciences, Charing Cross Hospital, London, UK

John M Stevens
Consultant Neuroradiologist
MRI Unit, St Mary's Hospital, London, UK

Phillip D Swanson
Professor of Neurology,
Department of Neurology, University of Washington School of Medicine, Seattle, USA

E J Thompson
Professor of Neurochemistry
The National Hospital for Neurology and Neurosurgery, London, UK

Elizabeth K Warrington
Professor of Psychology
Psychology Department, The National Hospital for Neurology and Neurosurgery, London, UK

Introduction

Neurology will always reign pre-eminent as the medical specialty in which the clinical skills of history taking, observation of physical signs, pattern recognition, and deduction play the most important part in diagnosis. This book illuminates aspects of the clinical history taking and examination which perplex even experienced neurologists, especially testing higher cerebral function, the visual system, eye movements, and balance. However, most of the book is devoted to an explanation of the investigations with which the mechanisms and causes of many major neurological diseases have been and are being so excitingly revealed. This includes most of the important and interesting aspects of neurological investigation from the mysteries of the electroencephalogram to modern techniques of examining the CSF. Four chapters explain and illustrate the best methods for imaging the brain and spinal cord and their blood vessels. Clear guidelines are set out for the investigation of neurogenic bladder, peripheral neuropathy, muscle disease, and metabolic disorders. For the neurosurgeon as well as the neurologist there is an explanation of multimodal monitoring of the brain during coma. Each chapter should encourage a careful planned approach to investigation with minimum discomfort, time, and cost. We recruited a panel of international experts to take on this task. Each chapter was subjected to the peer review process and published in the *Journal of Neurology, Neurosurgery, and Psychiatry* during 1995–6.

This is the third in the series of *Journal of Neurology, Neurosurgery, and Psychiatry* books. The first two, *Neurological Emergencies*, and *The Management of Neurological Disorders*, destroyed any lingering myth that neurology is a specialty which is strong on diagnosis, weak on treatment. This book provides the comprehensive guide needed by all who look after neurological disease, especially neurologists, neurosurgeons, and psychiatrists, whether trainee or consultant, to provide a sound diagnostic basis for practice and research.

R A C Hughes
March 1996

1 Electroencephalography

C D BINNIE, P F PRIOR

Genesis of the electroencephalogram

The electroencephalogram (EEG) is a recording of cerebral electrical potentials by electrodes on the scalp. Cerebral electrical activity includes action potentials that are brief and produce circumscribed electrical fields, and slower, more widespread, postsynaptic potentials. The magnitude of the signal recorded from a neural generator depends on the solid angle subtended at the electrode. Consequently, the activity of a single neuron can be recorded by an adjacent microelectrode, but not at a distant scalp electrode. Synchronous activity in a horizontal laminar aggregate of neurons with parallel orientation may, however, constitute a generator of sufficient extent to be detectable on the scalp. Thus the EEG is a spatiotemporal average of synchronous postsynaptic potentials arising in radially oriented pyramidal cells in cortical gyri over the cerebral convexity. It is estimated that the smallest detectable generator has an extent of some 6 cm.[2] Tangentially oriented generators in the walls of sulci do not generally appear in the EEG, but are seen in recordings of the brain's magnetic field (magnetoencephalogram or MEG).[1]

Synchronous neuronal activity arises by various mechanisms. Isolated aggregates of interconnected neurons spontaneously adopt rhythmic synchronous firing patterns. Afferents, for instance, from the reticular formation, stimulate individual neurons into independent asynchronous activity. Thus synchrony is

1

reduced by arousal and cognitive activity and increases with reduced vigilance, both in normal sleep and in pathological states, reflected in the EEG by increased amplitude and slowing. Specific pacemakers also exist that produce rhythmic synchronous activity.[2] There is, for example, an inhibitory feedback loop involving thalamocortical neurons which produces oscillatory burst firing in drowsiness and sleep. Transitory synchronous activity can be elicited by afferent stimuli (evoked potentials), spontaneous arousal (producing such phenomena as vertex sharp transients in light sleep), and pathological neuronal discharges in epilepsy.

Interpretative principles

Abnormalities on the EEG reflect general pathological processes and are rarely of specific diagnostic significance. Thus slowing may arise from causes as diverse as cerebral oedema or hypoxia, or systemic disorders such as hepatic insufficiency. The most reliable abnormal EEG sign is reduction of normal activity, ranging from reduced amplitude over a past cerebral infarct or a subdural haematoma, to electrocerebral silence in brain death. Spiky waveforms (epileptiform activity) occur in epilepsy and in some patients with cerebral disorder but without seizures. Rhythmic slow activities may occur bilaterally over the frontal or posterior temporal regions in patients with dysfunction of diencephalic or brainstem structures.

The EEG is profoundly influenced by alterations in vigilance and it also changes with age, most noticeably during childhood. Interpretation must take account of the range of normal findings at different ages and in different states of awareness. The slower components diminish with maturation and increase in sleep and drowsiness. As slowing is a common EEG abnormality, it may be difficult to distinguish the effects of immaturity, drowsiness, and pathology. This similarity between the immature and the abnormal EEG underlies an interesting approach to quantitative clinical EEG analysis by Matoušek and Petersén.[3] They developed a method of computing the subject's apparent age from spectral features and used the ratio of calculated to actual age as a measure of EEG abnormality.

Electroencephalography technology

Developments

Traditionally EEGs were written on electromechanical chart recorders; these are now being replaced by digital systems, which offer improved reliability and compact, accessible archives on optical discs. Within a few years clinical neurophysiology laboratories will be based on a local computer network, probably with generic data acquisition stations for recording EEG, EMG, and evoked potentials directly on to a file server, and workstations for reviewing the data and entering reports to form an integrated archive with the original signals.

These innovations have done little to reduce the inherent technological difficulties of obtaining satisfactory recordings of the EEG which, having an amplitude of only some 5 to 200 μV, is very susceptible to artifacts, from both bioelectric and physical sources. The problems can be largely overcome by good electrode technique, but this is particularly difficult to achieve in children and in others who may be distressed and uncooperative. Methods of constructing electrodes have changed little in recent decades, but a significant advance has been the development of improved adhesive pastes, which achieve secure electrode fixation and a low contact resistance without abrasion of the skin—an important consideration given current concerns with avoidance of cross infection.

Changes in vigilance may affect the occurrence of pathological phenomena; particularly in epilepsy, clinically relevant abnormalities may be found in sleep but not in wakefulness. Sleep recording is generally underused and is not routinely available in many departments.

Epilepsy monitoring

Arguably the most important recent development in epileptology has been long term EEG and video monitoring (see Binnie[4] and Gotman *et al*[5] for reviews). As the manifestations of epilepsy are intermittent, a routine EEG often fails to show epileptiform activity, which may occur only during seizures. Moreover, interictal epileptiform activity may be of doubtful clinical value, either for identifying the site of onset of seizures or for determining whether particular clinical events are epileptic.

3

The EEG can be telemetered over days through a cable or radio link, permitting limited mobility in hospital, while behaviour is documented by video. Alternatively, ambulatory monitoring can be carried out in an everyday environment with a portable cassette recorder, but behavioural documentation will be less reliable, depending on reports of carers. These technologies have different applications; telemetry is generally preferred, unless it is essential to record in a particular environment.

Brain mapping

A technical development that has generated recent enthusiasm is brain electrical activity mapping. Computer assisted EEG analysis has been used in research for more than 30 years, but has few clinical uses beyond monitoring (during surgery and intensive care and in metabolic disorders) and for automatic seizure detection during telemetry. Quantitative EEG information may be displayed topographically on a stylised head outline.[6-8] With development of personal computers these facilities have become commercially available and widely promoted for clinical use. The colourful displays invite comparison with neuroimaging, misleadingly, as EEG topography does not bear a simple relation to pathology. Artifacts are readily overlooked or generated in the process of analysis and mapping. Brain mapping extends expert analysis of the primary data,[9] and may highlight features which are difficult to detect,[10 11] but its general clinical utility has yet to be established and its promotion as a substitute for conventional EEG can only be deplored.[12 13]

Cerebral lesions

Electroencephalography provides information that primarily concerns disturbances of function rather than structure. Whereas clinical studies in the 1930s showed localised changes at the site of cerebral mass lesions, routine referral for EEGs on suspicion of intracranial tumour is no longer appropriate. Modern imaging techniques, although somewhat more costly, provide more precise identification of the presence, nature, and site of such lesions. It should also be noted that in this context the value of a negative EEG in excluding pathology may be somewhat illusory. The normal EEG does not exclude intracranial disorders; a more appropriate approach to the investigation is to recognise the relevance of EEGs with positive findings. The EEG only plays a relevant part when patients cannot, for various reasons, undergo scanning or when potential epileptogenicity,[14] possible postoperative recurrence of a tumour, or toxic effects of medical oncological drugs versus metastatic disease require evaluation. In these situations, clinical value accrues in the evolution of changes over serial recordings.

Vascular lesions may be more rewarding to investigate than tumours. The changes after a cerebral infarct will be most characteristic in the first hours and days, before those on CT become evident. Typically the appearances are of a localised reduction of normal cortical rhythms and a major surrounding slow wave abnormality with individual waves of less than 1 Hz. There is often a rapid evolution of the EEG abnormality that may resolve before the scan becomes positive.

Prognostic assessment of CT negative patients with transient or mild ischaemia depends on subtle abnormalities evident only when quantitative EEG techniques are used. These utilise computer analysis of the EEG frequency spectrum. A sensitivity of 50–70% and a specificity of 90–100% have been reported.[15-17] The topic is thoroughly reviewed by van Huffelen,[18] who also reminds us of the value of quantitative EEG techniques and somatosensory evoked potentials in monitoring patients at risk of cerebrovascular accidents during carotid[19 20] or open heart surgery.

Head injury is another condition where the detection of lesions by EEG has been rightly superseded by imaging, although its use for prognostication during coma has increased.[21 22] Quantitative methods, as with ischaemic lesions, can distinguish patients after mild head trauma from controls.[23]

Two groups of EEG phenomena in patients with cerebral lesions—periodic events and projected rhythms—sometimes cause confusion. The fascinating and distinctive range of periodic EEG phenomena merits particular attention. Periodic lateralised epileptiform discharges (PLEDs; figure 1.1) are acute, self limiting features with a repetition rate of 3–7 per 10 second period that reflect a sudden disturbance of blood supply at or near the cortex or cortical white matter junction.[24] They occur in obtunded patients, varying with fluctuations in consciousness, tending to decrease when the patient is alerted. The PLEDs are not specific to any particular disease (but confirm that local pathology is present),

5

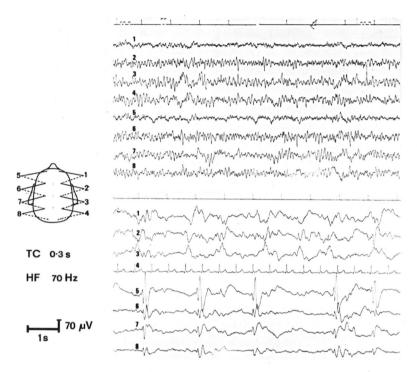

Figure 1.1   *Periodic lateralised epileptiform discharges (PLEDs): two samples of recording in a woman of 63 years being treated for lymphoma who developed a confusional state with loss of memory and a single grand mal fit two weeks before the upper sample. This showed bilateral slow waves underlying the faster cortical rhythms. The second sample three weeks later was four days after onset of left hemiparesis and right sided Jacksonian seizures starting in her right foot. It shows a clear asymmetry with repetitive complexes at irregular intervals over the left hemisphere with some lower voltage spread to the right. These periodic discharges had virtually disappeared at follow up two days later. An astrocytoma was found, extending from the right hemisphere via the corpus callosum to the left hemisphere*

being seen with—for example, extracerebral haematomas, metastases, infarcts, infections. They run a one to two week course, disappearing even when the underlying lesion is progressive. Although described as epileptiform, any focal clinical events may be subtle and transient. The PLEDs may be bilateral—for exam-

6

ple, in herpes simplex encephalitis when they evolve with different periodicity over each temporal lobe. They appear, often unilaterally, on the second or third day of the illness, and become evident contralaterally by the next day. The independent timing or repetition rate of the PLEDs over each hemisphere is an important diagnostic feature in herpes simplex encephalitis, implying separate localised areas of pathology arising in the temporal lobes rather than a generalised encephalitic disorder. If PLEDs arise elsewhere—for example, in frontal or parietal regions—they should be interpreted with caution: most patients turn out to have other disease. The EEG in herpes simplex encephalitis shows a parallel, progressive, loss of normal cortical rhythms and may show prolonged seizure discharges waxing and waning over one or other temporal lobe, with or without clinical accompaniment. With antiviral agents, PLEDs can resolve rapidly; it is thus important to consider the value of an emergency EEG to establish the likely diagnosis at an early stage before antibody titres become available.

Generalised periodic discharges in the EEG occur in subacute sclerosing panencephalitis in children and teenagers and in Creutzfeldt-Jakob disease in the middle aged. In subacute sclerosing panencephalitis the discharges may be subtle initially and consist of simultaneous bilateral complexes of slow and faster components, each stereotyped morphologically in a particular region, repeating at about 10–20 second intervals. By contrast, those of Creutzfeldt-Jakob disease occur at about 1–2 second intervals and are more likely to be confused with ECG pickup on the scalp. In both conditions there is a gradual loss of cortical rhythms until the repetitive complexes appear on a near silent background. Periodic EEG complexes have not been found in Kuru; they were also absent in the 46 patients with progressive dementia and myoclonus considered as possible Creutzfeldt-Jakob disease but in whom neither transmissibility nor prion protein could be demonstrated.[25] Similarly, in Gerstmann-Sträussler-Scheinker disease periodic complexes are limited to patients with clinical manifestations resembling Creutzfeldt-Jakob disease.[26] Although associated with spectacular EEG changes at a fairly early stage (often before the conditions have been considered diagnostic possibilities), Creutzfeldt-Jakob disease and subacute sclerosing panencephalitis are rarities. More common causes for generalised periodic EEG features are mentioned with the systemic disorders.

7

The projected rhythms or so called "rhythms at a distance" are another potential cause of confusion when assessing EEG reports. As already described, cortical rhythms are generated locally but modulated by deeper pacemakers at both thalamic and brainstem reticular activatating system levels. Lesions or biochemical dysfunction in subcortical structures may produce projected effects on the EEG via thalamocortical and other pathways. Two forms of projected abnormality are commonly encountered and have somewhat different mechanisms.

The first is the paradoxical slow wave arousal response[27] in which a noxious stimulus in a lightly or moderately comatose patient produces a massive and prolonged run of slow delta activity starting at less than 1 Hz and gradually increasing in frequency. It may last for several minutes and be accompanied by tachycardia, tachypnoea, increase in arterial blood, and intracranial pressures and motor activity ranging from a few muscle potentials on the ECG or EEG tracing to a massive extensor decerebrate response. It represents an abnormal arousal response, most commonly due to dysfunction or damage to the brainstem reticular activiting pathways. It is common in young people comatose in the first week after head injury and, although it indicates a reason for slow awakening from coma, it does not necessarily carry a poor prognosis.

The second type of projected slow wave abnormality, frontal intermittent rhythmic delta activity (FIRDA), and its occipital counterpart (generally confined to childhood or the early teens), are rhythmic bursts of bilaterally synchronous delta waves at 2 Hz which are attenuated on alerting the patient or on eye opening to command. They occur in metabolic or toxic disturbances and also with intracranial lesions involving or compressing subcortical structures.

The metabolic causes of FIRDA may be as benign as the typical response to routine "voluntary" hyperventilation in the healthy young subject during EEGs or reflect, for example, a serious disturbance of calcium or glucose metabolism. A typical toxic cause for this EEG pattern is phenytoin toxicity.

Intracranial lesions producing FIRDA include subdural haematomas, carotid occlusion, frontal or subfrontal or callosal "butterfly" tumours, thalamic lesions, and basal infiltrations or exudates (for example, tuberculous meningitis). Evolution may be complex from lateralised or asymmetric, to symmetric, then contralateral as, for example, a butterfly tumour grows across the midline.

Distinguishing between intracranial lesions and encephalopathies when FIRDA presents the main EEG abnormality rests on careful inspection of both the delta bursts and the background on which they appear.

Epilepsy

Pathophysiology

Epilepsy is characterised by excessive and hypersynchronous neuronal activity. Synchronous activity in a small neuronal aggregate at the onset of a partial seizure is often of high frequency (12–70 Hz) and may be recordable only by depth electrodes.[28] As larger populations are recruited, slower, rhythmic, spiky activity appears more widely, often showing a progressive increase in amplitude and diminution of frequency, and may be detected with EEG electrodes on the scalp. In generalised seizures, or after propagation of those of focal origin, normal thalamocortical oscillatory burst firing mechanisms[29] may be entrained, producing repetitive spike wave activity,[30] recordable both over the cortex and in the thalamus. The spikes correspond to burst firing, the slow waves to periods of reduced neuronal activity due to hyperpolarisation of thalamocortical cells.

In the interictal state similar activities may briefly occur. Apart from generalised spike and wave activity, however, interictal discharges are generally slower and of greater amplitude than early ictal events. Interictal EEGs of patients with temporal lobe epilepsy thus typically show discrete anterior temporal spikes and sharp waves, unlike the faster, rhythmic activities at seizure onset.

Electrophysiological findings have contributed importantly to theoretical concepts and classifications of epilepsies and seizures, supporting for instance the central distinction between localised and generalised corticoreticular epileptogenesis.[31][32] Indeed the main clinical application of the EEG in epilepsy is for classification. It is, for instance, of practical use to distinguish the focal discharges of partial epilepsy from generalised epileptiform activity. As focal ictal and interictal events can undergo rapid propagation leading to secondarily generalised discharges and seizures, it is important to identify possible focal elements at the onset of a gen-

9

eralised discharge. The EEG also contributes to classification by detecting abnormalities of ongoing activity due to cerebral pathology, focal slowing, or asymmetries of normal activity in symptomatic partial epilepsy, and generalised abnormalities in symptomatic generalised epilepsy.

Spikes, sharp waves, and spike and wave activity are seen in some patients with cerebral disorders without epilepsy. There is no agreed name for this class of EEG phenomena; the phrase, "epileptiform activity", used here, acknowledges the association with epilepsy underlying the concept, while stressing that the term refers to the waveform, not its clinical correlates. Various sharp or episodic transients occur in normal subjects and are a source of misunderstanding. They are recognisable by characteristic waveform, topography, and circumstances of occurrence and should not be mistaken for phenomena supporting a diagnosis of epilepsy.[33][34] Most often misinterpreted are 6 and 14 per second positive spikes, rhythmic bursts which, unlike most epileptiform activity, are electropositive at the site where they are of greatest amplitude. They occur in many adolescents and young adults during drowsiness and light sleep and are not associated with epilepsy. Other non-epileptic spiky or episodic phenomena include benign epileptiform transients of sleep (short sharp spikes), rhythmic midtemporal discharge (formerly misleadingly termed psychomotor variant), and the bifrontal slow activity seen on hyperventilation in normal children, which too often is wrongly interpreted as evidence of epilepsy.

Diagnostic strategies

Such interpretative errors contribute to confusion about the sensitivity, specificity, and general utility of the EEG (boxes 1.1 and 1.2). Most routine EEGs are interictal and attention focuses chiefly on epileptiform activity. The EEGs of people with epilepsy show considerable spontaneous variation and may exhibit interictal discharges on one occasion and not on another. Serial studies indicate that only one third of patients with epilepsy consistently exhibit discharges in the interictal, waking state; one sixth never do so; in the remaining half the picture varies, with a probability of about one in three of epileptiform activity in any 30 minute waking record.[35] Drowsiness and sleep increase the probability of finding discharges, particularly in partial epilepsies.

These considerations suggest strategies for EEG investigation of epilepsy. Possibly as routine, certainly if an initial waking record shows no epileptiform activity, a sleep tracing should be obtained. The combination of a waking and sleep EEG shows epileptiform activity in 80% of adults with epilepsy and in a larger proportion of children. With repeated waking and sleep records the number approaches 92%.[36] If the interictal EEG is persistently negative and a clinical problem exists that may be resolved by EEG evidence, an ictal recording may be obtained by telemetry, provided that the seizures occur often enough to be captured within a reasonable period.

Regarding specificity of epileptiform activity to epilepsy, estimates of false positives are inflated by misinterpretation of the non-epileptic transients noted earlier. In neurologically screened adults the prevalence of rigorously defined epileptiform activity is some 3/1000[37 38]; comparable data for children are not available but the prevalence is probably higher. However, clinical EEG investigations are performed, not in normal subjects, but in patients with symptoms of possible cerebral origin. Here the incidence of EEG abnormalities, including epileptiform activity is much greater.[39] Overall 10% of patients who have undergone intracranial surgery and 3% of psychiatric patients without epilepsy exhibit epileptiform EEG activity.[40] The interpretation of a record containing spikes depends therefore on the clinical context. This finding, in a patient with mental handicap or a cerebral tumour, contributes little to the diagnosis of epilepsy. Conversely, the finding of epileptiform discharges in a patient with episodic symptoms and without evidence of cerebral pathology shifts the balance of probability in favour of epilepsy.

Owing in part to spontaneous variation of the EEG, a close relation is rarely found between the amount of epileptiform activity in routine records and current seizure frequency or response to medication. Repeated EEGs are, however, requested in the belief that they are of value for monitoring clinical progress.[41] Similarly, the EEG is of little value for deciding when to terminate medication in adults who have become seizure free[42] except in so far as it reflects different syndromes with different prognoses. In children, however, persistent epileptiform activity indicates a high probability of relapse.[43 44]

11

Box 1.1   Misconceptions about the EEG in epilepsy

It is not in general true that:
● The interictal EEG can:
  Prove the diagnosis of epilepsy
  Exclude epilepsy
● An ictal EEG almost always shows:
  Epileptiform activity
● EEG abnormality reflects severity as manifest by:
  Seizure frequency
  Therapeutic response to antiepileptic drugs
  Prognosis

Activation procedures

The importance of EEG activation by sleep has already been noted. Spontaneous sleep can often be achieved by a restful recording environment and a relaxed approach. Sleep can also be induced by medication or by prior deprivation of sleep. Sedative drugs modify the EEG, producing increased fast activity, but this is no disadvantage as it may highlight any local reduction of fast activity reflecting underlying pathology. Sleep deprivation increases seizure liability but there is little evidence that it specifically activates the EEG except by promoting sleep.[45] It is usually more convenient to induce sleep by medication than by sleep deprivation.

Two other activation procedures are routinely used: hyperventilation and photic stimulation. Three minutes of vigorous overbreathing induces a seizure accompanied by spike and wave activity in patients with absences, so consistently that the lack of such a response virtually excludes uncontrolled absence epilepsy (but not other epilepsies).[46] Other types of EEG abnormalities and seizures are less consistently provoked.

Rhythmic photic stimulation elicits generalised, self sustaining epileptiform discharges in some 5% of people with epilepsy, particularly in those with idiopathic syndromes, notably juvenile myoclonic epilepsy.[47 48] Photosensitivity is of practical importance:

Box 1.2   Utility of EEG in epilepsy

The interictal EEG is of value to:
- Support diagnosis if other cerebral disease can be excluded
- Exclude or identify specific epilepsy syndromes
- Classify epilepsies and syndromes
- Detect or confirm photosensitivity
- Detect non-convulsive status epilepticus
- Detect antiepileptic drug intoxication
- Detect possible epileptogenic lesion
- Monitor status epilepticus
- Locate epileptogenic zone in preoperative assessment by ictal recording

Ictal recording, by long term monitoring if necessary, is of value to:
- Distinguish epileptic from non-epileptic attacks
- Classify seizures
- Determine incidence of frequent minor seizures
- Detect subtle seizures causing transient cognitive impairment
- Identify seizure precipitants including self induction

---

most photosensitive subjects found in clinical EEG practice have epilepsy[49] and have seizures induced by environmental visual stimuli such as television and flickering sunlight. In about 50% it seems that no spontaneous seizures occur, all attacks being visually induced.[47 50] Avoidance of precipitating stimuli rather than medication is an important therapeutic option.

Monitoring

Long term monitoring is most used for differential diagnosis of epileptic and non-epileptic attacks.[51 52] The presence of ictal EEG changes will generally confirm the epileptic nature of an event (as cardiogenic seizures also produce EEG changes, simultaneous ECG monitoring may be necessary[53]). However, interpretation of a negative ictal EEG may be difficult. Abnormal activity in small or deep neuronal populations may not be reflected in the EEG, or may produce only minor changes in ongoing rhythms. Various different seizure types are consistent in this respect. Absences, for instance, are accompanied by spike-and-wave activity; a staring attack without this cannot be an absence. The EEG signatures of

13

some seizure types are usually not epileptiform: low amplitude fast activity occurs during tonic seizures, an electrodecremental event during an infantile spasm, or an atonic seizure, and bitemporal theta activity during many complex partial seizures. Simple partial seizures, particularly with psychic or viscerosensory symptoms, often produce no EEG change.[54] Interpretation of an apparently negative ictal EEG thus depends on the nature of the seizure and coregistration of the EEG and behaviour to facilitate detection of minimal EEG changes.

Close comparison of the EEG with behaviour may also show subtle ictal events, or show these to be more frequent than supposed.[55 56] Thus a momentary arrest of activity may be identified as ictal because of consistent accompanying EEG change. Conversely, seemingly interictal EEG discharges may be shown to be accompanied by subtle clinical events. If no changes are evident during unconstrained behaviour, transitory cognitive impairment may be shown by more structured tasks, including formal psychological testing.[57] This is a possibility to be considered in any patient with frequent EEG discharges and unexplained cognitive difficulties.

Ictal recording, sometimes with foramen ovale,[58] subdural, or depth electrodes,[59-61] forms an important component of preoperative assessment as an aid to identifying the site of seizure onset. Here too, simultaneous behavioural monitoring is essential, as electrographic localisation of seizure onset cannot be claimed if clinical events precede the first detected electrical changes.

Ambulatory monitoring without video documentation of behaviour is not a substitute for telemetry in detecting minor seizures, locating ictal onset, or deciding whether subtle events are epileptic. It is, however, the preferred method for investigating a known EEG phenomenon in a particular setting—for instance, to determine the frequency of absence seizures at school.

Psychiatry

Ironically, although the human EEG was discovered by a psychiatrist, and many pioneering EEG laboratories were in psychiatric hospitals, the contribution of the EEG to psychiatry has proved disappointing. Quantitative EEG analysis (and particularly cognitive evoked potentials) tantalisingly show group differences between patients with various psychiatric disorders, their relatives, and control populations. These features generally fall within the range of normal variation, are difficult to detect except by computer assisted analysis, and have no diagnostic value in the individual patient.

Psychoses

In the functional psychoses there may be group EEG differences from controls or changes with clinical state. Amount and frequency of alpha activity are decreased in depression and increased in mania.[62-64] There is generally a raised incidence of non-specific EEG abnormalities in bipolar affective disorder.[65] Schizophrenic patients typically exhibit low amplitude irregular EEGs, aptly described as "choppy" by Davis,[66] but these too fall within normal limits resembling records of anxious, healthy subjects. Findings of positive diagnostic value by EEG are confined to those psychiatric syndromes with an overtly organic basis.

Confusional states

Delirium can be distinguished from psychoses presenting with disturbance of consciousness (for example, mania, acute schizophrenia, and puerperal psychosis) by the finding of EEG abnormalities, which increase with clinical deterioration (box 1.3). In organic confusional states the EEG typically shows progressive slowing: firstly, reduced alpha frequency, then increasing theta and loss of alpha and beta activity, then diffuse or bifrontal delta

---

Box 1.3   EEG in acute delirium

- *Slowing:* consider – infective, toxic or metabolic cause, including drug overdose
- *Excess fast activity:* delirium tremens or tranquilliser overdose
- *Continuous epileptiform activity:* non-convulsive status epilepticus (confirm by EEG response to intravenous diazepam)
- *Unexplained intermittent epileptiform activity especially with photosensitivity:* drug or alcohol withdrawal.
- *Normal:* psychiatric cause most likely but repeat EEG if condition deteriorates

---

activity with onset of coma. The differential diagnosis includes toxic and metabolic disorders (notably hypocalcaemia and hypercalcaemia, hepatic encephalopathy, metabolic alkalosis, and water intoxication—which may occur in schizophrenia), overdosage with psychotropic drugs, and meningitis. Widespread excessive fast activity occurs in delirium tremens[67] and benzodiazepine or barbiturate intoxication. Epileptiform activity, generalised or focal, appears virtually continuously in non-convulsive status epilepticus, and intermittently, often in association with photosensitivity, after acute withdrawal of barbiturates, alcohol, or benzodiazepines.

Dementia

The commonest organic differential diagnosis in old age psychiatry is between the vascular and various non-vascular dementias, and the commonest organic and functional differential diagnosis is between the various dementias and depressive pseudodementia. A normal EEG is compatible with any dementia, especially early in the condition and serial recording is therefore often required. In Alzheimer's disease,[68 69] there is early decrease in alpha frequency and amplitude; later generalised irregular slow activity appears with a frontal emphasis and fast activity disappears. Serial quantitative EEG studies show a high correlation between the degree of dementia and theta power and mean frequency.[70] Focal EEG changes, with or without generalised slowing, suggest either multi-infarct dementia[71] or normal pressure hydrocephalus.[72]

Among the less common dementias, Huntington's chorea is characterised by a tracing of conspicuously low amplitude; this is of little clinical value, being rarely seen in atypical or early cases.[73 74] Changes in the EEG are uncommon and mild in alcoholic dementia[75] and in Pick's disease,[76 77] contrasting with the severe clinical picture. In the course of Creutzfeldt-Jakob disease, diffuse or focal slowing develops, with characteristic stereotyped, bilaterally synchronous sharp waves. Regular slow triphasic bursts on slow background activity usually appear at advanced stages.[77] Serial recordings when awake and sleeping may be required to detect these but it is claimed that if periodic discharges have not appeared within 10 weeks a diagnosis other than Creutzfeldt-Jakob disease is unlikely.[78] Later the record consists of diffuse slow activity of progressively diminishing amplitude.[79]

Cerebral tumour and psychiatry

Before the advent of neuroimaging the yield of unsuspected cerebral tumours from routine EEGs in psychiatric hospitals was about 1%.[80] Abnormal findings were not uncommon but mostly mild, non-specific, and often inexplicable (possibly iatrogenic), rarely providing evidence of localised structural abnormality. Now, with appropriate use of CT, the contribution of EEG to the detection of lesions underlying psychiatric symptoms should be negligible. However, meningiomata are over represented in psychiatric patients and often present with epilepsy; occasionally EEG investigation of a patient with atypical auditory or olfactory hallucinations with absent or atypical psychotic symptoms will lead to the detection of a tumour.

Post-traumatic syndromes

A range of psychological disabilities and psychiatric conditions occurs after head injury, particularly in cases of post-traumatic epilepsy.[81] Late EEG changes are not closely related to the chronic psychiatric morbidity after head injury. After brain injury the affected neurons either die or recover and the EEG then becomes normal apart from possible amplitude reduction or changes related to epilepsy. Paradoxically, a normal EEG is an adverse sign: post-traumatic symptoms that remain after the EEG returns to normal are likely to persist.[82]

Epilepsy and psychiatry

Preictal or postictal EEG changes may elucidate the relation between seizures and psychiatric symptoms in patients with psychoses associated with epilepsy. Rarely, the finding of epileptiform activity establishes unrecognised epilepsy as a cause of psychiatric symptomatology—for instance, in the Landau-Kleffner syndrome. There are often requests for EEGs to investigate epilepsy as a possible cause of episodic behavioural disturbances in mentally handicapped children, or of hallucinosis in patients likely to be psychotic. Such investigations rarely serve any useful purpose unless performed during the behaviour in question, and in any event the yield of diagnostically useful information is small.

17

Sleep

The EEG is probably the most sensitive measure available for detecting changes in alertness. It changes profoundly during sleep, has played an important part in the development of concepts concerning sleep, and is an essential component of accepted sleep staging systems. That described by Dement and Kleitman[83] has been employed for almost 40 years, generally by experienced observers with standardised rating criteria. Automatic, or more usually computer assisted sleep staging systems are now available, making quantitative sleep studies less labour intensive and more accessible as clinical and research tools. As well as the classic stages of light, deep, and rapid eye movement (REM) sleep, other patterns have been recognised, notably the cyclic alternating pattern of deep and lighter sleep with a period of only 40 seconds.[84] This in turn is related to other regulatory mechanisms and there is hope that it may be of value in the investigation of, for instance, cardiac and autonomic dysfunction.

Sleep provides a valuable means of activating the EEG to obtain clinically significant information—for instance, to elicit epileptiform activity, as noted earlier. In various encephalopathies, even without seizures, characteristic EEG abnormalities may appear more readily during sleep, at certain phases of evolution of the disease. Thus sleep recording may be necessary to show the repetitive complexes of Creutzfeldt-Jakob disease and of subacute sclerosing panencephalitis, particularly in the early stages.

Recording of EEG during sleep has a special role in the investigation of the dysomnias and parasomnias. For nightlong "polysomnography" in patients with possible disturbances of ventilatory function, the EEG is recorded in combination with other variables—namely, EMG, ECG and oculogram, oxygen saturation, air flow, and thoracoabdominal movement. These are required for sleep staging or investigating ventilatory disturbances.

Polysomnography, including respiratory studies and sleep oximetry, has a major role in the investigation of sleep apnoea and during the establishment of treatment with continuous positive airway pressure. Sleep apnoea is common, with a prevalence variously estimated as 1 to 10%.[85 86] Oximetry alone may be adequate to identify more than 50% of patients,[87 88] but in many patients with a high clinical suspicion of the condition, oximetry results are equivocal or normal, and polysomnography is then necessary for proper evaluation. The condition of high upper airway resistance is characterised by snoring and frequent arousals but without apnoea and here polysomnography is essential for diagnosis. Although costly and not widely available, nocturnal polysomnography is therefore the most satisfactory method of investigating patients with diurnal drowsiness or who report unexplained sleep disturbances.[89] Unlike oximetry alone, it will also help to identify those whose symptoms have some other cause, such as nocturnal epileptic seizures.

For the investigation of sleepiness, notably in such conditions as narcolepsy, the multiple sleep latency test (MSLT) is used. The subject is repeatedly placed in a quiet dark environment during the daytime and allowed to fall asleep. The mean time to onset of sleep provides a measure of sleepiness (five to 10 minutes represents moderate, and less than five minutes, severe sleepiness). In addition, the electrophysiological pattern at sleep onset is noted. In normal subjects there is a gradual progression through sleep stages of increasing depth, whereas in narcolepsy, and rarely in subjects with sleep apnoea, there may be a rapid progression to deep sleep or to the REM stage, not normally seen until after some 90 minutes of sleep. In many sleepy patients both nocturnal polysomnography and a multiple sleep latency test will be required for a full evaluation.

HIV and AIDS

Both HIV infection and full blown AIDs present a new range of neurodiagnostic problems. With strict assessment criteria, it seems that EEGs are normal in patients infected with HIV who have unimpaired neuropsychological status.[90] In those with AIDs or AIDs related complex, the incidence and severity of abnormal EEGs increased with development of AIDs related dementia, 65% showing diffuse and 22% focal slowing, and 11% paroxysmal slow and sharp activity.[91] Current patterns of disease and use of prophylactic treatment against infections are associated with a preponderance of diffuse encephalopathic EEG abnormalities over focal changes from localised lesions or multifocal leucoencephalopathies. Diffuse slowing is correlated with slowed reaction times[92] and, together with quantitative methods in longitudinal studies, provides a sensitive warning of impending neurological disease in asymptomatic patients.[93]

19

Systemic disorders

The encephalopathies form an indication par excellence for systematic EEG studies and the use of simple quantitative methods. In general terms there is a fairly consistent sequence of global EEG changes, often quantitatively related to the severity of the underlying metabolic or toxic process. These comprise slowing of the normal ongoing posterior (alpha) rhythm, gradual loss of its reactivity to eye opening or auditory stimulation, further slowing to theta and delta frequency ranges (figure 1.2) with loss of faster components, then a terminal state in which intermittent suppression of activity progresses to total electrical silence.

With certain exceptions, such as the triphasic waves of hepatic precoma and coma, there are few specific EEG features and the contribution of the investigation is to indicate the presence and severity of abnormality rather than a particular diagnosis. This is especially important in the confused patient for distinguishing between an organic cause such as an encephalopathy, non-convulsive status epilepticus (which may even mimic hepatic encephalopathy with repetitive stereotyped diphasic or triphasic complexes; figure 1.3), and some psychogenic causes.

The consistent sequential EEG changes in metabolic and toxic encephalopathies, their quantitative relation to severity of causal factors, their independence of patient responses, and their objective nature, provide valuable clinical tools. This has led to the development of various electronic methods for measurement of EEG changes.[94] The value of such methods is in the rapid and continuing feedback to the clinician for guidance in management—for example, in an acute crisis where complex medical or surgical intervention may be required.

Exclusion of an acute or subacute encephalitic illness may be a reason for the EEG in a patient admitted in coma with little available history concerning antecedent events. Repetitive EEG transients may occur in encephalitis, but also unfortunately with several alternative conditions such as hepatic encephalopathy ("triphasic waves"; see Fisch and Klass[95] regarding diagnostic specificity), severe posthypoxic encephalopathy, and occasionally in uraemia, electrolyte disorders, and barbiturate overdose.

Whereas acute cerebral hypoxic damage leads to diffuse repetitive transients, an episode of profound arterial hypotension or perfusion failure usually produces changes localised to arterial

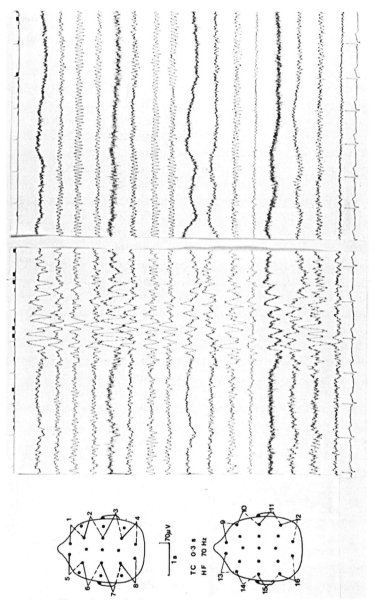

Figure 1.2   *Hypoglycaemia: two samples from EEGs in a man of 37 with an insulinoma. At the time of the first EEG (left hand sample) after a 36 hour fast there were episodes of high voltage frontally accentuated delta waves on a slightly irregular background; blood glucose was 2·4 mmol/l. The second EEG (right hand sample) two days later when he was normoglycaemic was normal*

21

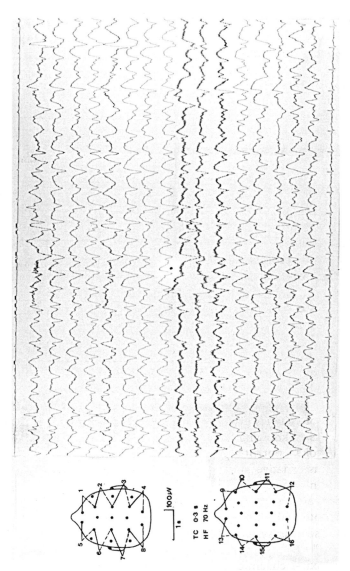

Figure 1.3   *Triphasic waves in hepatic encephalopathy: EEG in a 26 year old woman who was withdrawn, drowsy and restless, two weeks after appendicectomy. Previous reconstructive surgery as a child included ureterocolic anastomosis. Typical triphasic waves with clear anteroposterior time lag are shown. In view of the clinical possibility of non-convulsive status epilepticus 3 mg diazepam was given cautiously intravenously in fractionated doses but had no effect on the EEG. Liver function tests were grossly abnormal*

boundary zone or "watershed" regions.[96] These may include PLEDs together with local flattening and surrounding localised slow waves. Such changes may also occur with raised intracranial pressure, or when hypotension occurs in patients with occlusive vascular disease in the neck. Apart from causal attribution, differentiation between ischaemic and hypoxic abnormalities is of clinical importance as outcome in patients with boundary zone infarcts may be improved by reduction of surrounding oedema and control of epileptiform activity.

Intensive care

The neurophysiology team is closely involved in many aspects of intensive care. Only limited clinical neurological assessment is possible in unconscious, sedated and ventilated, or traumatised patients with problems from inaccessibility of limbs because of traction or vascular lines and impossibility of examining pupils, optic fundi, and caloric responses because of local trauma or swelling. A carefully planned EEG can help by demonstrating a global cerebral response to systematic stimulation in peripheral and cranial nerve territories.

Unfortunately, the EEG itself may be extinguished by major sedatives and anaesthetics commonly used in intensive care units, albeit in higher doses than commonly used in the United Kingdom. In high dose barbiturate treatment of major head injuries short-latency evoked potential recordings may provide the only means of knowing if the brain is alive.[97] Conveniently, short latency evoked potentials are not appreciably affected by major intravenous sedative and anaesthetic agents and have predictive value even when the EEG has been rendered isoelectric.[98] Prognosis after severe trauma may be helped by multimodality evoked potential studies,[99 100] and in the absence of significant sedation, scoring systems based upon EEG features retain a useful place.[101]

In hypoxic-ischaemic coma burst suppression patterns and isoelectric EEGs, unless caused by CNS depressant drugs or hypothermia, are of adverse prognostic import. Total EEG silence occurs during asystole but with resuscitation intermittent and then continuous activity return by three and 10·5 hours respectively in patients who will recover from coma.[102] In a comparison of recovery times for brainstem reflexes and EEG in a series of 125

23

patients, a stereotyped sequence of returning brainstem reflexes preceded the first appearance of EEG activity (from respiratory movements and pupillary light reflex by seven to 12 minutes, to stereotyped reactivity by 3·3 hours). Full recovery was only seen in patients in whom intermittent EEG had returned within three hours, consciousness within two days, speech within 6·5 days, and activities of daily living by two weeks.[102] From EEGs predictors, based on systematic scoring compared with a computerised "knowledge-base" derived from patients with established outcome, have long proved powerful tools.[103] Prognostic systems based on quantitative EEG analysis[104] and additional somatosensory evoked potentials[105] extend the basis for prognostic assessment in posthypoxic coma.

Monitoring of severity scores based on EEG features has also proved of prognostic value in sepsis associated encephalopathies when severe but reversible abnormalities occur and require differentiation from effects of major sedatives.[106]

Quantitative EEG methods are presently limited in detection of some prognostically important patterns (for example, FIRDA, triphasic waves, and burst suppression patterns). Indeed, overall patterns of function, including long term cyclic variability and reactivity,[107] are of more fundamental importance than simple quantitative or "present or absent" measures. Neurophysiological measures are always of much more value when showing positive evidence of function than in assessing possible significance of its absence. None the less despite a wide consensus concerning the primacy of proper clinical testing, there is still occasional controversy over the role of neurophysiological investigations in brainstem death. The arguments for and against are comprehensively reviewed by Chatrian[108] and Pallis.[109]

Purpose built continuous EEG monitoring devices have become a standard part of the intensive care of comatose or sedated patients[110-112] and are used to detect seizure discharges in ventilated patients with status epilepticus,[113] to assist management of sedation in ventilated head injured patients,[114] and in detection of arousals.[115] Now, in addition, evoked potential monitors will allow continuous observation of auditory or somatosensory function to the level of brainstem and primary cortical potentials,[116] some being combined with displays of quantitative EEGs.[117]

The problems of assessing patients in the intensive care unit have been highlighted in a series of nerve conduction and electromyographic studies concerned with difficulties in recovery attributable to myopathies, neuropathies, and neuromuscular problems in the critically ill.[118] [119] It is therefore naive to think of EEG as an isolated investigation in unresponsive patients in intensive care units but it may be highly rewarding to approach each individual problem with the appropriate battery of EEG, evoked potential, and EMG diagnostic and monitoring tools.

Service provision in the United Kingdom

The favoured pattern for optimal delivery of services in the United Kingdom parallels that for other neurosciences, comprising a "hub and spoke" model with the main resources at neuroscience centres, while smaller linked departments in peripheral hospitals provide basic services to local communities. The Association of British Clinical Neurophysiologists[120-122] and the American Electroencephalographic Society[123] have issued recommendations on standards for clinical neurophysiology and guidance to purchasers about the indications for and selection of different investigations. Local services must not be devolved to such a degree that individual departments are too small to be cost effective or to maintain standards. Even a basic EEG laboratory cannot be expected at the site of every neurology outpatient clinic.

An Association of British Clinical Neurophysiologists survey in the four Thames Health Authority regions reported 5500 neurophysiological investigations per million population per year, more than doubling 1968 levels; EEG comprised half the workload, EMG one third, and evoked potential studies and special techniques the remainder. Two thirds of the investigations were in outpatients; only half the referrals were from neuroscience disciplines, the remainder from other specialties, notably paediatrics, orthopaedics, and rheumatology, but also general medicine, endocrinology, psychiatry, and geriatrics, and other surgical specialties.

The direct cost of a waking EEG is about £70, the total, £100 with ancillary costs in a neurosciences department. Unit costs will be higher in smaller units. Special EEG examinations range from £200 (drug induced sleep) to £400 per 24 hours for telemetry. Waiting lists for neurophysiology tests now average 4·9 weeks in the United Kingdom (Association of British Clinical

25

Neurophysiologists, 1992–94 surveys). They are longer for procedures requiring active involvement of physicians such as EMG, telemetry, and intraoperative monitoring, and unlikely to fall without an increase in consultant staffing levels.

"Usefulness" of investigations

Diagnostic utility of investigations may be assessed in terms of yield of positive findings or by the effect on management. Perhaps not unexpectedly the cost : benefit ratio is most favourable for costly complex investigations considering specific problems such as telemetry,[124] and worst for "routine" examinations used for screening purposes.[41]

The St Bartholomew's Hospital medical staff round audit for November 1990 was based on a detailed study of all clinical neurophysiological investigations performed in the first three months of that year. It provides an example of how EEG and evoked potentials are used (tables 1.1 and 1.2). The data from the audit suggested that "usefulness" criteria could be derived for EEG (table 1.3).

Table 1.1 Data on EEG from St Bartholomew's Hospital medical staff round audit (1990)

	EEGS		
		Results (%)	
Diagnosis	Workload (%)	Abnormal	Doubtful	Normal
---	---	---	---	---
Attacks epilepsy?	38	25	9	66
Epilepsy	28	60	8	32
Coma/encephalitis/ encephalopathy	11	94	4	2
Psychiatric	6	16	16	68
Intracranial lesions	5·3	55	0	45
Neonatal problems	2·4	70	0	30
Migraine/headaches/ sleep disorders etc	1·2	20	0	80
Other, uncertain diagnosis	8			

Table 1.2   Data on evoked potentials from St Bartholomew's Hospital medical staff round audit (1990)

Referral diagnosis	Workload (%)	Evoked potentials		
		Results (%)		
		Abnormal	Doubtful	Normal
Pituitary/chiasmal lesions	7	64	36	0
Demyelinating disease	56	50	13	36
Other pathology (trauma, vascular, tumours, toxic, metabolic etc)	18	52	11	37
Neonatal and paediatric	19	(follow up incomplete)		

Table 1.3   "Usefulness" criteria for EEG derived from the St Bartholomew's Hospital medical staff round audit (1990)

Referred problem	% "useful*"	comments
● Coma/encephalitis/	94	Very useful, often as emergency
● Neonates/infants brain damage? fits? encephalitis? spasms etc	70	Increasingly useful, often as emergency
● Epilepsy: classification of seizure type	60	May need sleep EEG or ambulatory/video EEG
● Structural brain lesions	55	Main use to assess function and complications such as fits
● Epilepsy? and "funny turns"	25	Normal EEG of no real value but simultaneous ECG monitoring may be
● Psychiatric disorders	16	Low yield of specific diagnostic information

*Usefulness was inferred when positive findings were present which actually altered or could have influenced decisions on changes in clinical management.

Summary

Notwithstanding recent advances in neuroimaging, EEG remains a major technique for investigation of the brain. Its main applications are in assessment of cerebral function rather than for detecting structural abnormalities. The principal clinical applica-

27

tions are in epilepsy, states of altered consciousness including postanoxic and traumatic coma, the parasomnias, dementias, toxic confusional states, cerebral infections, and various other encephalopathies.

Abnormalities in EEG reflect—for example, general pathophysiological processes, raised intracranial pressure, cerebral anoxia, or oedema, and epileptogenesis, and show little specificity for a particular disease. Consequently, they need to be interpreted in a particular clinical context; the use of routine EEG examination for screening purposes is rarely of value. Conversely, the investigation becomes most cost effective when applied to specific problems—for instance, monitoring serial changes in postanoxic coma or during open heart surgery, differential diagnosis (by telemetric ictal recordings) of epileptic and non-epileptic attacks, and providing early prediction of outcome after stroke.

High technological standards and an individualised problem solving approach are prerequisites of a cost effective, reliable clinical EEG service. These are most likely to be achieved by a considered, selective referral policy, the use when necessary of prolonged complex procedures such as telemetry, and the avoidance of routine examinations of dubious clinical relevance.

1 Hari R, Lounasmaa OV. Recording and interpretation of cerebral magnetic fields. *Science* 1989;244:432–6.
2 Steriade M, Gloor P, Llinas RR, Lopes da Silva FH, Mesulam M-M. Basic mechanisms of cerebral rhythmic activities. *Electroencephalogr Clin Neurophysiol* 1990;76:481–508.
3 Matoušek M, Petersén I. Automatic evaluation of EEG background activity by means of age-dependent EEG quotients. *Electroencephalogr Clin Neurophysiol* 1973;35:603–12.
4 Binnie CD. Telemetric EEG monitoring in epilepsy. In: Pedley TA, Meldrum BS, eds. *Recent advances in epilepsy*. I. Edinburgh: Churchill Livingstone, 1983;155–78.
5 Gotman J, Ives JR, Gloor P. Long-term monitoring in epilepsy. *Electroencephalogr Clin Neurophysiol* 1985; suppl 37:444.
6 Duffy FH, Burchfiel JL, Lombroso CT. Brain electrical activity mapping (BEAM): a method for extending the clinical utility of EEG and evoked potential data. *Ann Neurol* 1979;5:309–21.
7 Duffy FH, Bartels PH, Burchfiel JL. Significance probability mapping: an aid in the topographic analysis of brain electrical activity. *Electroencephalogr Clin Neurophysiol* 1981;51:455–62.
8 Lehmann D. Human scalp EEG fields: evoked, alpha, sleep and spike-wave patterns. In: Petsche H, Brazier MAB, eds. *Synchronization of EEG activity in the epilepsies*. New York: Springer, 1972:307–26.
9 Duffy FH. Brain electrical activity mapping: ideas and answers. In: Duffy FH, ed. *Topographic mapping of brain electrical activity*. Boston: Butterworths, 1986:401–98.
10 Gregory DL, Wong PK. Topographical analysis of the centrotemporal discharges in benign Rolandic epilepsy of childhood. *Epilepsia* 1984;25:705–11.
11 Ebersole JS. Equivalent dipole modelling—a new EEG method for localisation of epileptogenic foci. In: Pedley TA, Meldrum BS, eds. *Current problems in epilepsy*, London: John Libbey, 1992:51–71.

28

12 Fisch BJ, Pedley TA. The role of quantitative EEG topographic mapping or "neuromet-rics" in the diagnosis of psychiatric and neurological disorders: the cons. *Electroencephalogr Clin Neurophysiol* 1989;73:5–9.

13 Binnie CD, MacGillivray BB. Brain mapping: a useful tool or a dangerous toy? *J Neurol Neurosurg Psychiatry* 1992;55:527–9.

14 Cabral RJ, Scott DF. EEG features associated with the occurrence of epilepsy after surgery for intracranial aneurysm and acoustic neuroma. *J Neurol Neurosurg Psychiatry* 1977;40:97–9.

15 Van Huffelen AC, Poortvliet DCJ, Van der Wulp CJM. Quantitative electroencephalog-raphy in cerebral ischemia. Detection of abnormalities in "normal" EEGs. In: Pfurtscheller G, Jonkman EJ, Lopes da Silva FH, eds. *Brain ischemia: quantitative EEG and imaging techniques.* Amsterdam: Elsevier, 1984:3–18.

16 Veering MM, Jonkman EJ, Poortvliet DCJ, De Weerd AW, Tans JThJ, John ER. The effect of reconstructive vascular surgery on clinical status, quantitative EEG and cerebral blood flow in patients with cerebral ischemia, a three month follow-up study in operated and unoperated stroke patients. *Electroencephalogr Clin Neurophysiol* 1986;64:383–93.

17 Oken BS, Chiappa KH, Salinsky M. Computerized EEG frequency analysis: sensitivity and specificity in patients with focal lesions. *Neurology* 1989;39:1281–7.

18 Van Huffelen AC. EEG and cerebral pathology. In: Osselton JW, Binnie CD, Cooper R, Fowler CJ, Mauguière F, Prior PF, eds. *Clinical neurophysiology.* Vol 2. Oxford: Butterworth-Heinemann, 1996 (in press).

19 Messick JM, Casement B, Sharbrough FW, Milde LN, Michenfelder JD, Sundt TM. Correlation of regional cerebral blood flow (rCBF) with EEG changes during isoflurane anesthesia for carotid endarterectomy: critical rCBF. *Anesthesiology* 1987;66:344–9.

20 Kearse LA, Brown EM, McPeck K. Somatosensory evoked potentials relative to elec-troencephalography for cerebral ischaemia during carotid endarterectomy. *Stroke* 1992;23:498–505.

21 Bricolo AP, Turella GS. Electrophysiology of head injury. In: Braakman H, ed. *Handbook of clinical neurology.* Vol 13 (57) *Head injury.* Amsterdam: Elsevier Science Publishers BV, 1990:181–206.

22 Dusser A, Navelet Y, Devictor D, Landrieu P. Short- and long-term prognostic value of the electroencephalogram in children with severe head injury. *Electroencephalogr Clin Neurophysiol* 1989;73:85–93.

23 Thatcher RW, Walker RA, Gerson I, Geisler FH. EEG discriminant analyses of mild head trauma. *Electroencephalogr Clin Neurophysiol* 1989;73:94–106.

24 Schwartz MS, Prior PF, Scott DF. The occurrence and evolution in the EEG of a later-alised periodic phenomenon. *Brain* 1973;96:613–22.

25 Brown P, Kaur P, Sulina MP, Goldfart LV, Gibbs CJ Jr, Gajdusek DC. Real and imag-ined clinicopathological limits of "prion dementia". *Lancet* 1993;341:127–9.

26 Prusiner SB. Prion diseases of humans and animals. *J R Coll Physicians Lond* 1994;28 (suppl):1–30.

27 Schwartz MS, Scott DF. Pathological stimulus-related slow wave arousal responses in the EEG. *Acta Neurol Scand* 1978;57:300–4.

28 Babb TL, Wilson CL, Isokawa-Akesson M. Firing patterns of human limbic neurons dur-ing stereoencephalography (SEEG) and clinical temporal lobe seizures. *Electroencephalogr Clin Neurophysiol* 1987;66:467–82.

29 Deschênes M, Roy JP, Steriade M. Thalamic bursting mechanism: an inward slow cur-rent revealed by membrane hyperpolarization. *Brain Res* 1982;239:289–93.

30 Avoli M, Kostopoulos G. Participation of corticothalamic cells in penicillin induced spike and wave discharges. *Brain Res* 1982;247:159–63.

31 Dreifuss FE (Chairman, Commission on Classification and Terminology of the International League Against Epilepsy). Proposal for revised clinical and electroen-cephalographic classification of epileptic seizures. *Epilepsia* 1981;22:489–501.

32 Dreifuss FE (Chairman, Commission on Classification and Terminology of the International League Against Epilepsy). Proposal for revised classification of epilepsies and epileptic syndromes. *Epilepsia* 1989;30:389–99.

33 Naquet R. The clinical significance of EEG in epilepsy. In: Nistico G, De Perri R, Meinardi H, eds. *Epilepsy: an update on research and therapy.* New York: Alan R Liss, 1983:147–64.

34 Riley TL. Normal variants in EEG that are mistaken as epileptic patterns. In: Gross M, ed. *Pseudoepilepsy.* Lexington: Heath, 1983:25–7.

35 Ajmone Marsan C, Zivin LS. Factors related to the occurrence of typical paroxysmal abnormalities in the EEG records of epileptic patients. *Epilepsia* 1970;**11**:361–81.

36 Binnie CD. Electroencephalography. In: Laidlaw J, Richens A, Chadwick D, eds. *A Textbook of epilepsy*. 4th ed. Edinburgh: Churchill Livingstone, 1992:277–8.

37 Robin JJ, Tolan JD, Arnold JW. Ten-year experience with abnormal EEGs in asymptomatic adult males. *Aviation Space Env Med* 1978;**49**:732–6.

38 Gregory RP, Oates T, Merry RTG. Electroencephalogram epileptiform abnormalities in candidates for aircrew training. *Electroencephalogr Clin Neurophysiol* 1993;**86**:75–7.

39 Zivin L, Ajmone Marsan C. Incidence and prognostic significance of "epileptiform" activity in the EEG of non-epileptic subjects. *Brain* 1968;**91**:751–78.

40 Bridgers SL. Epileptiform abnormalities discovered on electroencephalographic screening of psychiatric inpatients. *Arch Neurol* 1987;**44**:312–6.

41 Binnie CD. EEG audit: increasing cost efficiency of EEG investigations in epilepsy. *Electroencephalogr Clin Neurophysiol* 1990;**76**:29P.

42 Overweg J, Binnie CD, Oosting J, Rowan AJ. Clinical and EEG prediction of seizure recurrence following antiepileptic drug withdrawal. *Epilepsy Res* 1987;**1**:272–83.

43 Shinnar S, Vining EPC, Mellits ED, et al. Discontinuing antiepileptic medication in children with epilepsy after two years without seizures. A prospective study. *N Engl J Med* 1985;**313**:976–80.

44 Holowach J, Thurston DL, O'Leary JL. Prognosis in childhood epilepsy: follow-up study of 148 cases in which therapy had been suspended after prolonged anticonvulsant control. *N Engl J Med* 1972;**286**:169–74.

45 Veldhuizen R, Binnie CD, Beintema DJ. The effect of sleep deprivation on the EEG in epilepsy. *Electroencephalogr Clin Neurophysiol* 1983;**55**:505–12.

46 Browne TR, Penry JK, Porter RJ, Dreifuss FE. Responsiveness before, during and after spike-wave paroxysms. *Neurology* 1974;**24**:659–65.

47 Jeavons PM, Harding, GFA. *Photosensitive epilepsy*. London: Heinemann, 1975.

48 Binnie CD, Jeavons PM. Photosensitive epilepsies. In: Roger J, Dravet C, Bureau M, Dreifuss FE, Perret A, Wolf P, eds. *Epileptic syndromes in infancy, childhood and adolescence*. 2nd ed. London and Paris: John Libbey, 1992:299–305.

49 Reilly L, Peters JF. Relationship of some varieties of electroencephalographic photosensitivity to clinical convulsive disorders. *Neurology* 1973;**13**:1050–7.

50 Kasteleijn-Nolst Trenité DGA. Photosensitivity in epilepsy: electrophysiological and clinical correlates. *Acta Neurol Scand* 1989 (suppl 125):80.

51 Ramani, V. Intensive monitoring of psychogenic seizures, aggression and dyscontrol syndromes. In: Gumnit RJ, ed. *Advances in neurology*. Vol 46: *intensive neurodiagnostic monitoring*. New York: Raven Press, 1986:203–17.

52 Binnie CD. Nonepileptic attack disorder. *Postgrad Med J* 1994;**70**:1–4.

53 Blumhardt LD. Ambulatory ECG and EEG monitoring in the differential diagnosis of cardiac and cerebral dysrhythmias. In: Gumnit RJ, ed. *Intensive neurodiagnostic monitoring. Advances in neurology*. Vol 46. New York: Raven Press, 1987:183–202.

54 Wieser HG. "Psychische Anfalle" und deren stereoelektroenzephalographisches Korrelat. *Z EEG EMG* 1979;**10**:197–206.

55 Browne TR, Penry JK, Porter RJ, Dreifuss FE. A comparison of clinical estimates of absence seizure frequency with estimates based on prolonged telemetered EEGs. *Neurology* 1974;**24**:381–2.

56 Penry JK, Porter RJ, Dreifuss FE. Simultaneous recording of absence seizures with video tape and electroencephalography: a study of 374 seizures in 48 patients. *Brain* 1975;**98**:427–40.

57 Aarts JHP, Binnie CD, Smit AM, Wilkins AJ. Selective cognitive impairment during focal and generalized epileptiform EEG activity. *Brain* 1984;**107**:293–308.

58 Wieser HG, Elger CE, Stodieck SRG. The "foramen ovale electrode": A new recording method for the preoperative evaluation of patients suffering from mesiobasal temporal lobe epilepsy. *Electroencephalogr Clin Neurophysiol* 1985;**61**:314–22.

59 Spencer SS, Williamson PD, Bridgers SL, et al. Reliability and accuracy of localization by scalp ictal EEG. *Neurology* 1985;**35**:1567–75.

60 Spencer SS, Williamson PD, Spencer DD, Mattson RH. Combined depth and subdural electrode investigation in uncontrolled epilepsy. *Neurology* 1990;**40**:74–9.

61 Sperling MR, O'Connor MJ, Tougas P. Utility of depth and subdural electrodes in recording temporal lobe seizures. *Epilepsia* 1988;**29**:679.

62 Perris, C. A study of bipolar (manic depressive) and unipolar recurrent depressive psy-

choses. *Acta Psychiatr Scand* 1966;42:118–52.

63 Anderson W McC, Dawson J, Margerison JH. Serial biochemical, clinical and electroencephalographic studies in affective illness. *Clin Sci* 1964;26:323–36.

64 Hurst LA, Mundy-Castle AC, Beerstecher DM. The electroencephalogram in manic depressive psychosis. *Journal of Mental Science* 1954;100:220–40.

65 Hays P. Etiological factors in manic depressive psychoses. *Arch Gen Psychiatry* 1976;33:1187–8.

66 Davis PA. Evaluation of the electroencephalogram of schizophrenic patients. *Am J Psychiatry* 1940;96:851.

67 Kelly JT, Reilly EL. EEG, alcohol and alcoholism. In: Hughes JR, Wilson WP, eds. *EEG and evoked potentials in psychiatry and behavioural neurology.* London: Butterworths, 1983.

68 Letemendia F, Pampiglione G. Clinical and electroencephalographic observations in Alzheimer's disease. *J Neurol Neurosurg Psychiatry* 1958;21:167–72.

69 Harner RN. EEG evaluation of the patient with dementia. In: Benson DF, Blumer D, eds. *Psychiatric aspects of neurologic disease.* New York: Grune and Stratton, 1975:63–82.

70 Coben LA, Danziger W, Stotandt M. A longitudinal EEG study of mild senile dementia of Alzheimer type: changes at 1 year and 2·5 years. *Electroencephalogr Clin Neurophysiol* 1985;61:101–12.

71 Soininen H, Partanen VJ, Nelkala EL, Riekinen PJ. EEG findings in senile dementia and normal aging. *Acta Neurologica Scand* 1982;65:59–70.

.72 Brown DA, Goldensohn ES. The electroencephalogram in normal pressure hydrocephalus. *Arch Neurol* 1973;29:70–1.

73 Foster DB, Bagchi BK. Electroencephalographic observations in Huntington's chorea. *Electroencephalogr Clin Neurophysiol* 1949;1:247–8.

74 Shista SK, Troupe A, Marszalek KS, Kremer LM. Huntington's chorea: an electroencephalographic and psychometric study. *Electroencephalogr Clin Neurophysiol* 1974; 36:387–93.

75 Newman SE. The EEG manifestations of chronic ethanol abuse: relation to cerebral cortical atrophy. *Ann Neurol* 1978;3:299–304.

76 Gordon EB, Sim M. The EEG in presenile dementia. *J Neurol Neurosurg Psychiatry* 1967;30:285–91.

77 Johannesson G, Brun A, Gustafson L, Ingvar DH. EEG in presenile dementia related to cerebral blood flow and autopsy findings. *Acta Neurol Scand* 1977;56:89–103.

78 Chiappa K, Young R. The EEG as a definitive diagnostic tool early in the course of Creutzfeldt-Jakob disease. *Electroencephalogr Clin Neurophysiol* 1978;45:26P.

79 Terzano MG, Mancia D, Calzetti S, Zacchetti O, Maione R. Diagnostic value of EEG periodic discharges and cyclic changes in Creutzfeldt-Jakob disease. *Electroencephalogr Clin Neurophysiol* 1981;52:52P.

80 Waggoner RW, Bagchi BK. Initial masking of organic brain changes by psychic symptoms: clinical and electroencephalographic studies. *Am J Psychiatry* 1954;110:904–11.

81 Lishman WA. Brain damage in relation to psychiatric disability after head injury. *Br J Psychiatry* 1968;114:373–410.

82 Williams D. The electroencephalogram in chronic post-traumatic states. *J Neurol Psychiatry* 1941;4:131.

83 Dement W, Kleitman N. Cyclic variations in EEG during sleep and their relation to eye movements, body motility, and dreaming. *Electroencephalogr Clin Neurophysiol* 1957;9:673–90.

84 Terzano MG, Mancia D, Salati MR, et al. The cyclic alternating pattern as a physiological component of normal NREM sleep. *Sleep* 1985;8:137–45.

85 Lavie P. Incidence of sleep apnoea in a presumably healthy working population: a significant relationship with excessive daytime sleepiness. *Sleep* 1983;6:312–8.

86 Gilason T, Lindholm C-E, Almqvist M, et al. Uvulopalatopharyngoplasty in the sleep apnoea syndrome. *Arch Otolaryngol Head Neck Surg* 1988;114:45–51.

87 Rajagopalan N, Douglas NH. Diagnostic pick-up rate of polysomnography. *Thorax* 1990;45:788.

88 Williams AJ, Yu G, Santiago S, Stein M. Screening for sleep apnoea using pulse oximetry and a clinical score. *Chest* 1991;100:631–5.

89 Rutherford R, Popkin J, Nguyen HK, et al. Reliability of respiratory sleep studies versus polysomnography in the investigation of suspected obstructive sleep apnoea. *Am Rev Respir Dis* 1987;135:A48.

90 Nuwer MR, Miller EN, Visscher BR, et al. Asymptomatic HIV infection does not cause

31

EEG abnormalities: results from the multicenter AIDs cohort study (MACS). *Neurology* 1992;**42**:1214–9.

91 Gabuzda DH, Levy SR, Chiappa KH. Electroencephalography in AIDs and AIDs-related complex. *Clin Electroencephalogr* 1988;**19**:1–6.

92 Jabbari B, Coats M, Salazar A, Martin A, Scherokman B, Laws WA. Longitudinal study of EEG and evoked potentials in neurologically asymptomatic HIV infected subjects. *Electroencephalogr Clin Neurophysiol* 1993;**86**:145–51.

93 Parisi A, Di Perri G, Strosselli M, Nappi G, Minoli L, Rondanelli EG. Usefulness of computerised electroencephalography in diagnosing, staging and monitoring AIDs-dementia complex. *Aids* 1989;**3**:209–13.

94 Amiel SA, Pottinger RC, Archibald HR, Chusney G, Cunnah DTF, Prior PF, Gale EAM. Effect of antecedent glucose control on cerebral function during hypoglycemia. *Diabetes Care* 1991;**14**:109–18.

95 Fisch BJ, Klass DW. Diagnostic specificity of triphasic wave patterns. *Electroencephalogr Clinical Neurophysiol* 1988;**70**:1–8.

96 Brierley JB, Prior PF, Calverley J, Jackson SJ, Brown AW. The pathogenesis of ischaemic neuronal damage along the cerebral arterial boundary zones in Papio anubis. *Brain* 1980;**103**:929–65.

97 Marshall LF, Smith RW, Shapiro HM. The outcome with aggressive treatment in severe head injuries. Part II. Acute and chronic barbiturate administration in the management of head injury. *J Neurosurg* 1979;**50**:26–30.

98 Ganes T, Lundar T. The effect of thiopentone on somatosensory evoked responses and EEGs in comatose patients. *J Neurol Neurosurg Psychiatry* 1983;**46**:509–14.

99 Narayan RK, Greenberg RP, Miller JD, *et al*. Improved confidence of outcome prediction in severe head injury: a comparative analysis of the clinical examination, multimodality evoked potentials, CT scanning and intracranial pressure. *J Neurosurg* 1981;**54**:751–62.

100 Choi SC, Ward JD, Becker DP. Chart for outcome prediction in severe head injury. *J Neurosurg* 1983;**59**:294–7.

101 Rae-Grant AD, Barbour PJ, Reed J. Development of a novel EEG rating scale for head injury using dichotomous variables. *Electroencephalogr Clin Neurophysiol* 1991;**79**:349–57.

102 Jørgensen EO, Malchow-Møller A. Natural history of global and critical brain ischaemia. *Resuscitation* 1981;**9**:133–88.

103 Binnie CD, Prior PF, Lloyd DSL, Scott DF, Margerison JH. Electroencephalographic prediction of fatal anoxic brain damage after resuscitation from cardiac arrest. *BMJ* 1970;**4**:265–8.

104 Young WL, Ornstein E. Compressed spectral array during cardiac arrest and resuscitation. *Anesthesiology* 1985;**62**:535–8.

105 Rothstein TL, Thomas EM, Sumi SM. Predicting outcome in hypoxic-ischemic coma. *Electroencephalogr Clin Neurophysiol* 1991;**79**:101–7.

106 Young GR, Bolton CF, Archibald YM, Austin TW, Wells GA. The electroencephalogram in sepsis-associated encephalopathy. *J Clin Neurophysiol* 1992;**9**:145–52.

107 Evans BM. Periodic activity in cerebral arousal mechanisms—the relationship to sleep and brain damage. *Electroencephalogr Clin Neurophysiol* 1992;**83**:130–7.

108 Chatrian GE. Coma, other states of altered consciousness and brain death. In: Daly DD, Pedley TA, eds. *Current practice of clinical electroencephalography*. New York: Raven Press Ltd, 1990:425–87.

109 Pallis, C. Brainstem death. In: Braakman H, ed. *Handbook of clinical neurology*. Vol 13 (57) *Head injury*. Amsterdam: Elsevier Science Publishers BV, 1990: 441–96.

110 Maynard D, Prior PF, Scott DF. Device for continuous monitoring of cerebral activity in resuscitated patients. *BMJ* 1969;**4**:545–6.

111 Bricolo A, Turazzi F, Faccioli F, Odorizzi F, Sciarreta G, Eruliani P. Clinical applications of compressed spectral array in long-term EEG monitoring of comatose patients. *Electroencephalogr Clin Neurophysiol* 1978;**45**:211–25.

112 Maynard DE, Jenkinson JL. The cerebral function analysing monitor. Initial clinical experience, application and further development. *Anaesthesia* 1984;**39**:678–90.

113 Tasker RC, Boyd S, Matthew DJ. EEG monitoring of prolonged thiopentone administration for intractible seizures and status epilepticus in infants and young children. *Neuropediatrics* 1989;**20**:147–53.

114 Procaccio F, Bingham RM, Hinds CJ, Prior PF. Continuous EEG and ICP monitoring as a guide to the administration of Althesin sedation in severe head injury. *Intensive Care*

Medicine 1988;**14**:148–55.

115 Prior PF. The EEG and detection of responsiveness during anaesthesia and coma. In: Lunn JN, Rosen M, eds. *Consciousness, awareness, pain and general anaesthesia.* London: Butterworths, 1987:34–45.

116 Garcia-Larrea L, Bertrand O, Artru F, Pernier, J, Mauguière F. Brain-stem monitoring II. Preterminal BAEP changes observed until brain death in deeply comatose patients. *Electroencephalogr Clin Neurophysiol* 1987;**68**:446–57.

117 Pfurtscheller G, Schwarz G, Schroettner O, *et al.* Continuous and simultaneous monitoring of EEG spectra and brainstem auditory and somatosensory evoked potentials in the intensive care unit and the operating room. *J Clin Neurophysiol* 1987;**4**:389–96.

118 Coakley JH, Nagendran K, Honavar M, Hinds CJ. Preliminary observations on the neuromuscular abnormalities in patients with organ failure and sepsis. *Intensive Care Medicine* 1993;**19**:323–8.

119 Zochodne DW, Ramsay DA, Saly V, Shelley S, Moffatt S. Acute necrotising myopathy of intensive care: electrophysiological studies. *Muscle Nerve* 1994;**17**: 285–92.

120 Association of British Clinical Neurophysiologists. Clinical neurophysiology services. London: Royal College of Physicians, 1989:1–14.

121 Association of British Clinical Neurophysiologists. The future for clinical neurophysiology in the reorganised health service. London: Royal College of Physicians, 1991:1–4.

122 Association of British Clinical Neurophysiologists. Guidelines for the neurophysiological investigation of patients. London: Royal College of Physicians, 1994:1–4.

123 American Electroencephalographic Society. Guidelines in electroencephalography, evoked potentials and polysomnography. *J Clin Neurophysiol* 1994;**11**:21–47.

124 Binnie CD, Rowan AJ, Overweg J, *et al.* Telemetric EEG and video monitoring in epilepsy. *Neurology* 1981;**31**: 298–303.

2 Imaging the adult brain

IVAN MOSELEY

The techniques which form the neuroradiologist's armamentarium depend in one form or another on transformation of energy waves; with the exception of ultrasonography, those of the electromagnetic spectrum. None of these energy forms is free from potentially noxious biological effects, and this is particularly true of the so-called ionising radiations, x, β, and γ waves. It is probably true that, as in the case of new drugs vis-à-vis the formulary, attempts to introduce x ray based techniques as innovative procedures today might well fail. It is therefore realistic to consider diagnostic imaging procedures primarily in relation to the energy source employed: x rays and other ionising radiations, radiofrequency, and sound waves.

Plain radiographs

The neuroradiologist's use of x ray techniques has changed considerably over the past 20 years. "Radiographic" (x ray) procedures register the differential absorption of a beam of x rays by the various tissues of the body. They differ greatly in the manner in which that registration is effected so as to preserve anatomical relations and maximise clinically useful data, while attempting to limit radiation exposure. In the classic radiograph or "plain film" the patient is simply placed between a source of x rays and a film sensitive to radiation. Because most of the unabsorbed radiation is emitted in a straight line, anatomical relations are maintained and spatial distortion is minimal unless the film is not orthogonal to the beam; most modern radiographic tables ensure that obliquity is avoided.

Contrast media in plain radiography

Contrast media can be employed to increase radiographic contrast between anatomical structures, demonstrating some not normally visible. They are usually introduced into pre-existing body spaces, such as the alimentary tract or subarachnoid space (for myelography or cisternography) or into the vascular system, where their flow within (in arteriography or phlebography) or excretion from it (in urography) can be followed with a suitably timed series of x ray exposures, otherwise similar to those when no contrast medium is used.

Computed tomography

In x ray tomography of all kinds, some motion occurs between the three elements, x ray tube-patient-film. In x ray computed tomography (CT) the beam emerging from the patient is registered not on a film but by an array of radiation detectors, as the x ray tube passes around the part being examined (in this case, the head). A computer is used to transform the intensity of the emergent beam relative to the incident beam into measures of x ray attenuation, to identify in two dimensions the site of the tissue causing that attenuation, and to construct a two dimensional map of attenuation analogous to an anatomical section. The planes of section of the head given by CT are effectively limited by the construction of the gantry bearing the x ray tube and detectors to axial and coronal planes. Reformatted images in other planes can be constructed by analysing the data from a series of contiguous sections. One of the latest developments in CT is "spiral", or more correctly "helical", scanning, in which the tube rotates continuously around the head while the patient is moved through the gantry. The rapidly acquired, continuous sequence of attenuation measurements can be "cut up" into segments, corresponding to two dimensional sections the thickness of which is determined by the operator. The merits of this method are speed, which makes it more useful for examination of children and uncooperative adults, and greater spatial resolution in images reconstructed in planes other than that of acquisition.

35

The relative "attenuation coefficients" of certain structures can also be modified by contrast media, usually containing iodine, introduced into the vascular system or subarachnoid space. Other types of contrast medium, such as inhaled stable xenon gas, are rarely used in clinical practice.

Digital radiography

The third main method of registering x ray attenuation data is by using a high speed camera to scan a screen coated with a phosphor that emits light when radiation falls on it. If the camera transforms the light energy into an electronic signal, this can be digitised and a computer employed to compare the results of one scan of the phosphor screen with that of those which precede or follow it. A digital to analogue converter can then store and display only the difference between two sets of attenuation data— before and after arrival of contrast medium, for example—in a format similar to that of the original phosphor screen picture, but with unwanted detail removed. This is the basis of digital subtraction techniques, used particularly in angiography to produce images in which only the blood vessels are displayed. The major advantages of this technique are that the detection system is much more sensitive than plain film angiography to minor changes in intensity of the emergent beam, and that, because the data are stored on a computer, they are amenable to interrogation and postprocessing.

Radionuclide studies

The other techniques using ionising radiations generally consist of the introduction into the body of a radionuclide—namely, a source of radiation, usually β or δ rays—and registration of the radiation it emits with external detectors. Originally, these detectors gave no spatial information, but with the development of scanning methods subsequently applied to CT, and the gamma camera, a scintillation detector similar to the phosphor screen device referred to earlier, anatomical localisation became possible, although spatial resolution is inferior to that of most of the techniques described. Modern techniques such as single photon emission computed tomography (SPECT) use a combination of scanning and scintillation detection. Positron emission tomography (PET), as discussed in Chapter 3, uses the same fundamental principles, but with some technical modifications.

The great potential merit of the radionuclides used in these nuclear medicine studies is that they can be attached to chemical compounds which have a greater or lesser degree of tissue specificity, and provide metabolic or dynamic information.

Nuclear magnetic resonance methods

These exploit the behaviour of nuclei with unpaired electrons (paramagnetic nuclei) within the body in a strong magnetic field. The basic principle is very simple: some of these nuclei align themselves with that external field and can be displaced by a pulse of radiofrequency energy. The extra energy imparted to the system is dissipated, also as radiofrequency waves, once the radiofrequency pulse ceases and the nuclei return to their previous position. The speed at which the energy is given up, and thereby the strength of the radiofrequency signal at any given moment, depend on the biophysical characteristics of the tissue in which the nuclei (typically hydrogen protons in clinical imaging) lie; the decay of energy release is exponential, the curve being determined mainly by two "relaxation time constants", T1 and T2. For many biological tissues T1 is of the order of 1000 ms and T2 75 ms. The intensity of the energy released from a given tissue depends on the number of susceptible nuclei: water has numerous mobile protons, whereas dense bone has very few. As the frequency of the radio signal emitted also depends on the strength of the magnetic field, a "gradient"—that is, a variation in strength of the field across the region being examined—enables localisation of the nuclei in one plane of space. Thus by examining the intensity and the rate of decay of a radiofrequency signal of known frequency, some of the characteristics of the proton emitting it can be assessed. Simple though the principle may be, the electronic switching and computation required for three dimensional localisation and tissue characterisation are exceedingly complex.

The characterisation can be refined by modifying the way in which the nuclei are excited, applying a "sequence" of radiofrequency pulses instead of simply one, and by sampling the emitted signal after varying delays. Consideration of how this is achieved

37

is beyond the scope of this article; suffice it to say that most clinical MR images are maps of water distribution, but that they can be modified to show mainly differences in T1 (T1 weighted images) or T2 (T2 weighted images) of the tissues being studied. As a simple guide, the T1 weighted images give more morphological data, whereas the T2 weighted images provide more information about the constitution of the tissues. A full MRI study usually combines at least these types of image. Some of the unsatisfactory diagnostic applications noted in the early days of MRI resulted from the use of a limited number of sequences, or sequences which did not provide sufficient contrast between normal and pathological tissues. Intravascular contrast media, mainly containing the paramagnetic rare earth gadolinium, can be used, as with *x* ray CT.

Flow imaging

Because electromagnetic waves travel at the speed of light, techniques which employ them are essentially instantaneous. Because in MRI there is a finite delay between the application of the excitatory radiofrequency pulse and reception of the emitted magnetic resonance signal, however, protons which are moving through the tissue being imaged have different properties from those which are macroscopically stationary. This enables the relatively gross movement in blood vessels and the CSF to be characterised and imaged with specially designed sequences.

Magnetic resonance angiography (MRA) was first presaged in the imaging literature almost a decade ago,[1] but has been available in clinical practice and of a quality which makes it a useful investigation for about five years; image quality is still improving. A more detailed account of the technique and its applications is found in Chapter 4. In combination with MRI, clinical application of MRA will bring about a major change in the investigation of at least those patients in whom information about the cervical or intracranial vessels is useful, but not central to their management—for example, patients with parasellar tumours. In the long term, it may completely replace diagnostic angiography.

The present and future role of CSF imaging is less unambiguous. A number of research papers have been published concerning motion and pulsatility of the intracranial fluid in such puzzling conditions as normal pressure hydrocephalus[2] and benign intracranial hypertension,[3] but without as yet casting any clear light on pathophysiology. One reviewer[4] identified other applications for phase contrast MRI of CSF movement: assessment of the functional significance of drainage via extra-arachnoid structures or the central canal of the spinal cord; investigating why some arachnoid cysts enlarge; and characterisation of obstructive hydrocephalus "without having to introduce contrast agents into the subarachnoid space"—a practice which virtually disappeared with the introduction of CT! In another study, a fast field echo technique, applied to determination of the patency of ventricular shunts, was shown to be fallible, despite which the authors claimed that the technique "may be useful".[5] The future clinical utility and, indeed, adoption of these applications are at present questionable.

Diffusion weighted MRI

Magnetic resonance imaging techniques can be used to show other physical characteristics of tissues. One method which has been developed over the past five years is diffusion weighted imaging.[6] Depending on the gradients used, the contrast in the images can depend on magnetic susceptibility, perfusion, and diffusion. To date the genuine clinical applications of this technique have also not been clarified, although research has been carried out on brain myelination, stroke, and some tumours.[7]

Magnetic resonance spectroscopy

The phenomena of nuclear magnetic resonance were originally employed for in vitro chemical analysis. In vivo analysis of body tissues can be carried out with magnetic resonance spectroscopy (MRS), which relies on the same variation in the resonant frequency of given nuclei due to their physicochemical environment to create spectra which reflect the concentration of chemical compounds containing them. In the brain, spectra from both hydrogen and phosphorus containing compounds have been investigated; much clinical research on proton spectroscopy is currently oriented towards relative concentrations of choline, creatine, n-acetyl aspartate, and lactate in normal and pathological brain tissues. Magnetic resonance spectroscopy is not strictly an imaging technique, although it employs essentially the same imager; it is combined with MRI to localise the volume of brain from which the spectrum is obtained. Until recently, a major problem with clinical applications of MRS has been the low signal to noise ratio, which has entailed large volumes of interest and long acquisition times. Smaller volume spectra have, however, shown, for example, that choline tends to be increased in solid brain tumours, whereas alanine concentration is high in meningiomas; however, even though such information might be useful in cases in which the imaging features were otherwise inconclusive, spectroscopic results are by no means diagnostic.[8] Wider application to cerebral metabolic disease is awaited.[9]

Unlike MRA, for which the major future contribution to clinical neurology and neurosurgery seems unequivocal, these other techniques are perhaps still in search of clinical applications.

Sonography

An ultrasound probe contains a "transducer" which emits 1–20 MHz sound waves and, when they bounce back off the tissues, converts the reflected energy into an electrical signal, which is analysed, usually to form an image. Bone, however, is not a good medium for transmission, so that current applications of sonography to the brain are confined to small children, in whom the fontanelles act as "acoustic windows", patients with skull defects (including intraoperatively[10]), and examination of the eye and the major arteries in the neck. The major arteries are considered in chapter 4.

The use and utility of imaging procedures

An article in May 1994[11] considered the possibility and utility of "periodically updated reviews of all randomised controlled trials relevant to neurology and neurosurgery". Virtually none of the trials referred to was primarily concerned with imaging the brain, and the unfortunate truth is that many clinicians appropriately guided by controlled trials of treatment approach imaging in what seems to their radiological colleagues to be a decidedly aleatoric way, guided by personal prejudices and what their chiefs used to do rather than by the latest audit on best practice. That radiologists are also prone to promote procedures that they enjoy ("cath time"[12]) and that far too many radiological publications are uncritical in their praise for recently developed procedures[13] is unhelpful.

My intention is to review, very broadly, categories of disease, and to attempt to indicate which imaging tests are the most likely to provide the information most appropriate for management of the patient; in general, I shall not dwell on how imaging research has clarified disease processes. I shall not look at patients likely to have cerebrovascular disease, as this is the subject of another review in this series. Neither shall I attempt to review all the imaging literature of recent years. Regrettably, in the countries from which the bulk of this literature arises there are strong motives for both promoting the use of medical facilities and for publishing one's work, which may explain the remarkable, and sometimes lamentable absence of outcome studies. To my knowledge, there is, for example, very little evidence that the outcome for patients with even the "surgical" neurological diseases (intracranial tumours, abscesses, haematomas, etc) has been appreciably improved by the most recent advances in imaging, except when these are indissolubly wedded to a surgical technique, as in image guided stereotaxic surgery. Indeed, such studies as have been performed have produced very disheartening results, showing no long lasting improvement in the quality of our patients' lives.[14]

Outcome in this sense is, of course, not the only measure. The great advantage of many modern imaging methods is that the patient endures far less unpleasant experiences, or runs less risk, to achieve the outcome, albeit identical. In this sense, CT represented a considerable advance over its predecessors, not necessarily improved on by progression to MRI, with the notable exception of MRA. Even short term outcome may not be affected much. Thus in MRI studies of the brain in patients with AIDS, there is no clear benefit for the large majority if contrast medium is given intravenously,[15] but some radiologists would defend its routine use. "Some of us are willing to pursue diagnostic accuracy with imaging studies to greater lengths than others, and each of us is likely to have some diseases to which we are willing to devote more time than others. This phenomenon (the "compulsiveness factor"), rooted in human nature, will survive even the current rage for outcome analysis".[16] One may counter this by observing that radiologists, like too many other doctors, become so accustomed to sticking sharp objects into their patients that they cease to regard it as an assault. Were the doctor injecting a patient to explain that his main motive was diagnostic compulsiveness rather than any expectation of altering management, he might well expose himself to a charge of battery![17]

With the advent of CT about 20 years ago, followed less than a decade later by MRI, the range of methods by which neuroradiologists make diagnoses and carry out follow up studies has paradoxically decreased. Both these cross sectional imaging techniques have led to a very significant fall in the number of other investigations performed, both plain radiographic and invasive, something which did not occur with the introduction of radionuclide examinations into neuroradiology in the years preceding the introduction of CT.[18] We are still going through the phase, familiar to radiologists, in which patients are submitted to multiple tests which yield essentially the same information, as occurred with CT and some of the older invasive investigations.[19] Thus many patients currently undergo both CT and MRI when either (or even neither) would suffice, but one may hope that this is a temporary phenomenon.

The choices of imaging procedure(s) the clinician has to make when confronted with a given clinical problem were summarised by the Royal College of Radiologists in a booklet *Making the best use of a department of clinical radiology. Guidelines for doctors*,[20] the second edition of which appeared at the end of 1993. Its recommendation was that every time someone thinks of requesting an examination they ask themselves "Do I need it?"; "Do I need it now?"; "Has it been done already?"; "Have I explained the problem?"—that is, do the radiographer and radiologist understand what I need to know and why?; and "Is this the best study?". The answers to several of these questions are different in Britain in 1995 from what they might be in an ideal world. Most neurologists and neurosurgeons acknowledge that they are perforce tempered by considerations of cost and availability, as well as inconvenience and risk to the patient (from radiation and other hazards), but they should also be informed by the answers to the implied questions "Is this test really likely to have any impact on my management of this patient? If not, will it nevertheless give data which will genuinely help my understanding of this disease and management of other patients with similar problems?", and, one might add "If so, does the patient who will suffer the inconvenience and risk of this test—a threat to life of 1 in 40 000 in contrast enhanced CT studies, for example[21]—know that?"

Head injuries

The controversy over the optimal imaging approach to head injuries continues to burn and, regrettably, the Royal College of Radiologists' booklet only serves to fan the flames. A major problem with rational management in Britain is that, more than in any other group of potentially neurological patients, the primary care of those with acute head injuries is largely entrusted to inexpert junior doctors who lack both the necessary maturity of judgement and a clear knowledge of the facts. The confusion over the relative roles of plain radiography and other tests, which in this context means essentially CT, pervades the Royal College's recommendations. Complex non-invasive techniques should not be employed to identify fractures of the cranial vault in patients with significant intracranial injuries. The presence of a linear fracture itself is irrelevant to the patient's management. It is often said that lawyers place great emphasis on injuries having been severe enough to cause a fracture; if this is so, it should be the clinician's task to re-educate them. If plain radiographs have any part to play it is in the assessment of complex fractures and, more debatably,[22] in raising suspicion of an underlying injury which may require treatment. Thus the advice that a patient "disorientated or worse . . . drunk/difficult to assess [or having] stable focal neurological signs" should have a skull radiograph and be admitted for observation seems like recourse to both belt and braces; that consultation with the neurosurgeons be immediate if the skull film shows a fracture but only after 12 hours if the patient fails to improve is questionable at best. Even more debatable is the suggestion that for a patient developing focal signs or whose conscious level is deteriorating, even for one whose pupil is dilating, pulse slowing, and blood pressure rising CT *or a skull film* is appropriate—as though the two were equivalent! A nationwide survey in the United States, reported in 1991, indicated that skull radiographs were obtained for trauma rarely or never in almost half of the hospitals surveyed, and performed less often in larger hospitals, with free access to CT, and at the behest of neurologists or neurosurgeons.[23]

As indicated earlier, CT would at present seem to be the primary investigation for detecting the intracranial complications of head injuries for several reasons: cheapness and general availability, lack of the logistic problems posed by carrying out MRI in emergency situations with a patient on a ventilator, etc, the ready detection of acute haemorrhage, and the fact that the management and prognostic relevance of the changes shown is understood. Magnetic resonance imaging is more sensitive to contusion or shearing injuries, but currently the therapeutic consequences of their demonstration are less well defined. This point applies not only in head injury. Because more intracranial lesions can be shown by MRI than by other techniques in patients with suspected disseminated malignancy, etc, staging of these patients, based on the sensitivities of older techniques, may have to be revised.

A late consequence of head injury which can lead to longstanding problems is the CSF fistula, usually giving rise to rhinorrhoea. A number of investigations, some of which (conventional tomography of the skull base, radionuclide cisternography) deliver a hefty radiation dose for little or no return, have been proposed in the past. For patients who are surgical candidates because of persistent problems, however, CT with intrathecal water soluble contrast medium, performed in the active phase of leakage,[24] is often the only radiological investigation required.

Brain death

Innumerable techniques have been proposed for use in the diagnosis or recognition of brain death, often with little or no regard to the relevant national or international recommendations. Indeed, many of the suggestions seem to be predicated on the presumed inability of neurologists to make the diagnosis reliably. The *Guidelines for the determination of death* drawn up in the United States by the *President's Commission* almost 15 years ago indicated that the diagnosis is indeed clinical, and that paraclinical tests, including imaging, might be used firstly to determine the cause of irreversible coma and secondly to shorten the period of observation required for definitive diagnosis.[25] There is little or no evidence that these imaging procedures are in practice used to supplement clinical examination in *earlier* determination of brain death, their only putative merit. One should not forget that, as Griner and Glaser[26] observed, diagnostic tests may be useful in four ways; two of these—screening and diagnosis—may be of direct utility to the patient. The third—assessment of treatment— is just as likely to be beneficial, if at all, only to the doctor, whereas the fourth—income generation—is uniquely so. The presumably self interested claim in the Royal College of Radiologists' *Guidelines* that in brain death radionuclide investigations have a "first line" role for "confirmation of neuronal loss" (!) seems as inappropriate as factually incorrect.

Acute lesions of cranial nerves

The plain film has no part to play in the initial assessment of patients with visual loss, except when this is thought to be due to an intraocular foreign body[27]; neither are there any indications for optic foramen views.[28] Should examination suggest an ocular cause other than intrinsic disease of the lens or retina, sonography of the globe (a specific technique best reserved for experts) may be employed. Magnetic resonance imaging may produce images which are more readily interpreted by the non-specialist, but it is doubtful that it has much to contribute when expert sonography is available.

When the signs suggest involvement of the intraorbital optic nerve, sonography is contraindicated; CT is probably as useful in most cases as MRI, and may show some significant abnormalities such as calcified, buried drusen of the optic disc or small, or even large,[29] plaques of calcification in a meningioma of the sheath of the optic nerve, to which MRI is insensitive; MRI may, however, be more informative when CT shows a mass lesion with a questionable anatomical relation to the optic nerve (and therefore its amenability to resection), or when it is important to determine whether a tumour arising from the nerve itself or its sheath extends intracranially.

Lesions within the substance of the anterior optic pathways that are not space occupying, essentially inflammatory, or degenerative, can be shown only by MRI. Thus pronounced swelling and contrast enhancement of the nerve-sheath complex may be shown in sarcoidosis. With high resolution coronal sections, it may be clear that the inflammatory process involves the meninges rather than the nerve itself, and the same contrast enhanced MRI study may show multifocal intracranial meningeal involvement as a bonus. The genuine utility of demonstrating plaques of demyelination, signal change in Leber's optic neuropathy, etc, is debatable, unless the presence and extent of a lesion within the optic nerve could influence the decision whether to treat the patient

45

with high dose steroids. In Britain, about two thirds of patients presenting with classic retrobulbar neuritis will go on to develop multiple sclerosis, and there is evidence that the large majority of those at risk can be identified by the presence of lesions in the brain at the time of initial presentation with visual disturbance[30]; if this knowledge is considered important, a stronger argument can be made for requesting MRI of the brain rather than the optic nerves. There are nevertheless some conditions, such as radiation neuropathy, in which imaging may be used not only to exclude a compressive lesion (a recurrent skull base tumour, for example) but also to establish a positive diagnosis, by showing pathological contrast enhancement within the nerve(s). Moreover, as damage to the blood-brain barrier is evanescent, follow up studies showing its restitution can resolve any diagnostic doubts.[31]

Mass lesions confined to the optic canal or affecting solely the adjacent bone are very rare. Magnetic resonance imaging would be the best technique for showing such masses, although CT often shows the bone to better effect. Evidence that surgical or other treatment is effective for visual loss due to trauma to the optic canal region is largely unconvincing, and a recent authoritative review suggests that it should be the subject of a serious controlled trial.[32] Recommendations about radiological attempts to show fractures, etc, must therefore be viewed critically. It may, however, be important for the faciomaxillary surgeon to be forewarned of the presence of a fracture through the canal when a visually intact patient is to undergo treatment for other facial injuries; this would be best documented by CT. As indicated, MRI is the examination of choice for demonstrating intracranial extension of a primary tumour of the optic pathways, manifest as signal change or expansion of the optic chiasm. With the addition of intravenous contrast medium, it is also the best way of demonstrating spread to the intracranial meninges of an optic nerve sheath meningioma.[33]

If the pattern of field loss localises the visual pathway disturbance to the intracranial optic nerve (by virtue of a contralateral junctional scotoma) or to the optic chiasm, MRI is in general superior to CT not only for detection, but even more so for effective preoperative characterisation. Images can be obtained in multiple planes, and MRA, which adds only a few minutes to the duration of the examination, can adequately show the parasellar arteries. An important study showed that aneurysms of sufficient size to compress the proximal intracranial optic pathways were unlikely not to be visible on MRI or CT.[34] The investigation of lesions affecting the optic chiasm is essentially similar to that of pituitary tumours, and is considered below. Patients with retrochiasmal visual loss can be divided clinically into two groups: those in whom the visual deficit is isolated and those with other evidence of a cerebral lesion. For a cerebral lesion the role of imaging is to show the presence or absence of a mass lesion, plaques of demyelination, etc, and these are considered elsewhere. An isolated homonymous hemianopia is usually due to an infarct involving the optic radiations or visual cortex, and CT or MRI are adequate for its demonstration. Angiography is not required unless some form of intervention would be contemplated.

Papilloedema

When patients presenting with longstanding headaches or visual disturbances are found to have bilateral disc swelling, the assumption is that they have papilloedema due to raised intracranial pressure until proved otherwise. From a strictly pragmatic viewpoint, a simple CT study without intravenous contrast medium only is required to establish firstly that there is no intracranial space occupying lesion, and secondly that lumbar puncture, indispensable for the diagnosis of benign intracranial hypertension, may be performed safely. It should be unnecessary to add that the cerebral ventricles are of *normal* size in this condition.[35] Demonstration of an empty sella turcica and dilated optic nerve sheaths is a bonus. Magnetic resonance imaging will show the sheaths in more detail, which may conceivably be useful if visual impairment is such that operative decompression of the sheaths is considered. It can also give additional information on the patency or otherwise of the dural venous sinuses, but the true value of that information in someone with chronic disease is highly questionable; the employment of invasive angiography can scarcely be justified.

Acute ocular motor nerve palsies

The investigation of acute cranial nerve palsies presumed to be due to structural vascular lesions, specifically aneurysms, is discussed in chapter 9. Many of the larger non-vascular lesions, particularly those amenable to treatment, will be visible on CT but, in as much as isolated acute cranial nerve lesions may be a manifestation of demyelination, MRI is clearly preferable.[36] Even then, no causative lesion will be shown in most patients presenting in this way; modern imaging has largely failed so far to elucidate such lesions as the "microvascular" third nerve palsy.

Extending the CT or MRI study to the orbit can be of value in identifying lesions of the superior oblique or lateral rectus muscles that mimic fourth or sixth nerve palsies.

Acute facial palsy

There have been reports of positive findings on MRI, particularly with gadolinium contrast enhancement, in patients with isolated acute facial weakness, and their relation to prognosis.[37] In typical cases of Bell's palsy, however, the genuine therapeutic utility of these expensive investigations may be on a par with that of showing uncomplicated rib fractures with a chest radiograph, and it seems entirely reasonable to reserve imaging for atypical cases. One must be aware that, as with some inflammatory lesions—cerebral abscess being a prime example—contrast enhancement may persist once clinical resolution has occurred. One must remember that imaging can disclose only a relatively small range of abnormalities (swelling, shrinkage, change in density or intensity, etc); it cannot interpret images without the clinical picture firmly in mind, as a report of findings on contrast enhanced MRI in the Ramsay Hunt syndrome—in a patient with symptoms for two days—mimicking an intracanalicular vestibular schwannoma[38] emphasises.

Acute lower cranial nerve palsies are commonly either vascular or demyelinating and are therefore treated elsewhere.

Chronic lesions of the lower nerves

The number of patients presenting with disturbances of hearing or balance is very large, and were all to be intensively investigated, the imaging services would be in danger of being swamped. The number of patients referred for imaging can, however, be controlled so that the services are used much more appropriately if neuro-otological consultations precede imaging. This is particularly true in patients who have vertigo without hearing loss, in whom a positive diagnosis can often be made without recourse to imaging, and a structural lesion is rarely found. When the history, examination, and otological tests indicate the possibility of a vestibular schwannoma, there is now little justification for carrying out any test other than MRI. Plain films and conventional tomography have no part to play in the 1990s (and it was very difficult to rationalise their use in the preceding decade).[39] It is now evident that, when MRI is not available, CT is a poor second best, although it can demonstrate relatively large tumours. The promotion of gadolinium enhanced images for MRI demonstration of smaller tumours[40] was always questionable, as most could be shown with adequate clarity by a combination of T1 and T2 weighted images, except perhaps on the least satisfactory machines. The recommendations for the use of contrast medium by the 1991 NIH Consensus Development Panel, not published until 1994,[41] have been overtaken by technical developments: it is now widely accepted that high resolution T2 weighted images of the region of the internal auditory meatus in a single plane are adequate for exclusion of even small tumours[42] (figure 2.1); when the results are equivocal, addition of a second plane is quicker, kinder, and much cheaper than subjecting the patient to an intravenous injection. Optimal techniques may, of course, vary depending on local factors such as machine strength, availability of specific coils, high resolution programmes, etc; discussion with the radiologist may be necessary to achieve the optimal results in any given unit.

"Vascular compression syndromes" in the posterior fossa continue to stir up debate. If one believes that compression of the fifth or seventh cranial nerves by relatively small vessels can produce facial pain or twitching respectively, and that surgery is the answer, high resolution MRI similar to that used for investigation of the VIIIth nerve is the optimal imaging technique. It is the only one which shows clearly the cranial nerves and the adjacent vessels: it may be supplemented by MRA showing the whole course of the "offending" artery,[43] but if the surgical approach does not depend on the detailed vascular anatomy, this may be redundant.

The diagnostic yield of CT in patients with palsies of the lower cranial nerves (IX-XII) is sufficiently low compared with that of MRI that the older technique should be foregone whenever feasible. Intrinsic lesions—neoplastic, vascular, or inflammatory—of the lower brain stem, often quite small, can often be identified

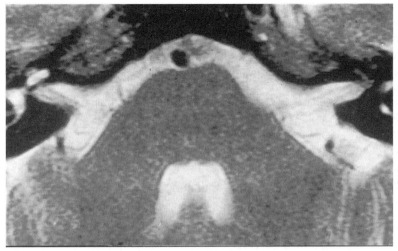

(A)

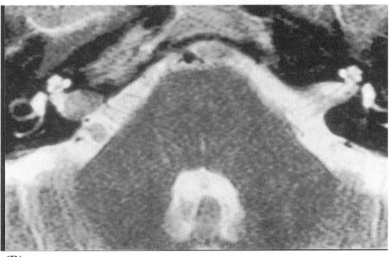

(B)

Figure 2.1   *The value of high resolution T2 weighted MRI in diagnosis of tumours in the cerebellopontine angle. (A) Normal axial section: the individual nerve bundles are clearly seen within each internal auditory meatus. No further imaging is required to exclude even a small vestibular Schwannoma. (B) Right intracanalicular tumour: the widened right meatus is almost filled by tissue giving signal similar to that of the brain*

only with MRI.[44] Most extra-axial lesions are also clearly visible, with the exception of malignant or inflammatory basal meningitis, in which even quite extensive lesions may be evident only on images after intravenous gadolinium.

When extra-axial masses are identified in the lower part of the posterior cranial fossa, MRI will confirm the nature of aneurysms or provide preoperative vascular mapping in the case of soft tissue lesions. When MRI discloses a lesion in the region of the foramen magnum, however, particularly one showing inhomogeneous contrast enhancement that suggests the presence of large vessels in a glomus tumour, an intra-arterial study with the aim of proceeding to therapeutic preoperative embolisation is indicated.

Magnetic resonance imaging is also the prime investigation for patients in whom brain stem or cerebellar disorders are thought to be due to anomalies at the foramen magnum. Numerous studies have suggested that the cerebellar tonsils may, in normal subjects, extend a few millimetres below the foramen magnum, whereas older studies, usually myelographic, suggested that this was not the case. More recent work suggests that the older data, although obtained with a technique liable to alter the craniospinal hydrodynamics, were indeed correct, and that it is the normal biventral lobules extending through the central part of the foramen, which lie higher than its lateral borders, which give the impression of cerebellar ectopia.[45] In practice this means that it is not abnormal for a midline sagittal image to show the inferior part of the cerebellum extending slightly below the plane joining the anterior and posterior lips of the foramen magnum. More important pathological observations are that the neuraxis seems to pack the foramen and that the anterior surface of the medulla seems compressed against the odontoid peg. Needless to say, the appearances of "cerebellar ectopia" in a patient without appropriate symptoms or signs are usually irrelevant. Imaging for suspected foramen magnum lesions should include the upper cervical spine, as an asymptomatic associated syrinx may be detected. Plain films or CT may be required before surgery for foramen magnum abnormalities, because of their superior demonstration of the bone.

Acute cerebral and cerebellar lesions

It is only a few years since editorials published in several neuroscience journals emphasised that, despite the inroads of MRI, the diagnosis of multiple sclerosis was essentially clinical, backed up by neurophysiological and CSF testing.[46] The same can be said of many diseases, especially those in which initial clinical presentation is protean and subsequent course equally variable. In pragmatic terms, however, one may question this judgement. *In the appropriate clinical context*, particularly in young people, the demonstration of multiple, characteristic lesions, usually in the brain, but occasionally solely in the spinal cord, gives a sufficiently strong clue to the diagnosis to obviate further investigation. For example, the predictive value of a positive MRI study of the brain in patients presenting with retrobulbar neuritis or myelitis as an initial neurological disturbance is so strong that extensive additional investigations would seem meddlesome unless there are discordant features. Whether the patient with optic neuritis *should* undergo MRI of the brain is an ethical question; in purely pragmatic terms, the efforts of the popular press in drawing attention to this condition as the harbinger of multiple sclerosis are such that many young women consider themselves inadequately investigated without MRI.

It is certainly no longer effectively the case that multiple sclerosis is a diagnosis of exclusion. For both clinical and technical reasons, however, routine MRI is more likely to show lesions in the head than in the spinal cord; indeed, the detection of lesions in the spinal cord is one of the most stringent tests of the quality of the imager. Estimates of the proportion of patients in whom MRI will show spinal lesions when images of the brain appear normal vary, but in the most reliable series the percentage is small. This being the case, a strong argument can be made for imaging the head first and foregoing images of the spine in young patients with relapsing symptoms, when cranial MRI clearly shows typical, disseminated disease. Even when a spinal cord episode is the first neurological illness, demonstration of brain lesions increases the relative risk of progression to multiple sclerosis in less than two years by 36 times, or by about 15 times if patients with complete transverse myelitis are excluded.[47] The proportion of this group, when attacks involve different spinal levels, in which an additional structural lesion will be found is minuscule. As an analogy, when a patient with multiple enlarged lymph nodes is shown by biopsy to have classic sarcoidosis, one does not proceed to sample all the other nodes in case one might show Hodgkin's disease. In older patients with progressive symptoms, which might be due to superimposed spondylosis, for example, the situation is obviously different.

It is axiomatic that on MRI the lesions of multiple sclerosis are not pathognomonic. Some of the diseases that may simulate multiple sclerosis, including sarcoidosis and tropical spastic paraparesis,[48] may produce very similar radiological appearances. Clinical features, together with CSF analysis, are therefore paramount in a proportion of cases. Fortunately, these conditions are rare, as are the often suggested but rarely documented cerebral vasculitides, although these tend to produce more peripheral and basal ganglion lesions,[49] as does Behçet's disease, which also shows a predilection for the brain stem.[50] Small vessel ischaemia, however, is ubiquitous, and in the individual patient, for whom statistical analyses are unhelpful, it may be difficult to make a firm diagnosis on imaging grounds. Lesions which are predominantly periventricular, involving the corpus callosum, and with transverse diameter greater than their anteroposterior extent, favour multiple sclerosis, as does finding multiple, apparently asymptomatic supratentorial and infratentorial abnormalities in a young patient. None of these characteristics is absolute; I am not convinced that statistical analysis of lesion numbers, etc[51] helps any more than an experienced radiologist's impression in any given case. Once the diagnosis of multiple sclerosis is established or strongly suggested, repeated MRI studies to demonstrate the appearance of new lesions are rarely indicated, particularly in establishing a differential diagnosis between, for example, small vessel ischaemic disease and multiple sclerosis in a middle aged person. Occasionally, the finding of new lesions may facilitate the differentiation of acute disseminated encephalomyelitis, a monophasic illness, and multiple sclerosis; whether this is worthwhile clinically is, however, debatable. In established multiple sclerosis, there is little point in repeat MRI studies charting the course of the individual patient's disease, unless there are strong reasons for thinking that a new neurological episode is due to some other condition.

Before the advent of MRI, some workers proposed double dose, delayed contrast enhanced CT for detection of cerebral plaques,[52] but this was always of doubtful value as most of the patients with positive results had diagnostic changes in the CSF. Accepting the caveat that the diagnosis of multiple sclerosis is essentially clinical, and that the role of radiology before the advent of MRI was largely exclusory, the use of this technique in patients who cannot for some reason undergo MRI is highly debatable. In general it is also true that when MRI studies are positive in patients with suspected multiple sclerosis, recourse to gadolinium enhancement is unnecessary. Occasionally, however, when alternative diagnoses seem likely, the absence of contrast enhancement of any lesion may strengthen the suspicion of multiple sclerosis, particularly when the patient is not in an acute relapse, whereas enhancement of all or most of the lesions visible on T2 weighted images may point to acute disseminated encephalomyelitis—in which some of the lesions are often large,[53]—or an inflammatory condition such as sarcoidosis.

Intracranial infections

There is little doubt that CT revolutionised the neurologists' and surgeons' approach to many intracranial infections, including cerebral abscesses, empyemas, granulomatous disease, etc. It is also clear that for certain types of infection, notably encephalitis, MRI is significantly more sensitive, particularly in the early stages of the disease (figure 2.2).[54] This is also true of other conditions, such as meningitis and AIDS, but the added sensitivity in some of these may simply allow observation of disease progression rather than conferring any benefit on the individual patient, much though they may advance medical knowledge.

Many subacute or chronic infections produce changes that can be identified on CT, or with greater ease on MRI. Unfortunately, as in so many situations, the radiological findings are non-specific; thus the diagnosis of intracranial Whipple's disease, Lyme disease,[55] etc, is invariably based as much on clinical and epidemiological factors as on imaging. This also applies to opportunistic infections in AIDS: although in many parts of the world the major organism is toxoplasma, cryptococcus may be relatively common in some areas,[56] whereas in Spain, for example, tuberculosis is an important consideration.[57] Differentiation of toxoplasmosis from lymphoma by means of MRI is sufficiently unreliable for antimicrobial treatment or biopsy to be the recommended course[58] rather than reliance on the radiologist's diagnostic "compulsiveness".

Chronic and progressive syndromes

Cerebral lesions

Historically, one of the fields to which most effort has been directed in imaging the head is that of progressive focal or generalised neurological deficit—that is, detection and characterisation of intracranial tumours. This is not, however, a single task, and for practical purposes, it can be subdivided as follows[59]:

- Detecting a mass lesion within the head
- Indicating whether it lies within or without the brain
- Whether it requires biopsy for tissue characterisation
- Indicating the best means of intervention
- Directing that intervention
- Monitoring the natural history of untreated lesions
- Secondary effects of the lesion
- The effects of treatment.

It is a truism that skull radiographs and radionuclide investigations are not indicated, even as non-invasive screening tests, for *detection* of intracranial masses; both have unacceptably high false negative rates.[60 61] Magnetic resonance imaging yields a significantly higher detection rate than CT, especially in the anatomical sites to which CT is known to be relatively blind—namely, the anteroinferior part of the middle cranial fossa and the posterior cranial fossa, particularly the brain stem. Studies carried out when MRI was first introduced, however, gave conflicting results as regards the detectability of supratentorial neoplasms other than in the temporal lobes.[62] Some of these were methodologically questionable, and more recent scientifically conducted comparisons are few, but a clinical impression is that, with modern equipment, the detection rate for tumours in or adjacent to the cerebral hemispheres with the two techniques is not greatly different. Even clinicians' awareness of this does not, however, prevent many patients having both tests.

Contrary to a widespread belief, numerous studies have confirmed the radiologists' impression that there is only a very small (less than 1%) decrease in detection rate of primary cerebral tumours if intravenous contrast medium is not given; furthermore, this was true even when image quality was much inferior to that available today.[63] It is recognised that "false negative" CT studies occur with fast growing malignant gliomas, particularly in patients presenting with seizures; a second examination months later, by which time neurological signs have often developed, may show a large tumour genuinely invisible on the first[64]; the same may also occur with MRI. Not surprisingly, contrast enhanced MRI has been found to be more effective than CT for detection of intracranial metastases. This applies particularly to extra-axial deposits, to

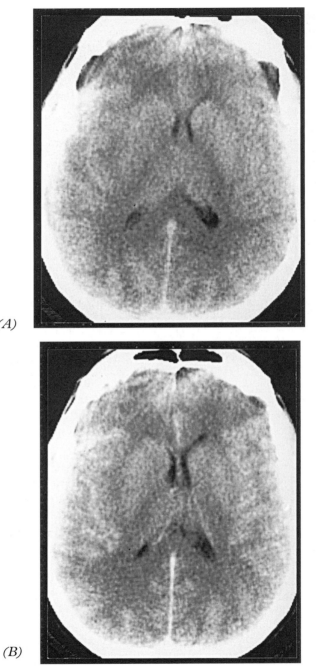

(A)

(B)

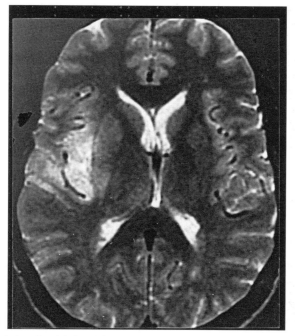

(C)

Figure 2.2   *Sensitivity of MRI in suspected encephalitis. Computed tomography (A) before and (B) after intravenous contrast medium shows only mild diffuse low density in the right external capsular region, with minor swelling. (C) On T2 weighted MRI a focal temporal and insular lesion is shown sufficiently clearly to enable biopsy, if required*

which CT is notoriously insensitive,[65] but is also true when only parenchymal lesions are present[66]; there seems to be little or no benefit in delaying the postinjection imaging, a manoeuvre claimed to increase the detection rate in CT.

Once the radiologist has decided that an intracranial mass is neoplastic, which is not difficult in most cases, his long term aim would clearly be to be able to provide a tissue diagnosis sufficiently reliable to obviate biopsy. Until we reach that happy state, it can be argued that the neuroradiologist should rather "ask himself whether or not a precise diagnosis is really useful",[67] and throw in the towel. Situations which engender negative answers to that question are almost certainly more common than otherwise. Exceptions include the fundamentally important, but often rather

57

low level decision, as to whether a mass lies within or outside the brain, as in the former case it is potentially resectable; whether multiple or less commonly single masses are likely to be part of disseminated metastatic disease, in which case surgery on the head, even biopsy, may not be the preferred option; or whether it might be a lymphoma, in which case one should abstain from steroid treatment before biopsy.[68] It seemed at one time that immunolocalisation of brain tumours, using tissue specific antibodies labelled with radionuclides[69] or some compound detectable by magnetic resonance, would obviate radiological diagnostic guesswork, but that promise does not seem as yet to have been fulfilled.

Similar remarks apply to attempts to grade degrees of malignancy by imaging (figure 2.3). Considerable effort has been devoted to establishing correlations between malignancy and radiological criteria derived from angiography, CT, MRI, and isotope studies. When these involve complex formulae or multifactorial analyses which barely achieve statistical significance,[70] their clinical utility is effectively nil. Simple Gestalt analyses of some of these tests, however, can contribute to prognosis when biopsy is either unhelpful or patently at variance with the radiological data, indicating that atypical tissue has been obtained. These should be the minority of cases, as histological examination is in general more reliable. Unfortunately, many recent enthusiastic reports on radiological differential diagnosis of intracerebral or intraventricular[71] tumours have the same fatal flaw; the differential diagnostic game may be entertaining for the radiologist to play, but clinical features may be equally important and the images rarely supplant biopsy. It is perhaps puzzling that a report showing a close correlation between grades of malignity of intracranial tumours and the methyl and methylene peaks of peripheral blood on MRS[72] seems to have engendered little excitement among neurosurgeons—or perhaps not!

Where extracerebral tumours are concerned, the value of current imaging techniques in general is in similarly providing morphological detail rather than refining diagnosis. Magnetic resonance signal characteristics, for example, do not seem particularly useful for assessing preoperatively the likely consistency of meningiomas.[73]

Surgical use of imaging technology for localisation of lesions to be removed or biopsied has progressed in less than 20 years from

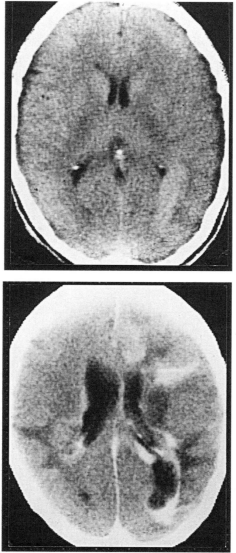

(A)

(B)

Figure 2.3 *Pitfalls of attempting to grade cerebral tumours on imaging characteristics. (A) A well defined, homogeneously dense area within the left occipital white matter shows no features, such as accompanying vasogenic oedema or contrast enhancement, to indicate that it should not be classed as low grade. (B) Six months after excision, the tumour has manifested its malignancy by spreading throughout the cerebrum; it now shows both oedema and contrast enhancement*

59

the complex but rather crude, using very rough data given by air studies and angiography, to the highly sophisticated, using a variety of techniques and combining the information into computer generated images which often contain more information than the surgeon can use. The ways in which CT or MRI guided stereotaxy are currently performed are almost as various as the institutions involved. Suffice it to say that by the time these words are published routine intracranial surgery carried out, perhaps by remote control, within a dedicated MR imager, with effectively real time data presentation, may no longer be science fiction.

Angiography remains part of the preoperative investigation of patients with intracranial tumours in some institutions, although the benefits it confers are debatable. There would seem to be no justification for using an invasive technique with a known morbidity for localisation of masses, particularly when, as in the large majority of cases, non-invasive procedures are more reliable. Grading of intrinsic tumours on the basis of pathological vessels, etc, has not been shown to be more sensitive than grading by CT or MRI. When information about patency of dural sinuses, etc, is thought necessary before surgery, this can be acquired by intravenous digital subtraction angiography or MRA, and the same may be said for the demonstration of large vessels before stereotaxic biopsy. Virtually the only firm indication for preoperative intra-arterial angiography is when intravascular intervention is foreseen. Presurgical embolisation of some vascular neoplasms, especially those around the skull base such as glomus jugulare tumours or juvenile angiofibromas, is today generally considered the best practice, but surgeons' universal enthusiasm for intra-arterial treatment of, for example, convexity meningiomas, seems to have waned as doubt has been cast on the real benefits.[74] Unfortunately, meningiomas arising from the skull base, in which surgical access to the feeding vessels is less straightforward and haemostasis would be a real gain, are often not strikingly vascular on angiography.[75]

If cerebral tumours are treated by biopsy and radiotherapy (with or without other types of treatment) rather than by excision, it is important to know the extent of brain involvement, as it is undesirable to expose normal brain to therapeutic doses of radiation. There is evidence from surgical biopsies, postmortem examinations, and correlation with PET studies of cerebral metabolism that CT underestimates tumour spread,[76] and the same is almost certainly true of MRI. There have been a number of accounts of treatment of cerebral[77] and brain stem neoplasms by intra-arterial infusion of cytotoxic agents. Theoretically at least, delivering the noxious agent close to the vascular bed of the tumour has advantages, but it remains to be proved that these outweigh the morbidity of the technique.

Computed tomography or MRI are excellent methods of following up patients with cerebral tumours, treated or untreated. It is, however, reasonable to restrict the use of these or any other investigations to clinical situations in which there is some realistic likelihood that they will modify management. When surgery seems inappropriate for a patient with a low grade intrinsic tumour, imaging follow up is required only when a significant change in clinical status occurs, which might tip the balance in favour of surgery, or in the unlikely event that some new operative technique renders intervention a better choice. Much the same applies in many situations; imaging as occupational therapy for the outpatient whose recent clinical status is unchanged some months or even years after total removal of a meningioma, for example, is fruitless.[77a].

Differentiating recurrent tumour from radionecrosis remains difficult with imaging; neither CT nor MRI is sufficiently reliable. There have been several reports of the use of PET for this purpose, but its expense and limited availability tend to exclude it from routine use; SPECT techniques, which are considerably cheaper, may be informative, however, in at least some cases.[78]

Headache

Some surveys have confirmed the very low diagnostic yield of imaging in patients with either non-specific headache unaccompanied by neurological disturbances or recognisable forms of migraine, migrainous neuralgia, etc. This is one area in which sensible clinical assessment is invaluable, given the frequency of complaints of headache and the desire of many patients to be investigated. The other side of the coin is that CT is now a cheap and almost completely anodyne test, provided that contrast medium is avoided. When CT was considerably less widely available and relatively more expensive than today, one audit of its utility suggested that an EEG might be a good pre-CT screening test in patients with chronic headache[79]; one could probably reverse this argument on cost-benefit grounds today. Plain films of the skull are an even cheaper way of confirming the diagnosis in unusual conditions in which the skull itself is the source of pain, such as Paget's disease. In a more common situation, films of the paranasal sinuses will usually show or exclude inflammatory or other changes severe enough to cause chronic headache, although they may not suffice for further management. Conversely, plain films of the craniocervical junction or cervical spine hardly ever elucidate isolated occipital pain; moreover, they are so often abnormal in elderly people[80] that they cannot genuinely support a diagnosis of cervicogenic pain.

Investigation of types of headache known to be associated with intracranial or craniocervical lesions—as in subarachnoid haemorrhage or cough headache—will depend on the presumed nature of the underlying lesion: an intracranial aneurysm or cerebellar tonsillar ectopia, for example. Because, save for such cases, there is little to indicate that MRI is superior to CT in the investigation of headache, it is probably unjustifiable to use the more expensive method as a primary imaging test.

Epilepsy

The contribution of imaging to investigation of patients whose illness is dominated by or consists primarily of epileptic attacks has traditionally been the detection of potentially treatable causes, typified by intracranial tumours or vascular malformations. With the advent of CT, causative lesions not amenable to such treatment—small cortical infarcts, or the effects of previous trauma— could be identified. This may have satisfied the neurologist's curiosity, but positive effects on management were minor.[81] When the increased sensitivity of MRI to parenchymal pathology first became evident, it was suggested that the detection rate for lesions responsible for epilepsy was very much higher than when using CT. This has not been entirely borne out by subsequent experience and, with some exceptions, the abnormalities to which the newer technique is indeed more sensitive tend to be those in which their presence explains why the patient should have fits rather than those to which present surgical approaches are suited.

Thus when a patient presents with seizures, the aim of imaging should be firstly to determine whether he or she has a lesion that should be treated itself, and of which the fits are simply the clinical manifestation. A convexity meningioma is the paradigm; in a relatively young patient the likely morbidity of investigation and treatment is outweighed not merely by the presentation, but also by the natural history. When preliminary imaging shows a complex arteriovenous malformation in an eloquent area in someone of middle age, the equation is more finely balanced, but will depend to some extent on imaging data. Needless to say, plain films and radionuclide investigations are sufficiently insensitive as to be effectively useless, but there is little evidence that for detection of such "surgical" lesions MRI is superior to CT, although further investigations may be required before surgical decision making. When CT is normal in patients whose epilepsy is not so severe as to require more radical surgery, there is little or no justification for further investigation. There are some adults and children in whom MRI will show anomalies of cerebral cortication, or heterotopic grey matter, etc, but if, given today's surgical possibilities, a mildly affected patient would not be a candidate for cerebral resection surgery, this type of investigation cannot be justified in clinical practice, other than as research.

When the fits are so intractable, however, or the side effects of conservative treatment so onerous that the patient would be offered surgery as primary treatment, MRI is the examination of choice. This is particularly true when the presumed epileptogenic focus lies in the temporal lobe, to which CT is recognised to be relatively blind. Thin coronal T1 and T2 weighted images, which permit volumetric analysis and three dimensional reconstructions, can show not only hamartomas and indolent tumours, but minor degrees of hippocampal atrophy and signal change, indicating mesial temporal sclerosis. As always when images are used to generate measurements there are important methodological sources of error, from which a number of the most often cited publications may not be free.[82] Even when these are taken into consideration, for successful surgery the results must be considered in combination with clinical and electrophysiological data, including preoperative tests of cerebral dominance using intra-arterial sodium amytal. Possibly because of the expense of both techniques, the combination of MRI with magnetoencephalography,[83] to produce what at least one radiologist, possibly with political foresight, has termed "magnetic source imaging", has not become widespread as yet. It has been suggested that interictal or particularly ictal and peri-ictal functional radionuclide studies give more demonstrative lateralising data[84] but, even so, MRI demonstration of detailed anatomy greatly assists the neurosurgeon. A few years ago, some centres were reporting successful outcomes of surgery for mesial temporal sclerosis in as few as 60% of patients.[82] This should improve with current MRI techniques, and in the near future intraoperative MRI will almost certainly prove extremely valuable in guiding the extent of resection.

Movement disorders

Regrettably, static imaging methods, concerned with structure rather than function, have contributed little to clinical investigation of involuntary movements, except where these are symptomatic of structural disease, as in the rare meningioma causing tremor. Demonstration by high field MRI of putative changes in brain iron distribution in parkinsonism variants was very enthusiastically promoted some years ago,[85] but has since spectacularly failed to change clinical practice.

Some disorders, such as Hallervorden-Spatz disease, have highly suggestive MRI findings (the "eye of the tiger" globus pallidus).[86] The findings in Wilson's disease, however, are variable, inconstant (although much less so than with CT), and do not necessarily correlate with clinical status or response to treatment[87]; they may serve to strengthen a clinical diagnosis, but clearly do not replace metabolic investigations. The atrophic changes seen in "multiple system atrophy" are similarly non-specific and bolster clinical impressions rather than throwing up unsuspected diagnoses.[88]

Dementia

Investigation of patients presenting with or found to have dementia is highly variable in practice, although the underlying controversy is rarely articulated. Published evidence is certainly contradictory. On the one hand, there are studies, often initiated by radiologists, which show the very poor cost-benefit gains from imaging in such patients, especially those without neurological signs and that, contrary to widespread belief, the proportion of patients with genuinely treatable lesions does not increase greatly with earlier onset of dementia.[89] On the other hand, hardly an issue of a self respecting neurological journal appears without an article on changes that may be shown by detailed analysis of

expensive investigations (CT, MRI, SPECT, or PET) in demented patients. Few, if any, of these have shown any useful, reliable
correlation between structural or even functional imaging and specific causes of dementia (rather than dementia in general); indeed,
in most published studies the accepted diagnosis is that made on
clinical and psychometric grounds. This is especially regrettable,
as, despite some claims to greater accuracy, at least one series, in
which clinical, radiological, and neurophysiological assessments
were compared with postmortem findings, revealed only 47% sensitivity and 65% specificity in diagnosing Alzheimer's disease.[90] It
may be true that other neuropsychologists are better at clinical differential diagnosis, but those who have not put themselves to the
test should not assume this to be the case. Nevertheless, the frequency and "scientific" tone of such studies seem to have convinced some neurologists that they should be carrying out these
tests as diagnostic aids on their patients. Were some specific treatment for Alzheimer's disease, for example, to become available, it
would be comprehensible that an imaging test of high specificity
and sensitivity might be used to select which demented patients
were treated. But unless that test were quick, cheap, freely available, and virtually infallible, it would seem unethical not to extend
treatment to other demented patients, unless it proved unacceptably toxic or expensive; and neither that test nor the treatment are
currently to hand. It has been suggested that simple linear measurement of the distance between the medial border of the uncus
on the two sides might be useful for identifying patients with
Alzheimer's disease, but some groups have been unable to distinguish patients with mild to moderate dementia from normal subjects of the same age with this criterion.[91] A recent update on the
OPTIMA group's suggestion that measurement of the minimum
width of medial temporal lobe tissue at the level of the brain stem[92]
indicates that this simple test does have high discriminant value;
however, it is by definition not useful until the disease has already
reached a stage at which structural changes have occurred.

It cannot be overemphasised that loss of brain volume is a normal phenomenon in elderly people, and its demonstration cannot
be assumed to have advanced the investigation of dementia. For
this reason many radiologists prefer the term "cerebral involution", because of the traditionally "pathological" overtones of
"atrophy". It should also be understood that correlations between
the lesions due to small vessel ischaemia which can be shown by

CT or, with greater sensitivity by MRI, and cognitive decline is sufficiently vague to be of no clinical value in the individual case, particularly in the elderly, mildly demented patient.[93] In a number of brain diseases known to be associated in some cases with dementia (such as parkinsonism), although some workers have suggested focal atrophy of the medial frontal lobes and around the third ventricle,[94] others have found no good correlation with specific imaging changes.[95] Not surprisingly, some correlation between cognitive decline and the extent of brain disease has been identified in multiple sclerosis.[96]

It was to be hoped that modern imaging might prove more helpful than invasive techniques in diagnosis of early Huntington's disease, but clinical features and, of course, family history and DNA analysis seem to be better guides. It has been suggested, however, that the degree of atrophy of the caudate nucleus may be a guide to prognosis.[97]

A persistent controversy concerns the frequency (perhaps even the existence) of normal pressure hydrocephalus. In Britain this is a rather infrequent diagnosis in patients without a clear antecedent history of intracranial bleeding or infection, and very small numbers are subjected to shunt procedures on the basis of a diagnosis of idiopathic normal pressure hydrocephalus, but one report describes 22 patients in whom normal pressure hydrocephalus had been diagnosed undergoing a non-standard MRI procedure before operation in a relatively short time at a single German university hospital.[98] When the clinical and laboratory criteria for the diagnosis seem so geographically variable, assessment of claims about the therapeutic significance of putative radiological signs is virtually impossible. With recent reports about the relevance of MRI findings of concomitant white matter disease and arterial hypertension to the pathophysiology,[99] water on the brain is probably at its muddiest ever, at least in the imaging literature.[100]

Other neuropsychiatric disorders

Several imaging studies in recent years have applied CT, MRI, and radionuclide methods to patients with schizophrenia, autism, psychosis, etc.[101] The range of imaging features examined has been extensive and various, and few groups have used widely accepted criteria. In addition, many workers have published the statistical analyses of their findings rather than the measurements themselves, which are essential for replication and comparison. The main thrust seems to have been to show that people with psychiatric disorders do indeed have structural abnormalities, a fact which some psychiatrists, presumably battling with their psychoanalytical colleagues, find "exciting".[102] As yet, the data are too soft and contradictory for any clue to pathophysiology to have emerged, and their clinical relevance is doubtful.

Neuroendocrine disease

The history of the application of imaging to the investigation of neuroendocrine disease, specifically to small but hormonally active pituitary tumours, makes entertaining reading. As each of a series of techniques has become available, it has made clear the high level of self deception by both radiologists and endocrinologists necessary for the use of its predecessor. Thus plain radiography, conventional tomography, and even CT[103] have all been shown to be extremely unreliable in the light of later technology; the particularly high inaccuracy of CT was recognised even before comparisons were made with MRI.[104] Although MRI is also not infallible, it would seem to be by far the best investigation currently available. As I have pointed out previously, however, "the desirability of locating the tumour within the pituitary gland of a patient with hyperprolactinaemia is predicated solely and absolutely on surgery being the treatment of choice"; it is otiose when chemotherapy will be employed.

When larger pituitary region tumours are present, the multiplanar capacity of MRI, linked to MRA for demonstration of the vascular anatomy, renders this the technique of choice. Combining image quality with economy, in ideal circumstances, it is probably necessary to use only a fat suppressed contrast enhanced T1 weighted volume acquisition but once again this will depend to some extent on the technical possibilities of the apparatus available. This simple technique can also be used for follow up after surgery, although, as I have indicated elsewhere, clinicians' fondness for follow up studies may have to yield to audits showing their lack of cost or benefit effectiveness. This would seem to be particularly true when women being treated with, for example, bromocriptine are asymptomatic as regards both their hormonal status and vision.

The greater sensitivity to both the internal structure of pituitary tumours and their relations with the anterior optic pathways make

67

MRI the ideal method for investigating suspected pituitary apoplexy, and for deciding which patients actually need treatment, as the apoplectic episode may itself result in involution of tumour usually found to underlie it.[105]

Magnetic resonance imaging has opened doors to other endocrine disturbances to which CT was effectively blind. As an example, the normal posterior lobe of the pituitary gives high signal on T1 weighted MRI, for reasons not entirely clear. This is absent in most patients with central or nephrogenic diabetes insipidus, but not in those with primary polydipsia.[106]

Conclusions

It is difficult to draw overall conclusions from the foregoing, as I have tried to indicate in each case the sort of selection process that the neurologist or neurosurgeon should make when thinking of referring a patient for imaging. To best use his services to the patient's advantage, the clinician should: (*a*) refrain from any imaging for which there is no clear clinical indication and (*b*) prefer anodyne to invasive, cheap to expensive, but (*c*) not perform a harmless, low cost examination if it will not obviate a more aggressive or expensive one.

In Britain the legal power to determine whether *any* imaging investigation is carried out is unequivocally vested in the radiologist.[107] This gives force to the Royal College of Radiologists' uncontentious recommendation that "if you are in doubt as to whether an investigation is required or which investigation is best, it makes sense to ask the radiologists who, like other consultants, will know much more about their specialty than those whose primary interests are in other fields".[20]

1 Dumoulin CL, Hart HR. MR angiography. *Radiology* 1986;**161**:717–20.
2 Nitz WR, Bradley WG, Watanabe AS, Lee RR, Burgoyne B, O'Sullivan RM, *et al.* Flow dynamics of cerebrospinal fluid: assessment with phase-contrast velocity MR imaging performed with retrospective cardiac gating. *Radiology* 1992;**183**:395–405.
3 Gideon P, Sorensen PS, Thomsen C, Ståhlberg F, Gjerris F, Henriksen O. Assessment of CSF dynamics and venous flow in the superior sagittal sinus by MRI in idiopathic intracranial hypertension: a preliminary study. *Neuroradiology* 1994;**36**:350–4.
4 McComb JG. The usefulness of phase-contrast MR measurement of cerebrospinal fluid flow. *AJNR Am J Neuroradiol* 1993;**14**:1309–10.
5 Castillo M, Hudgins PA, Malko JA, Burrow BK, Hoffman JC Jr. Flow-sensitive MR imaging of ventriculo-peritoneal shunts: in vitro findings, clinical applications, and pitfalls. *AJNR Am J Neuroradiol* 1991;**12**:667–71.
6 Le Bihan D, Breton E, Lallemand D, Grenier P, Cabanis E, Laval-Jeantet M. MR imaging of intravoxel incoherent motions: applications to diffusion and perfusion in neurological disorders. *Radiology* 1988;**161**:401–7.

7 Henkelman RM. Diffusion-weighted MR imaging: a useful adjunct to clinical diagnosis or a scientific curiosity? *AJNR Am J Neuroradiol* 1990;**12**:932–4.
8 Dorothee O, Henning J, Ernst T. Human brain tumors: assessment with in vivo proton spectroscopy. *Radiology* 1993;**186**:745–52.
9 Vion-Dury J, Meyerhoff DJ, Cozzone PL, Weiner MW. What might be the impact on neurology of the analysis of brain metabolism by in vivo magnetic resonance spectroscopy? *J Neurol* 1994;**241**:354–71.
10 Rubin JM, Mirfakhree M, Duda EE, Dohrmann GJ, Brown F. Intraoperative ultrasound examination of the brain. *Radiology* 1980;**137**:831–2.
11 Counsell CE, Fraser H, Sandercock PAG. Archie Cochrane's challenge: can periodically updated reviews of all randomised controlled trials relevant to neurology and neuro-surgery be produced? *J Neurol Neurosurg Psychiatry* 1994;**57**:529–33.
12 Daves ML. Radiologic overkill. *JAMA* 1967;**200**:999–1000.
13 Kent DL, Larson EB. Magnetic resonance imaging of the brain and spine: is clinical efficacy established after the first decade? *Ann Intern Med* 1988;**108**:402–24.
14 Dixon AK, Southern JP, Teale A, Freer CEL, Hall LD, Williams A, *et al*. Magnetic resonance imaging of the head and spine: effective for the clinician or the patient? *BMJ* 1991;**302**:79–82.
15 Friedman D, Rapaport R. Routine use of contrast-enhanced MR scans in AIDS. *AJNR Am J Neuroradiol* 1993;**14**:1324.
16 Zimmerman RD. Routine use of contrast-enhanced MR scans in AIDS. *AJNR Am J Neuroradiol* 1993;**14**:1326–84.
17 McLean SAM. *A patient's right to know. Information disclosure, the doctor and the law.* Aldershot: Dartmouth, 1989:**14.**
18 Moseley IF. Long term effects of the introduction of noninvasive investigations in neuro-radiology. Part 1: overall trends. *Neuroradiology* 1988;**30**:187–92.
19 Tatler GLV, Moseley IF. Use of invasive neuroradiological investigations in patients with normal computerised tomography. *BMJ* 1982;**ii**:1026–8.
20 Roberts GM, ed. *Making the best use of a Department of Clinical Radiology. Guidelines for doctors.* 2nd ed. London: Royal College of Radiologists, 1993.
21 Ansell G. Clinical considerations in the administration of contrast media to high-risk patients. In: Carr DH, ed. *Contrast media.* Edinburgh: Churchill Livingstone, 1988: 78–88.
22 Feuerman T, Wackym PA, Gade GF, Becker DP. Value of skull radiography, head computed tomographic scanning, and admission for observation in cases of minor head injury. *Neurosurgery* 1988;**22**:449–53.
23 Hackney DB. Skull radiography in the evaluation of trauma: a survey of current practice. *Radiology* 1991;**181**:711–4.
24 Colquhoun IR. CT cisternography in the investigation of cerebrospinal fluid rhinorrhoea. *Clin Radiol* 1993;**47**:403–8.
25 Anon. Guidelines for the determination of death: report of the medical consultants on the diagnosis of death to the President's Commission for the study of ethical problems in medicine and biomedical and behavioral research. *JAMA* 1981;**246**:2184–6.
26 Griner PF, Glaser RJ. Misuse of laboratory tests and diagnostic procedures. *N Engl J Med* 1982;**207**:1336–9.
27 Moseley IF. The plain radiograph in ophthalmology: a wasteful and potentially danger-ous anachronism. *J R Soc Med* 1991;**84**:76–80.
28 Moseley IF. The diagnostic value of "optic foramen views": experience from an eye hospital. *Br J Ophthalmol* 1990;**74**:235–7.
29 Lewis TT, Kingsley DPE, Moseley IF. Do bilateral optic nerve meningiomas exist? *Br J Neurosurg* 1991;**5**:13–8.
30 Miller DH, Ormerod IEC, McDonald WI, ManManus DG, Kendall BE, Kingsley DPE, *et al*. The early risk of multiple sclerosis after optic neuritis. *J Neurol Neurosurg Psychiatry* 1988;**51**:1569–71.
31 Guy J, Mancuso A, Beck R, Moster ML, Sedwick LA, Quisling RG, *et al*. Radiation-induced optic neuropathy: a magnetic resonance imaging study. *J Neurosurg* 1991; **74**:426–32.
32 Steinsapir KD, Goldberg RA. Traumatic optic neuro-pathy. *Surv Ophthalmol* 1994;**38**:487–518.
33 Zimmerman C, Schatz NJ, Glaser JS. Magnetic resonance imaging of optic nerve menin-giomas. Enhancement with gadolinium-DPTA. *Ophthalmology* 1990;**97**:585–91.

34 Day AL. Aneurysms of the ophthalmic segment. A clinical and anatomical analysis. *J Neurosurg* 1990;72:677–91.

35 Jacobson DM, Karanja PN, Olson KA, Warner JJ. Computed tomography ventricular size has no value in diagnosis pseudotumor cerebri. *Neurology* 1990;40:1454–5.

36 Bronstein AM, Rudge P, Gresty MA, du Boulay G, Morris J. Abnormalities of horizontal gaze and magnetic resonance findings. II. Gaze palsy and internuclear ophthalmoplegia. *J Neurol Neurosurg Psychiatry* 1990;53:200–7.

37 Schwaber MK, Larson TC, Zealear DL, Creasy J. Gadolinium-enhanced magnetic resonance imaging in Bell's palsy. *Laryngoscope* 1990;100:1264–9.

38 Anderson RE, Laskoff JM. Ramsay Hunt syndrome mimicking intracanalicular acoustic neuroma on contrast-enhanced MR. *AJNR Am J Neuroradiol* 1990;11:409.

39 Anon. Imaging patients with suspected acoustic neuroma. *Lancet* 1988;ii:1294.

40 Welling DB, Glasscock ME, Woods CI, Jackson CG. Acoustic neuroma: a cost-effective approach. *Otolaryngol Head Neck Surg* 1990;103:364–70.

41 Consensus Development Panel. National Institutes of Health Consensus Development Conference statement on acoustic neuroma, 11–13 December 1991. *Arch Neurol* 1991;51:201–7.

42 Renowden SA, Anslow P. The effective use of magnetic resonance imaging in the diagnosis of acoustic neuromas. *Clin Radiol* 1993;48:25–8.

43 Bernardi B, Zimmerman RA, Savino PJ, Adler C. Magnetic resonance tomographic angiography in the investigation of hemifacial spasm. *Neuroradiology* 1993;35:606–11.

44 Bradley WG. MR of the brain stem: a practical approach. *Radiology* 1991;179:319–32.

45 Savy LE, Stevens JM, Taylor DJ, Kendall BE. Apparent cerebellar ectopia: a reappraisal using volumetric MRI. *Neuroradiology* 1994;36:360–3.

46 Asbury AK, Herndon RM, McFarland HF, McDonald WI, McIlroy WJ, Paty DW, *et al.* National Multiple Sclerosis Society working group on neuroimaging for the Medical Advisory Board. *Neuroradiology* 1987;29:119.

47 Miller DH, Ormerod IEC, Rudge P, Kendall BE, Moseley IF, McDonald WI. The early risk of multiple sclerosis following isolated syndromes of the brainstem and spinal cord. *Ann Neurol* 1989;26:635–9.

48 Rudge P, Ali A, Cruickshank JC. Multiple sclerosis, tropical spastic paraparesis, and HTLV-1 infection in Afro-Caribbean patients in the United Kingdom. *J Neurol Neurosurg Psychiatry* 1991;54:689–94.

49 Miller DH, Ormerod IEC, Gibson A, du Boulay EPGH, Rudge P, McDonald WI. MR brain scanning in patients with vasculitis: differentiation from multiple sclerosis. *Neuroradiology* 1987;29:226–31.

50 Banna M, El-Ramahi K. Neurologic involvement in Behcet disease: imaging findings in 16 patients. *AJNR Am J Neuroradiol* 1991;12:791–6.

51 Fazekas F, Offenbacher H, Fuchs S, Schmidt R, Niederkorn K, Horner S, *et al.* Criteria for an increased specificity of MRI interpretation in elderly subjects with suspected multiple sclerosis. *Neurology* 1988;38:1822–5.

52 Viñuela FV, Fox AJ, Debrun GM, Feasby TE, Ebers GC. New perspectives in computed tomography of multiple sclerosis. *Am J Radiol* 1982;139:123–7.

53 Kesselring J, Miller DH, Robb SA, Kendall BE, Moseley IF, Kingsley D, *et al.* Acute disseminated encephalomyelitis. MRI findings and the distinction from multiple sclerosis. *Brain* 1990;113:291–302.

54 Lunsford LD, Martinez AJ, Latchaw RE, Pazin GJ. Rapid and accurate diagnosis of herpes simplex encephalitis with computed tomographic stereotaxic biopsy. *Surg Neurol* 1984;21:249–57.

55 Fernandez RE, Rothberg M, Ferencz G, Wujack D. Lyme disease of the CNS: MR imaging findings in 14 cases. *AJNR Am J Neuroradiol* 1990;11:479–81.

56 Tien RD, Chu PK, Hesselink JR, Duberg A, Clayton W. Intracranial cryptococcosis in immunocompromised patients: CT and MR findings in 29 cases. *AJNR Am J Neuroradiol* 1991;12:283–9.

57 Mercader JM, Perich J, Berenguer J, Pujol T, Cardenal C. Intracranial tuberculoma in AIDS: neuroradiological findings. *Neuroradiology* 1991;33:569–70.

58 Dina TS. Primary central nervous system lymphoma versus toxoplasmosis in AIDS. *Radiology* 1991;179:823–8.

59 Moseley IF. Radiological investigation of cerebral masses. *Current Imaging* 1991;3:31–6.

60 Hillemacher A. Die Wert amnesticher and klinische Daten sowie apparativer

Intersuchundsbefunde bei der Diagnose von Hirntumoren. *Fortschr Neurol Psychiatr* 1982;**50**:93–112.

61 Baker HL, Houser OW, Campbell JK. National Cancer Institute study: evaluation of computed tomography in the diagnosis of intracranial neoplasms. I. Overall results. *Radiology* 1980;**136**:91–6.

62 Haughton HV, Rimm AA, Sobocinski KA, Papke RA, Daniels DL, Williams AL, *et al.* Blinded clinical comparison of MR imaging and CT in neuroradiology. *Radiology* 1986;**160**:751–5.

63 Kazner E, Wende S, Grumme T, Lanksch W, Stochdorph O. *Computed tomography in intracranial tumours.* Berlin: Springer-Verlag, 1982.

64 Bolender NF, Cromwell LD, Graves V, Margolis MT, Kerber CW, Wendling L. Interval appearance of glioblastoma not evident in previous CT examination. *J Comput Assist Tomogr* 1983;**7**:599–605.

65 Enzmann DR, Krikorian J, Yorke C, Hayward R. Computed tomography in leptomeningeal spread of tumours. *J Comput Assist Tomogr* 1978;**2**:448–55.

66 Sze G, Milano E, Johnson C, Heier L. Detection of brain metastases: comparison of contrast-enhanced MR with unenhanced MR and enhanced CT. *AJNR Am J Neuroradiol* 1990;**11**:785–91.

67 Ruggiero G, Picard L. The true value of computed tomography, angiography and pneumoencephalography for the precise diagnosis of the brain tumours. In: Wackenheim A, du Boulay GH, eds. *Choices and characteristics in computerized tomography.* Amsterdam: Kugler, 1980:13–21.

68 De Angelis LM. Primary nervous system lymphoma: a new clinical challenge. *Neurology* 1991;**41**:619–21.

69 Davies AG, Richardson RB, Bourne SP, Kemshead JT, Coakham HB. Immunolocalisation of human brain tumours. In: Bleehen NM, ed. *Tumours of the brain.* Berlin: Springer-Verlag, 1986, 83–99.

70 Asari S, Makabe T, Katayama S, Itoh T, Tsuchida S, Ohmoto T. Assessment of the pathological grade of astrocytic gliomas using an MRI score. *Neuroradiology* 1994;**36**:308–10.

71 Jelinek J, Smirniotopoulos JG, Parisi JE, Kanzer M. Lateral ventricular neoplasms of the brain: differential diagnosis based on clinical, CT and MR findings. *AJNR Am J Neuroradiol* 1990;**11**:567–74.

72 Peeling J, Sutherland G, Marat K, Tomchuk E, Bock E. 1H and 13C nuclear magnetic resonance studies of plasma from patients with primary intracranial neoplasms. *J Neurosurg* 1988;**68**:931–7.

73 Carpeggiani P, Crisi G, Trevisan C. MRI of intracranial meningiomas: correlations with histology and physical consistency. *Neuroradiology* 1993;**35**:532–6.

74 Brismar J, Cronqvist S. Therapeutic embolisation in the external carotid artery region. *Acta Radiologies* 1978;**19**:715–31.

75 Halbach VV, Hieshima GB, Higashida RT, David CF. Endovascular therapy of head and neck tumors. In: Viñuela F, Halbach VV, Dion JE, eds. *Interventional neuroradiology. Endovascular therapy of the central nervous system.* New York: Raven Press, 1992:17–28.

76 Bergstrom M, Collins P, Ehrin E, Ericson K, Ericsson L, Greitz T, *et al.* Discrepancies in brain tumour extent as shown by computed tomography and positron emission tomography using [⁶⁸Ga]EDTA, [¹¹C]glucose, and [¹¹C]methionine. *J Comput Assist Tomogr* 1983;**7**:1062–6.

77 Piani C, Pasquini U, De Nicola M, Bevilacqua F, Menichelli F, Salvolini U, *et al.* Intraarterial ACNU chemotherapy in malignant cerebral gliomas: preliminary results. *Neuroradiology* 1991;**33**:319–21.

77a Hodgson TJ, Kingsley DPE, Moseley IF. The role of imaging in the follow up of meningiomas. *J Neurol Neurosurg Psychiatry* 1995;**59**:545–7.

78 Schwartz RB, Carvalho PA, Alexander E III, Loeffler JS, Folkerth R, Holman BL. Radiation necrosis vs high-grade recurrent glioma: differentiation by using dual-isotope SPECT with ²⁰¹Tl and ⁹⁹ᵐTc-HMPAO. *AJNR Am J Neuroradiol* 1991;**12**:1187–92.

79 Larson EB, Omenn GS, Lewis H. Diagnostic evaluation of headache. Impact of computerised tomography and cost-effectiveness. *JAMA* 1980;**243**:359–62.

80 Heller CA, Stanley P, Lewis-Jones B, Heller RF. Value of x ray examinations of the cervical spine. *BMJ* 1983;**287**:1276–8.

81 Daras M, Tuchman AJ, Strobos RJ. Computed tomography in adult onset epilepsy. *Can*

J Neurol Sci 1987;14:286–9.

82 Morrell F. In vivo imaging of human anatomy in temporal lobe epilepsy. *AJNR Am J Neuroradiol* 1991;12: 948–9.

83 Orrison WW, Davis LE, Sullivan GW, Mettler FA Jr, Flynn ER. Anatomic localization of cerebral cortical function by magnetoencephalography combined with MR imaging and CT. *AJNR Am J Neuroradiol* 1990; 11:713–6.

84 Borbely K, Balogh A, Halasz P, Vajda J, Czirjak S, Nyary I. Reliability of ictal and peri-ictal SPECT investigations in localizing epileptogenic foci in patients undergoing epilepsy surgery. *Neuroradiology* 1994;36(suppl):S76.

85 Drayer BP, Olanow W, Burger P, Johnson GA, Herfkens R, Riederer S. Parkinsonism plus syndrome: diagnosis using high field MR imaging of brain iron. *Radiology* 1986; 159:493–8.

86 Savoiardo M, Halliday WC, Nardocci N, Strada L, D'Incerti L, Angelini L, et al. Hallervorden-Spatz disease: MR and pathological findings. *AJNR Am J Neuroradiol* 1993;14:155–62.

87 Nazer H, Brismar J, Al-Kawi MZ, Gunasekaran TS, Jorulf KH. Magnetic resonance imaging of the brain in Wilson's disease. *Neuroradiology* 1993;35:130–3.

88 Savoiardo M, Strada L, Girotti F, Zimmerman RA, Grisoli M, Testa D, et al. Olivopontocerebellar atrophy: MR diagnosis and relationship to multisystem atrophy. *Radiology* 1990;174:693–6.

89 Bradshaw JR, Thomson JLG, Campbell MJ. Computed tomography in the investigation of dementia. *BMJ* 1983;286:277–80.

90 Ettun TM, Staehelin HB, Kischka U, Ulrich J, Scollo-Lavizzari G, Wiggli U, et al. Computed tomography, electroencephalography and clinical features in the differential diagnosis of senile dementia. *Arch Neurol* 1989;46:1217–20.

91 Early B, Rodrigo Escalona P, Boyko OB, Doraiswamy PM, Axelson DA, Patterson L, et al. Interuncal distance in healthy volunteers and in patients with Alzheimer disease. *AJNR Am J Neuroradiol* 1993; 14:907–10.

92 Jobst KA, Smith AD, Szatmari M, Molyneux A, Esiri ME, King E, et al. Detection in life of confirmed Alzheimer's disease using a simple measurement of temporal lobe atrophy by computed tomography. *Lancet* 1992;340:1179–83.

93 Erkinjuntti T, Gao F, Lee DH, Eliasziw M, Merskey H, Hachinski VC. Lack of difference in brain hyperintensities between patients with early Alzheimer's disease and control subjects. *Arch Neurol* 1994;51:260–8.

94 Steiner I, Gomori JM, Melamed E. Features of brain atrophy in Parkinson's disease. *Neuroradiology* 1985;27:158–60.

95 Huber SJ, Shuttleworth EC, Christy JA, Chakeres DW, Curtin A, Paulson GW. Magnetic resonance imaging in dementia of Parkinson's disease. *J Neurol Neurosurg Psychiatry* 1989;52:1221–7.

96 Callanan MM, Logsdail SJ, Ron MA, Warrington ER. Cognitive impairment in patients with clinically isolated lesions of the type seen in multiple sclerosis. *Brain* 1989; 112:361–74.

97 Wardlaw JM, Sellar RJ. Early caudate nucleus atrophy in Huntington's disease: does it correlate with presenting symptoms? *Neuroradiology* 1991;33:238–40.

98 Wakhloo AK, Jüngling F, Krauss JK, Schumacher M, Hennig J. Measurements of pulsatile brain motion with MR-interferography in patients with NPH. *Neuroradiology* 1992;34(suppl):S47.

99 Bradley WG Jr, Whittemore AR, Watanabe AS, Davis SJ, Teresi LM, Homyak M. Association of deep white matter infarction with chronic communicating hydrocephalus: implications regarding the possible origin of normal-pressure hydrocephalus. *AJNR Am J Neuroradiol* 1991;12:31–9.

100 George AE. Chronic communicating hydrocephalus and periventricular white matter disease: a debate with regard to cause and effect. *AJNR Am J Neuroradiol* 1991;12:42–4.

101 Moseley I. Neuropsychiatric disease. *Curr Opin Neurol Neurosurg* 1990;3:884–9.

102 Andreasen NC. Neuroradiology and neuropsychiatry: a new alliance. *AJNR Am J Neuroradiol* 1992;13:841–3.

103 Johnson MR, Hoare RD, Cox T, Dawson JM, Maccabe JJ, Llewellyn DEH, et al. The evaluation of patients with a suspected pituitary microadenoma: computed tomography compared to magnetic resonance imaging. *Clin Endocrinol* 1992;36:335–8.

104 Marcovitz S, Wee R, Chan J, Hardy J. The diagnostic accuracy of preoperative CT scanning in the evaluation of pituitary ACTH-secreting adenomas. *AJNR Am J Neuroradiol*

1987;**8**:641–4.

105 L'Huillier F, Combes C, Martin N, Leclerc X, Pruco JP, Gaston A. MRI in the diagnosis of so-called pituitary apoplexy. *J Neuroradiol* 1989;**16**:221–37.

106 Moses AM, Clayton B, Hochhauser L. Use of T1-weighted MR imaging to differentiate between primary polydipsia and central diabetes insipidus. *AJNR Am J Neuroradiol* 1992;**13**:1273–7.

107 Moseley IF. *Diagnostic imaging in neurological disease.* Edinburgh: Churchill Livingstone, 1986:1–2.

3 Imaging the head: functional imaging

GUY V SAWLE

If asked to choose between a brain that looked nice, or one that functioned well, most of us would choose the second. Furthermore, the ultimate importance of cerebral disease is that it affects brain function, not appearance. Yet clinical neuroimaging has been built around the practice of imaging brain structure. Why so? Because structural images are easier to acquire, and structure and function are so inextricably linked that one might as well image one as the other. But is this necessarily so? To what extent are structural and functional imaging processes independent of one another? And are there any clinical situations where structural imaging "just won't do"?

In this chapter I discuss several approaches to cerebral imaging in which the principal aim is to derive information about brain function. Specifically, I discuss positron emission tomography (PET), single photon emission computed tomography (SPECT), and functional magnetic resonance imaging (fMRI). Other functional imaging methods, such as blood flow measurements using ^{133}Xe-enhanced CT[1] have been of considerable historical importance but are now seldom used in clinical or research practice and so will not be covered.

Principles of the techniques

Positron emission tomography (PET)[2]

In PET short lived isotopes are used to label molecules of biological interest. After inhalation or injection, they decay by

74

positron emission, each positron becoming annihilated within 1–2 mm of its parent nucleus by collision with an electron. This annihilation generates two γ rays (of 511 keV energy) which travel apart at 180° to one another. It is the nearly simultaneous detection of these γ ray pairs by a ring of detector crystals that ultimately leads to the reconstructed image of isotope density. The theoretical limit of spatial resolution is the distance that positrons travel from their parent nucleus before annihilation. The actual spatial resolution depends in part on the size of detector crystals used in the camera. After positron annihilation deep within the brain, a percentage of the emitted photons fail to reach the detector crystals due to signal attenuation by brain tissue. In PET it is possible to correct for this loss using a second set of image data collected before isotope injection or inhalation. For this transmission scan an external (ring or moving rod) germanium-68 source is used. Current generation PET machines have a resolution of around 5 mm in the reconstructed image. Commonly employed PET isotopes include oxygen-15, carbon-11, and fluorine-18, used to replace the naturally occurring oxygen-16, carbon-12, and hydrogen-1 respectively in various biological molecules. This exchange of a radioactive atom for a naturally occurring atom results in little (if any) change in chemical behaviour. The half lives vary from two minutes (oxygen-15) to 110 minutes (fluorine-18). Such short lives have both advantages (less radiation dose) and disadvantages (cost, dependence on an on site cyclotron for production, and the need for a tight time schedule). Measurements by PET take minutes to hours, depending on the particular brain function under scrutiny. Radiation considerations preclude frequent repeat measurements. Table 3.1 gives an overview of some of the strengths and limitations of the PET method, together with comparative data for SPECT and fMRI.

Single photon emission computed tomography (SPECT)[3]

The isotopes used in SPECT (such as technetium-99 or iodine-123) have longer half lives, obviating the need for on site production. This reduces cost and eases some of the timing restraints of PET. On the other hand, because they emit single γ rays (hence single photon ECT), coincidence detection cannot be used to yield spatial information, which must, therefore, depend on collimation alone. Furthermore, signal attenuation by surrounding tis-

Table 3.1 Strengths and limitations of imaging methods

	PET	SPECT	fMRI
Isotopes	Fluorine-18, carbon-11, oxygen-15	Technetium-99m, iodine-123	None
Time per image	Two minutes to two hours	Minutes to hours	0.01 Seconds to a few minutes
Spatial resolution	About 5–6 mm	About 8 mm	0·75 mm upwards
Repeated studies	Very few (limited by radiation)	Very few (limited by radiation)	Yes
Able to study	Metabolism, blood flow, receptor-ligand interactions	Blood flow, some receptor-ligand interactions	Blood flow/venous drainage
Useful technical references	Phelps[2]	Lassen and Holm[3]	Lufkin[4]; Stehling et al[8]

sues cannot be corrected by an exact solution with transmission scan data as utilised in PET. Partly for the foregoing reasons, SPECT has a lower spatial resolution than PET. Nevertheless, because of the lower cost of SPECT and the greater availability of machines, SPECT has found an altogether larger place in the clinical arena than PET. Measurements by SPECT take minutes to hours. As with PET, radiation considerations preclude frequent repeat measurements.

Functional magnetic resonance imaging (fMRI)

In magnetic resonance methods,[4] the divide between structural and functional imaging is precarious. For example, is magnetic resonance angiography (MRA) a functional or an anatomical measurement—because it shows the anatomy of the major cerebral vessels using a sequence that is specifically sensitive to the movement of the contained blood? In this review I use the term functional magnetic resonance imaging (fMRI) to refer to a range of MR sequences designed to acquire information about brain function. These techniques are newer than either PET or SPECT and the scientific literature concerned with their use has so far been more methodological than medical. Nevertheless, at least two fMRI approaches deserve mention—namely, echo planar imaging (EPI), and fast low angle shot (FLASH) techniques. Each is concerned with the generation of images in which a change in signal with time is most likely the consequence of changing neuronal

76

function, the mediator between the two being a change in small vessel flow, or at least an increase in localised venous return. The present possibilities and imminent potentials of fMRI have been described in several recent reviews.[5-7]

Whereas the basics of PET and SPECT methodology follow parallel processes in other techniques such as photography and *x* ray computerised tomography, MRI has no easy parallel in our other experiences. The fundamentals of magnetic resonance have been covered by Moseley in chapter 2; see also Lufkin.[4] Conventional MR sequences build up an image in steps, using a series of magnetic field gradients to specify anatomical positions within the tissue of interest. In EPI an image is recovered from the signal generated by a single free induction decay over a fraction of a second.[8] On the other hand, FLASH sequences limit the time taken for scanning by minimising the perturbation of the magnetisation from its equilibrium so that successive excitation pulses can follow each other more quickly. Reported data from EPI at high (3 Tesla) field strength include images acquired in 0·1 s with a spatial resolution of 0·75 mm.[9] Despite the large number of MRI machines available for diagnostic purposes, few have either EPI or high (2–3 Tesla) field strength. It is possible to acquire FLASH[10] fMRI images at a lower field strength (1·5 Tesla) with a "clinical" MRI system; although signal acquisition is in this case somewhat slower. All fMRI methods share one advantage over PET and SPECT—namely, the avoidance of ionising radiation.

Practicalities of the techniques (table 3.1)

Because functional imaging studies have yet to enjoy wide use as clinical tools in routine neurological practice, the following account describes elements of the basic principles, as well as the nuts and bolts practicalities of patient scanning.

PET

General principles

The general principle of the PET measurement requires a mathematical model that corresponds to the functional system under scrutiny. This model is an approximation of the processes that lie between the "input" (the activity administered to the patient and available to the brain via its arterial supply or by inhalation) and the "output" (the activity measured regionally during the course of the experiment).

Cerebral blood flow

One of the simplest PET models relates to the measurement of regional cerebral blood flow during continuous inhalation of $C^{15}O_2$. After a few minutes inhalation, an equilibrium is reached whereby the arterial supply of radioactivity to the brain is equal to the loss of activity from venous washout and radioactive decay (the so called steady state condition). In this situation a simple mathematical expression describes the regional cerebral blood flow in terms of known or measurable values—namely, the radioactive decay constant (fixed for ^{15}O), the arterial activity of $H_2^{15}O$ (in $\mu Ci/ml$, measured in an arterial blood sample with a well counter), and the regional brain concentration of tracer in units/ml (measured in the PET camera). The steady state measurement of regional cerebral blood flow takes about 15 minutes to complete.

On the practical side, these measurements (and all of those listed below) require that the patient be still during image acquisition. They require a venous line for tracer administration (except when $C^{15}O_2$, $C^{15}O$, or $^{15}O_2$ are given by inhalation). Most quantitative studies also require an arterial line to measure the level of radioactivity presented to the brain over the time course of the scan.

Blood flow can also be measured during the rise and fall of brain radioactivity surrounding a bolus inhalation or injection of tracer. The mathematical model required to unscramble the collected data to a measured value for rCBF is in this case very much more complicated,[11] but the method is faster (data acquisition takes only two to three minutes).

Oxygen metabolism

Oxygen metabolism can be calculated from cerebral blood flow after additional measurements of the oxygen extraction fraction (the percentage of the available blood oxygen extracted during its passage through the brain vasculature; usually measured after inhalation of $^{15}O_2$) and regional blood volume (a correction for the percentage of any cerebral region which contains blood rather than brain).[12] Such a (triple) measurement using steady state models takes about 40 minutes (including time for radioactive decay between scans).

Glucose metabolism

Glucose metabolism is measured after intravenous injection of 2-[^{18}F]fluoro-2-deoxy-D-glucose (FDG), which is metabolised by hexokinase to FDG-6-phosphate. As FDG-6-phosphate can neither proceed down the glycolytic pathway nor be metabolised to glycogen (the metabolic destinies for glucose-6-phosphate) it stays trapped within the tissue for the duration of the PET measurement. This compartmental trapping is the cornerstone of the FDG measurement. Further interpretation may be fully quantitative (requiring continuous arterial and regional cerebral radioactivity measurements) or semiquantitative (using normative data from other subjects, and a further series of constants and restraints in the employed mathematical model). On the practical side this means that for the most accurate measurement, a patient must be in the camera during tracer injection and for the next 60 to 90 minutes, with simultaneous arterial blood sampling. For a less quantitative scan (from which regional inequalities in glucose metabolism can yet be semiquantified) the tracer can be injected out of the camera and a "snapshot" image (lasting perhaps 15 minutes) can be taken about 30 to 40 minutes later.

Neurotransmitter precursor studies

Aside from blood flow and measures of tissue metabolism, the other principal application of PET to date has been in neuropharmacological studies; PET has a small repertoire for the study of neurotransmitter synthesis and storage, principally the decarboxylation of [^{18}F]dopa to [^{18}F]dopamine. Like the FDG method, the premise on which most of the [^{18}F]dopa analytical methods are based is the assumption that the injected tracer ([^{18}F]dopa) is transported into the brain and then specifically taken up by dopamine neurons where it is decarboxylated, concentrated, and then stored in nerve terminal vesicles for the duration of the measurement. A particular disadvantage of [^{18}F]dopa as a tracer of the dopamine synthetic pathway is that the concentration of the endogenous (dopa) pool is unknown. So if anybody ever discovers the perfect mathematical model to unravel [^{18}F]dopa scan data (an endeavour that has attracted much energy, even some disagreement) they will still only have measured the rate of metabolism of exogenous [^{18}F]dopa; the rate of endogenous dopamine production cannot be deduced without a knowledge of the endogenous dopa pool—which you cannot measure! Despite these caveats,

[^{18}F]dopa has been an excellent workhorse in the PET armamentarium.

Neurotransmitter receptor studies

Tracers of much larger variety have been employed as markers for particular classes of neurotransmitter receptor, including dopamine D1 ([^{11}C]SCH23390[13]) and D2 ([^{11}C]raclopride[14]) postsynaptic receptors, dopamine reuptake sites ([^{11}C]nomifensine[15 16] and [^{11}C]WIN-35,428[17]) opiate receptors (μ([^{11}C]carfentanil[18]), μ and κ ([^{18}F]cyclofoxy[19]), μ, κ, and δ ([^{11}C]diprenorphine[20])), central ([^{11}C]flumazenil[21]) and peripheral ([^{11}C]PK11195[22 23]) benzodiazepine receptors, muscarinic cholinergic receptors ([^{11}C]scopolamine[24]), histamine H1 receptors ([^{11}C]pyrilamine[25]), and MAO-B activity ([^{11}C]deprenyl[26]). These ligands have been used (some extensively) to study the changes in receptor numbers or affinity in some diseases including Parkinson's and other akinetic rigid syndromes, Huntington's disease, epilepsy, pain, and stroke. Quantitative measurements require continuous measurement of blood and brain activity during and after injection of tracer. A single PET scan may be sufficient for semiquantification, but if a full description in neuropharmacological terms is required (to calculate, for example, B_{max}, the total concentration of binding sites) repeat studies may be necessary in the same subject with injections of tracer having different specific activities, or coinjection of cold (unlabelled) tracer.

Functional mapping

Aside from neurotransmitter studies, the other growth area in recent years has been the development of functional mapping studies in which repeat measurements of blood flow are used as a means of identifying brain regions active in particular cognitive or other prescribed tasks. If a subject is scanned twice, once at rest and the second time during right arm movement, it is argued that any difference between the two images of blood flow may be accounted for either by noise, by artefact, by a general (global) effect of the activity on cerebral blood flow, or by a specific activation of a responsible brain region. Various methods have been developed to extract the specific information by removing the confounding effects.[27 28] In large part the published base of work in this area has employed between subject averaging to improve the signal to noise characteristics of the method. Newer scanners with

MRI coregistration allow more confident results in individual subjects with greater accuracy in the anatomical loci of activation related change.[29] The use of functional mapping studies has not so far been reported as a clinical procedure.

SPECT

General principles

The practicalities of SPECT measurements are for the most part simpler than for PET. In part this is because SPECT data are by necessity less quantitative than PET data. Another relevant factor may be the closer liaison and relation between SPECT and clinical medicine, with the restraining hand of clinical practicality curbing the imager's urge to add complexity in the pursuit of accuracy.

Cerebral blood flow

The SPECT approach to cerebral blood flow hinges on the finding that certain tracers are irreversibly taken up into the brain in a regional pattern that reflects localised differences in cerebral blood flow. After intravenous injection, [^{123}I]-n-isopropyl amphetamine ([^{123}I]-iodoamphetamine)[30] crosses the blood-brain barrier by passive diffusion with a high first pass extraction. It is then retained in the brain by non-specific binding to amine receptors. So signal intensity in a "snapshot" image taken 20 to 60 minutes after tracer injection is proportional to the perfusion dominated distribution of tracer in the brain.

Likewise, [^{99m}Tc]hexamethylpropyleneamine oxime ([^{99m}Tc] HMPAO) crosses the blood-brain barrier easily by passive diffusion. It is then trapped in the brain (after decomposition to a by-product that cannot pass back across the barrier), uptake and trapping being complete within 10 minutes. Images taken 90 to 120 minutes after injection (image acquisition typically taking about 20 minutes) still show the frozen image of regional cerebral blood flow at the time of tracer administration. [^{99m}Tc]HMPAO is preferred to [^{123}I]-iodoamphetamine on several accounts, including its optimum imaging energy and shorter half life. Unlike PET blood flow measurements, which require an on site cyclotron, [^{99m}Tc]HMPAO can be produced in a hospital nuclear medicine department with a molybdenum-99 generator. It must be used within about 30 minutes of production to avoid decomposition

81

before injection. [^{99m}Tc] labelled N,N''-1,2-ethylene-diylbis-L-cysteine diethyl ester dihydrochloride ([^{99m}Tc]ECD) is similar to but more stable than [^{99m}Tc]HMPAO.[31]

Patients undergoing SPECT measurement of cerebral blood flow with these techniques do not need to be in the camera during tracer injection. They should, however, be rested at this time because it is blood flow around the time of injection that is measured during the later scan, not blood flow at the time of the measurement, as in PET.

For the most part, the interpretation of SPECT flow images follows the radiological tradition—namely, interpretation of the image appearance by an expert in the field. As with the assessment of age related atrophy on structural images, the observer must take into account the known changes in cerebral blood flow that accompany the normal aging process. Such images are often reported alongside structural images to help in the differentiation between normal and pathological appearances.

Neurotransmitter receptor studies

Several neurotransmitter systems have been studied with SPECT. Specifically the dopamine D2 ligand [^{123}I]-(S-)-2-hydroxy-3-iodo-6-methoxy-N[(1-ethyl-2-pyrrolidinyl) methyl]-benzamide ([^{123}I]-iodobenzamide) has been extensively used in neurological disorders. This ligand binds reversibly to dopamine D2 receptors. The amount of specific striatal binding increases over about 40 minutes and then remains stable for up to two hours. Typically data are acquired during the period 60 to 120 minutes after tracer injection, image acquisition taking about 50 minutes. Because of the limitations of measurement, SPECT [^{123}I]-iodoamphetamine data are reported as a specific:non-specific ratio, such as striatum:cerebellar counts.

fMRI

General principles

Procedures for fMRI are very different from either PET or SPECT, being independent of ionising radiation. Aside from any activity that the patient might be asked to perform while in the magnet, the patient's experience of fMRI is unlikely to differ greatly from any other MR procedure (loud noises in a dark tunnel), although EPI is presently particularly noisy. Although rapid

MR sequences (such as EPI) yield clear images of moving structures (such as a beating heart or a waving head) fMRI methods rely on a comparison of successive scans of the same area. In this case, the head position must be identical for the acquisition of each of the images contributing to data analysis. Even the tiniest head movements can wreck havoc with fMRI analysis; indeed it has even been possible to create striking "functional" data as a result of head movement artefact alone.[32] As with PET, one approach to the problem of head movement between scans may be to realign the data in software after image acquisition.[33 34]

What has been learned with these techniques, and to what extent may they be used in clinical practice?

Both PET and SPECT have been used in neuroscience research to examine brain function in health and in disease. Thus far fMRI has been most closely applied to the study of healthy subjects, although this will certainly change. This review will concentrate on those studies designed primarily to answer questions about disease. When applicable, mention will be made of clinical situations in which functional imaging could provide valuable additional information. The United Kingdom has a single PET research institution (the Medical Research Council Cyclotron Unit at the Hammersmith Hospital) and a single dedicated clinical PET facility (at the St Thomas' and Guy's Hospitals). The former unit has a broad range of chemistry facilities, whereas the available ligands in the clinical PET centre are fewer. This pattern is generally true elsewhere—most PET centres with clinical services chiefly offer [18F]fluorodeoxyglucose scans; other more closely research based units typically have a more extended repertoire. In the United States there is now an Institute for Clinical PET. Furthermore, some United States health insurance schemes have approved a variety of clinical PET procedures for reimbursement. Presently, SPECT scanners are more widely distributed, both in the United Kingdom and elsewhere. Although many hospital radiology departments are equipped with magnetic resonance machines, few have the hardware and software on hand for the acquisition of an fMRI signal.

Cerebrovascular disease

Early PET studies measured regional cerebral blood flow, blood volume, oxygen extraction, and oxygen metabolism to examine the pathophysiology of stroke, particularly the mechanisms of cerebrovascular compensation in the face of falling and failing arterial perfusion pressure.[35][36] Currently PET and SPECT can both detect cerebral ischaemia in acute stroke at a stage when CT images are still normal. It has been shown that PET also has some ability to predict the extent of functional recovery from stroke[37] and in recovered patients (using functional mapping) it can show the anatomical and functional substrate of recovered function.[38][39] Likewise PET and SPECT can show evidence of hypoperfusion ("misery perfusion") in the absence of infarction,[40] and hyperperfusion ("luxury perfusion") at a site of previous infarction. Haemodynamic changes can be shown by PET in patients after extracranial-intracranial bypass operations.[41] Although this operation has not been shown to be of benefit in large interventional studies[42] it is possible that preoperative functional imaging could be used to identify patients more likely to gain from operation.

Basic research in cerebrovascular disease has given cause for guarded optimism over the possible use of cerebral protective agents such as glutamate antagonists and free radical scavengers; PET is waiting in the wings to be used to increase the pathophysiological and therapeutic gains from patient trials with these agents. Whether it will be called on remains to be seen.

Clinical indications

There are presently no consensus indications for the clinical use of functional imaging in cerebrovascular disease (but then there are no clinically proved treatments for acute stroke either[43]; both could change).

Dementia

Early PET studies showed regional metabolic changes in Alzheimer's disease and some other degenerative conditions, and these findings led to the notion that particular diseases might be recognisable by specific regional changes in cerebral function. As in the study of several other disease states, many of the early reports of functional imaging in Alzheimer's disease included small numbers of patients and employed loose diagnostic criteria. Results were sometimes contradictory. With the passage of time, however, consensus has been reached in some areas as follows. In Alzheimer's disease, the brunt of the early PET changes are centred around the posterior temporal and parietal cortices (figure 3.1).[44-47] Regional between patient differences may correlate with differences in neuropsychological test scores.[45 48 49] Changes in PET may antedate clinical dementia in patients presenting with mild memory deficits.[50] SPECT studies in Alzheimer's disease, have also shown reduced flow in posterior temporal and other cortical regions.[51-53] In patients with familial Alzheimer's disease [18F]fluorodeoxyglucose PET in affected family members shows the same pattern of parietotemporal hypometabolism. Scans in asymptomatic at risk relatives show a similar (but less severe) pattern.[54]

Most PET scans in patients with Pick's disease established by necropsy or biopsy have shown predominantly frontal hypometabolism.[55 56] This finding is not specific to Pick's disease, however, as it has also been reported in progressive supranuclear palsy[57-59] and SPECT studies have shown a reduction in frontal [99mTc]HMPAO uptake in patients presenting with dementia of the frontal lobe type.[60]

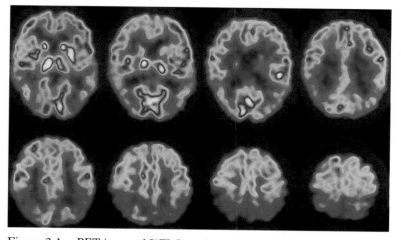

Figure 3.1   PET image of [18F] fluorodeoxyglucose metabolism in Alzheimer's disease. Note reduced tracer uptake in posterior temporal and parietal cortex (picture courtesy of Dr A Kennedy)

Patients with focal cortical degenerations presenting with slowly progressive apraxia or aphasia have been studied with PET and have been shown to have appropriate areas of cortical hypometabolism at a stage when structural imaging studies have been normal.[61][62] The pathology in these patients turns out to be variable. Much has been written about the identification of clinical and preclinical changes in PET metabolic indices in Huntington's disease.[63-66] Both striatal and cortical hypometabolism have been reported. After the demonstration of low caudate [18F]fluorodeoxyglucose metabolism in some at risk patients, considerable efforts were directed towards the development of PET as a preclinical disease marker.[65][66] Although genetic testing now provides a generally reliable means of making a positive diagnosis of Huntington's disease based on a blood sample alone,[67][68] it may be that PET still has a part to play in these patients. If, for example, neurotransplantation procedures become a practical proposition in this disorder, it may be that PET will provide a crucial means of identifying an appropriate preclinical or early clinical stage of disease for intervention. Gene positive at risk patients have lower striatal and pallidal volumes (a structural MR measurement) than gene negative at risk patients[69]; it has yet to be shown that either MRI or PET can indicate when an at risk subject will develop clinical problems. Neurotransmitter studies in the foregoing conditions are discussed in the next section.

Clinical indications

As with cerebrovascular disease, there are presently few if any treatment options that could reasonably be said to depend on diagnostic information which could only be gleaned from functional imaging studies. Both PET and SPECT may assist in the accurate diagnosis of these conditions presenting as a dementing illness; but such data cannot yet be regarded as mandatory in good patient care.

Movement disorders

In Parkinson's disease, early blood flow and metabolic studies[70-72] were soon upstaged by the demonstration of reduced striatal uptake of [18F]-6-L-fluorodopa ([18F]dopa) in affected patients.[73] Many [18F]dopa studies have now been reported in this disorder, considering issues such as the role of aging (most centres,[74 75] but not all,[76] have shown no effect of age on [18F]dopa uptake), the detection of presymptomatic disease (figure 3.2),[77] the rate of progression of clinically evident disease,[78–80] and the efficacy of neurotransplantation procedures (figure 3.3).[81 82]

Various other akinetic rigid conditions have been studied with [18F]dopa PET, including multiple system atrophy,[83–85] progressive supranuclear palsy,[57 83 84] corticobasal degeneration,[86] neuroacanthocytosis,[87] and 1-methyl-4-phenyl-1,2,3,6-tetrahydropyridine (MPTP) parkinsonism.[82 88] Some of these disorders have been reported to show characteristic patterns of striatal [18F]dopa uptake, such as severe asymmetric loss of caudate and putamen uptake (in corticobasal degeneration[86]) or severe bilateral early loss of both caudate and putamen signal (in progressive supranuclear palsy[84]). The difficulty in translating these patterns from research to clinical practice is that these studies have of course been undertaken in patients who carry a (fairly) confident clinical diagnosis. Even in such patients, if we move from a group to individual subjects and study their [18F]dopa PET data, it may be impossible to ascribe a particular diagnosis (for example Parkinson's disease v multiple system atrophy) with absolute certainty.[89]

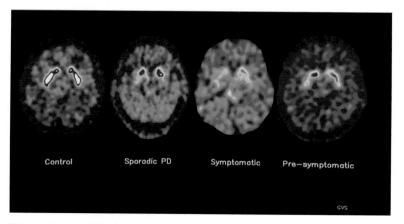

Figure 3.2   PET image to show [18F] dopa uptake in a normal subject (left), a patient with idiopathic (sporadic) Parkinson's disease, and two members of a sibship with familial parkinsonism. The symptomatic patient shows profoundly impaired fluorodopa uptake wheras the presymptomatic subject (who became clinically affected within months of the scan) shows fluorodopa uptake at a level intermediate between normal and parkinsonian values

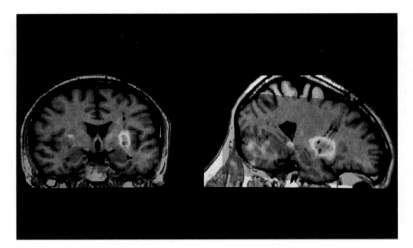

Figure 3.3   *Combined MRI (T1 weighted and PET ([¹⁸F] dopa) image from a parkinsonian patient who has undergone implantation of fetal material into the putamen. The MRI image shows the site of the burr hole and three needle tracks reaching down through the cortex and subcortical white matter into the putamen. The [¹⁸F] dopa image shows uptake at the graft site*

[¹⁸F]Dopa studies have also been performed in possibly less obvious disorders. It has been shown that the extrapyramidal symptoms in clinically diagnosed Alzheimer's disease seem not to be due to nigral degeneration.[90] The motor disorders in obsessional slowness[91] and manganese toxicity[92] are likewise unaccompanied by changes in [¹⁸F]dopa uptake, whereas in patients poisoned by cyanide [¹⁸F]dopa uptake is reduced, suggesting (direct or hypoxic induced) nigral toxicity.[93] Patients with parkinsonism resulting from neuroleptic or other dopamine blocking drugs may have either normal [¹⁸F]dopa uptake (suggesting a likely return to clinical normality after cessation of the offending agent) or low uptake (suggesting unmasking of otherwise subclinical parkinsonism).[94]

[¹⁸F]Dopa is not the only tracer to provide information about the presynaptic dopamine system. [¹¹C]Nomifensine has also been used (as a marker of catecholaminergic presynaptic reuptake sites) but in most cases the results of [¹¹C]nomifensine studies have closely paralleled those with [¹⁸F]dopa.[16 95] Cocaine analogues such as [¹¹C]CFT (also known as WIN 35, 428) have also been used to study the dopamine fibre system. In a primate model of parkinsonism, [¹¹C]CFT uptake was reduced in the striatum.[96] This ligand has the advantage of a substantially higher striatal to background signal than [¹⁸F]dopa, but the kinetics are, if anything, a little slow for use as a PET tracer. The related compound, CIT, has been used in SPECT as [¹²³I]β-CIT. Striatal uptake of this tracer was reduced in Parkinson's disease.[97]

In part, the answer to the problem of differential diagnosis using PET in individual patients might be helped by multiple tracer studies to examine receptor status in addition to (or in place of) [¹⁸F]dopa uptake. There are many publications concerning dopamine D2 receptors in akinetic rigid syndromes. On balance, PET and SPECT studies suggest relative upregulation of D2 receptors in patients with early Parkinson's disease, with normal or even lower levels later in disease; perhaps in part as an effect of treatment with dopaminergic drugs (PET[14 87 98–101]; SPECT[102–104]). Patients with multiple system atrophy are more likely to have low D2 ligand binding (PET[14 84]) and low tracer uptake in dopa naïve akinetic rigid patients may predict subsequent evolution to multiple system atrophy rather than Parkinson's disease (PET[14]; SPECT[105]) (figure 3.4). Unlike the D2 system, PET studies of dopamine D1 receptors have shown no evidence of upregulation in early levodopa naïve patients.[13] Other neurotransmitter receptors have also been studied in akinetic rigid syndromes. Specifically, striatal [¹¹C]diprenorphine binding has been shown to be impaired in patients with multiple system atrophy, but not in patients with Parkinson's disease.[106] In a study using [¹¹C]flumazenil as tracer to measure cerebellar GABA-A/benzodiazepine receptors, increased tracer binding was reported in patients with multiple system atrophy, whereas patients with sporadic and dominantly inherited olivopontocerebellar atrophy had increased and unchanged binding respectively.[107]

Although neurotransmitter studies occupy most of the literature on functional imaging in akinetic rigid syndromes, specific focused metabolic studies and more recent functional mapping papers are starting to redress the balance. In depressed parkinsonian patients, for example, a particular pattern of frontal hypometabolism has been found.[108] Also, with more complex statistical techniques, some correlations have been reported between regional metabolic changes, motor asymmetries, and fluorodopa uptake constants.[109] Functional mapping studies have shown failure of supplementary

89

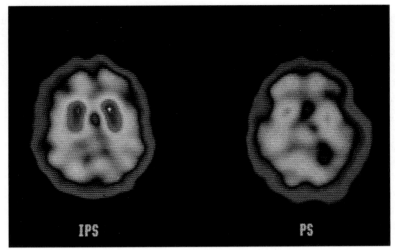

Figure 3.4   *SPECT [¹²³I] iodobenzamide binding in a patient with Parkinson's disease (left) and a patient with a non-dopa responsive parkinsonian syndrome (right) (picture courtesy of Drs K Tatsch and J Schwarz, Department of Nuclear Medicine and Neurology, University of Munich)*

motor cortex activation during internally generated movements in parkinsonian patients[110] with resolution towards the normal after dopamine agonist treatment (shown both with PET[111] and SPECT[112]). More recently, fMRI studies have begun to consider this same issue—namely, the identification of cortical areas responsible for the control of human movement.[113 114] Reported fMRI findings in this area include a positive relation between movement rate and the fMRI signal in the primary motor cortex,[114] and a greater signal intensity in supplementary motor areas during complex self paced movements than during externally paced movements.[113]

Although most PET studies in Huntington's disease have used [¹⁸F]fluorodeoxyglucose as the tracer, more recent attention has focused on the dopamine system. Dopamine D1 and D2 receptors have each been studied in affected patients (with [¹¹C]SCH23390 and [¹¹C]raclopride as tracers). Affected patients show a reduction of both D1 and D2 binding potentials (figure 3.5).[115] With [¹¹C]raclopride PET, asymptomatic gene positive subjects may show an intermediate reduction in binding potential (R Weeks, personal communication).

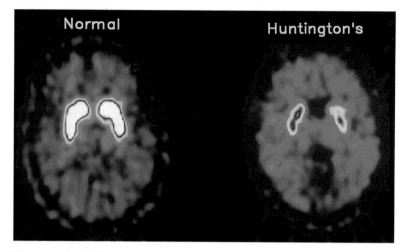

Figure 3.5 PET [¹¹C] raclopride images from a normal subject (left) and a patient with Huntington's disease (right). Note profoundly reduced tracer uptake in the striatum of the patient with Huntington's disease (picture courtesy of Dr R A Weeks)

At the time of writing, fMRI studies have yet to be reported in patients with Parkinson's disease or other movement disorders.

Clinical indications

What of the clinical utility of functional imaging in movement disorders? Despite the scientific findings discussed, no clear necessity for such imaging studies has yet been shown. In part, this relates to the lack of available treatment for many of these disorders. In akinetic rigid syndromes for example, some, but not all, patients respond to levodopa or dopamine agonists. Although there is little effective treatment for those patients who are resistant to such treatment, informed trial and error seems as good a therapeutic approach as functional imaging. A special exception to this rule might be argued for dopa responsive dystonia. Patients with this disorder gain long term benefit from levodopa without developing the side effects and complications that bedevil patients with Parkinson's disease,[116] particularly those with onset early in life.[117] Fluorodopa uptake in dopa responsive dystonia is close to normal,[118 119] but it is profoundly impaired in patients with young onset (age 20–40) or juvenile onset (before age 20) Parkinson's

91

disease.[120] A highly abnormal [18F]dopa PET scan in a young patient with an akinetic rigid syndrome would therefore imply a likelihood of early problems with levodopa treatment, whereas early treatment with levodopa would be appropriate in a patient in whom [18F]dopa PET showed uptake close to or in the lower normal range.

Patients undergoing experimental neurotransplantation procedures may also gain some direct personal benefit (graft site selection, for example)[81] but otherwise for now, the principal promise of functional imaging in movement disorders is in the advancement of our understanding of disease, causation, and treatment.

Epilepsy

In patients with focal epilepsy, a number of functional imaging studies (PET and SPECT) have shown evidence of interictal focal hypometabolism (figure 3.6).[121–123] In some cases it has been possi-

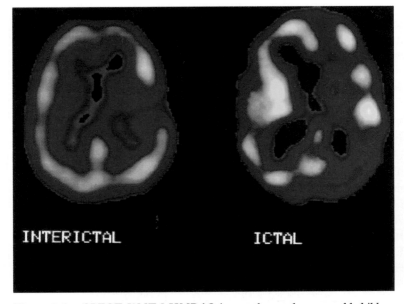

Figure 3.6   *SPECT [99MTc] HMPAO images from a four year old child with partial motor seizures. The interictal image shows hypometabolism in the left hemisphere. The ictal image shows an area of hypermetabolism corresponding to the seizure focus (picture courtesy of Dr J H Cross)*

ble to scan patients during seizures, in which case areas that are interictally hypometabolic may become ictally hypermetabolic or show high flow.[122 124 125] It has been reasonably argued that such regions represent epileptic foci, even in the absence of corroborative findings from structural imaging or EEG. In patients with intractable epilepsy, surgical excision of a definite seizure focus may radically improve clinical status. Current MRI techniques are able to identify structural abnormalities in an increasing number of such patients. There are, nevertheless, a significant number of patients in whom non-invasive means fail to clearly identify a seizure focus. Options in these patients include the placement of depth electrodes, and functional imaging studies.

In a comparative study of [^{18}F]fluorodeoxyglucose PET and [^{99m}Tc]HMPAO SPECT in patients undergoing investigation before surgery for temporal lobe epilepsy, different sensitivities were reported for the two techniques. In patients who had a normal MRI, PET with [^{18}F]fluorodeoxyglucose showed focal hypometabolism in 80% v 20% for SPECT with [^{99m}Tc]HMPAO.[126] The authors attributed this difference to the greater spatial resolution of the PET technique. Although PET is a potentially quantitative technique, it has been argued that for clinical epileptology purposes, image inspection by experienced eyes is generally sufficient.[127]

In another study of patients with intractable epilepsy, SPECT detected lateralising abnormalities in 19 of 30 patients; only two further lateralised abnormalities were found with CT or MRI.[128] As in many other areas of imaging the ground is shifting rapidly. With increasing structural resolution in MRI (including hippocampal volume measurements) the balance is swinging in favour of MRI having a greater chance of correct lateralisation than SPECT.[69]

A recent fMRI study of a four year old boy showed changes in image signal restricted to an area of structural abnormality during five seizures over a 25 minute period. Interictal SPECT showed reduced [^{99m}Tc]HMPAO uptake in the same region, whereas increased uptake was found during a seizure.[129]

Clinical indications

Both interictal and ictal functional imaging studies may show areas of abnormal signal in patients with focal epilepsy. This localisation is appropriately used to confirm or refute collateral evidence from structural MRI and EEG examinations in the assessment of patients with refractory epilepsy who are being considered for surgical treatment (usually a partial temporal lobectomy).

Oncology

Most cerebral tumours are easily seen by structural imaging, which typically shows the lesion location, morphological details, evidence of damage to the blood-brain barrier, and induced cerebral oedema. From these data it is often possible to reach an accurate prediction of tumour type and likely histology. Functional imaging studies can add further information. In patients with gliomas, PET [^{18}F]fluorodeoxyglucose studies have shown a relation between glucose metabolism and both histological grade[130] and survival.[131] It should not be assumed, however, that a lesion with high [^{18}F]fluorodeoxyglucose uptake is necessarily a tumour, as cerebral abscesses may also show increased uptake.[132] Use has also been made of SPECT in an effort to differentiate high from low grade gliomas. Thallium-201 (a tracer more familiarly used in myocardial studies) exhibits increased uptake in some tumours. In gliomas, uptake is greater in high grade lesions.[133]

A particular clinical problem in neuro-oncology is the management of patients presenting with recurrent lesions after radiotherapy for tumour. It can be difficult to differentiate recurrent tumour from radiation induced necrosis on the basis of clinical assessment and structural imaging alone. [^{18}F]Fluorodeoxyglucose PET is of clinical use in this situation,[134] as recurrent tumour has a high metabolic rate (figure 3.7), whereas low [^{18}F]fluorodeoxyglucose uptake suggests radionecrosis.[135] The measurement is not affected in the early postoperative period, nor by steroid treatment.[135]

Other aspects of tumour biochemistry have also been explored with PET, including measurements of amino acid uptake and protein synthesis. [^{11}C]Methionine accumulates readily in gliomas,[136] higher uptake usually occurring in high grade tumours.[137] Synthesis of DNA can also be followed with nucleosides such as deoxyuridine labelled with fluorine-18.[138] Peripheral benzodiazepine (ω3) receptors are expressed on human glioma cells; the presence of this tumour marker may be recognised with PET and the specific marker [^{11}C]-PK11195.[23]

94

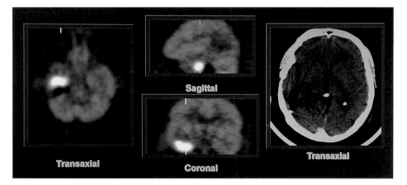

Figure 3.7   *PET [¹⁸F] fluorodeoxyglucose images from a patient with a recurrent glioma. The PET images (to the left) show increased metabolism indicative of recurrent tumour. (Illustration courtesy of Professor M Maisey.)*

Clinical indications

The principal consensus use of functional imaging in oncology is in the differentiation of recurrent cerebral glioma from postradiation necrosis.

Summary of clinical indications for functional imaging studies

As mentioned at the outset of this review, the cornerstone of clinical neuroimaging procedures has been the identification of broadly "structural" changes in neural tissue. The tools for such image acquisition (*x* ray, CT, and MRI) are widely available and of increasingly high quality and resolution. As we have so few functional imaging facilities, clinical indications for functional imaging studies must be restricted to situations where CT and MRI fail to answer the clinical question. All of these techniques are presently developing rapidly, with new MRI sequences blurring the structure and function divide, and newer PET and SPECT ligands pushing forward the capabilities of functional studies.

At the present time, I list the following sensible clinical indications for functional imaging. To my mind, these are clinical situations in which functional imaging studies can provide clinical information with important therapeutic implications:

95

- Differentiation of tumour recurrence from radionecrosis (PET/FDG)
- Contribution to presurgical assessment of patients with refractory epilepsy (PET/FDG, SPECT/flow tracers)
- Differentiation of juvenile Parkinson's disease from dopa responsive dystonia (PET/[^{18}F]dopa).

Further possibilities of substantial clinical use include:

- Identification of critical gyri/sulci before neurosurgical or neuroradiological procedures (fMRI)
- Neurochemical monitoring of patients undergoing neurotransplantation procedures (PET).

Functional imaging studies can also provide precise information contributing to diagnostic precision in, for example, the dementias and akinetic rigid syndromes. But whereas functional imaging touches on clinical practice, to my mind its principal strength lies in its position as one of our most powerful instruments for clinical research.

1 Mallett BL, Veall N. Investigation of cerebral blood flow in hypertension, using radioactive-xenon inhalation and extracranial recording. *Lancet* 1963;i:1081–2.
2 Phelps ME. Positron emission tomography (PET). In: Mazziotta JC, Gilman S, eds. *Clinical brain imaging principles and applications (contemporary neurology series No 39)*. Philadelphia: FA Davis, 1992:71–107.
3 Lassen NA, Holm S. Single photon emission computed tomography (SPECT). In: Mazziotta JC, Gilman S, eds. *Clinical brain imaging principles and applications (contemporary neurology series No 39)*. Philadelphia: FA Davis, 1992:108–34.
4 Lufkin RB. Magnetic resonance imaging. In: Mazziotta JC, Gilman S, eds. *Clinical brain imaging principles and applications (contemporary neurology series No 39)*. Philadelphia: FA Davis, 1992:39–70.
5 Prichard JW, Rosen BR. Functional study of the brain by NMR. *J Cereb Blood Flow Metab* 1994;14:365–72.
6 Cohen MS, Bookheimer SY. Localization of brain function using magnetic resonance imaging. *Trends Neurosci* 1994;17:268–77.
7 Turner R. Magnetic resonance imaging of brain function. *Ann Neurol* 1994;35:637–8.
8 Stehling MK, Turner R, Mansfield P. Echo-planar imaging: magnetic resonance imaging in a fraction of a second. *Science* 1991;254:43–50.
9 Mansfield P, Coxon R, Glover P. Echo planar imaging of the brain at 3·0T: first normal volunteer results. *J Comput Assist Tomogr* 1994;18:339–43.
10 Haase A, Frahm J, Matthaei D, Hänicke W, Merboldt KD. FLASH imaging: rapid NMR imaging using low flip-angle pulses. *J Magn Reson Imaging* 1986;67:258–66.
11 Lammertsma AA, Frackowiak RSJ, Hoffman JM, *et al*. The $^{15}CO_2$ build-up technique to measure regional cerebral blood flow and volume of distribution of water. *J Cereb Blood Flow Metab* 1989;9:461–70.
12 Lammertsma AA, Jones T. Correction for the presence of intravascular oxygen-15 in the steady-state technique for measuring regional oxygen extraction ratio in the brain. *J Cereb Blood Flow Metab* 1983;3:416–24.
13 Rinne JO, Laihinen A, Någren K, *et al*. PET demonstrates different behaviour of striatal dopamine D-1 and D-2 receptors in early Parkinson's disease. *J Neurosci Res* 1990;27:494–9.
14 Sawle GV, Playford ED, Brooks DJ, Quinn N, Frackowiak RSJ. Asymmetrical presynaptic and postsynaptic changes in the striatal dopamine projection in dopa-naïve parkinsonism: diagnostic implications of the D2 receptor status. *Brain* 1993;116:853–67.

15 Tedroff J, Aquilonius S-M, Hartvig P, et al. Monoamine re-uptake sites in the human brain evaluated in vivo by means of ¹¹C-nomifensine and positron emission tomography: the effects of age and Parkinson's disease. Acta Neurol Scand 1988;77:192–201.

16 Salmon E, Brooks DJ, Leenders KL, et al. A two-compartment description and kinetic procedure for measuring regional cerebral [¹¹C]nomifensine uptake using positron emission tomography. J Cereb Blood Flow Metab 1990;10:307–16.

17 Frost JJ, Rosier AJ, Reich SG, et al. Positron emission tomographic imaging of the dopamine transporter with ¹¹C-WIN 35,428 reveals marked declines in mild Parkinson's disease. Ann Neurol 1993;34:423–31.

18 Mayberg HS, Sadzot B, Meltzer CC, et al. Quantification of Mu and non-Mu opiate receptors in temporal lobe epilepsy using positron emission tomography. Ann Neurol 1991;30:3–11.

19 Carson RE, Channing MA, Blasberg RG, et al. Comparison of bolus and infusion methods for receptor quantitation: application to [¹⁸F]cyclofoxy and positron emission tomography. J Cereb Blood Flow Metab 1993;13:24–42.

20 Bartenstein PA, Duncan JS, Prevett MC, et al. Investigation of the opioid system in absence seizures with positron emission tomography. J Neurol Neurosurg Psychiatry 1993;56:1295–302.

21 Price JC, Mayberg HS, Dannals RF, et al. Measurement of benzodiazepine receptor number and affinity in humans using tracer kinetic modelling, positron emission tomography, and [¹¹C]flumazenil. J Cereb Blood Flow Metab 1993;13:656–67.

22 Ramsay SC, Weiller C, Myers R, et al. Monitoring by PET of macrophage accumulation in brain after ischaemic stroke. Lancet 1992;339:1054–5.

23 Junck L, Olson JMM, Ciliax BJ, et al. PET imaging of human gliomas with ligands for the peripheral benzodiazepine binding site. Ann Neurol 1989;26:752–8.

24 Frey KA, Koeppe RA, Mulholland GK, et al. In vivo muscarinic cholinergic receptor imaging in human brain with [¹¹C]scopolamine and positron emission tomography. J Cereb Blood Flow Metab 1992;12:147–54.

25 Yanai K, Watanabe T, Yokoyama H, et al. Mapping of histamine H₁ receptors in the human brain using [¹¹C]pyrilamine and positron emission tomography. J Neurochem 1992;59:128–6.

26 Lammertsma AA, Bench CJ, Price GW, et al. Measurement of cerebral monoamine oxidase B activity using L-[¹¹C]deprenyl and dynamic positron emission tomography. J Cereb Blood Flow Metab 1991;11:545–56.

27 Friston KJ, Frith CD, Liddle PF, Dolan RJ, Lammertsma AA, Frackowiak RSJ. The relationship between global and local changes in PET scans. J Cereb Blood Flow Metab 1990;10:458–66.

28 Friston KJ, Frith CD, Liddle PF, Frackowiak RSJ. Comparing functional (PET) images: the assessment of significant change. J Cereb Blood Flow Metab 1991;11:690–9.

29 Watson JDG, Myers R, Frackowiak RSJ, et al. Area V5 of the human brain: evidence from a combined study using positron emission tomography and magnetic resonance imaging. Cereb Cortex 1993;3:79–94.

30 Winchell HS, Baldwin RM, Lin TH. Development of I-123 labelled amines for brain studies: localization of I-123 iodophenylalkylamines in rat brain. J Nucl Med 1980;21:940.

31 Greenberg JH, Lassen NA. Characterization of ⁹⁹ᵐTc-bicasate as an agent for the measurement of cerebral blood flow with SPECT. J Cereb Blood Flow Metab 1994;14(suppl 1):S1–S3.

32 Hajnal JV, Myers R, Oatridge A, Schwieso JE, Young IR, Bydder GM. Artifacts due to stimulus correlated motion in functional imaging of the brain. Magn Reson Med 1994;31:283–91.

33 Woods RP, Cherry SR, Mazziotta JC. Rapid automated algorithm for aligning and reslicing PET images. J Comput Assist Tomogr 1992;115:565–87.

34 Tyszka JM, Grafton ST, Chew W, Woods RP, Colletti PM. Parceling of mesial frontal motor areas during ideation and movement using functional magnetic resonance imaging at 1·5 Tesla. Ann Neurol 1994;35:746–9.

35 Wise RJS, Bernardi S, Frackowiak RSJ, et al. Serial observations on the pathophysiology of acute stroke: the transition from ischaemia to infarction as reflected in regional oxygen extraction. Brain 1983;106:197–222.

36 Gibbs JM, Wise RJS, Leenders KL, Jones T. Evaluation of the cerebral reserve in patients with carotid artery occlusion. Lancet 1984;i:310–4.

37 Kushner M, Reivich M, Fieschi C, et al. Metabolic and clinical correlates of acute ischaemic infarction. Neurology 1987;37:1103–10.

38 Chollet F, DiPiero V, Wise RJS, Brooks DJ, Dolan RJ, Frackowiak RSJ. The functional anatomy of motor recovery after stroke in humans: a study with positron emission tomography. Ann Neurol 1991;29:63–71.

39 Weiller C, Chollet F, Friston KJ, Wise RJS, Frackowiak RSJ. Functional reorganization of the brain in recovery from striatocapsular infarction in man. Ann Neurol 1992; 31:305–14.

40 Baron JC, Bousser MG, Rey A, et al. Reversal of focal "misery-perfusion" by extra-intracranial artery bypass in haemodynamic cerebral ischaemia. Stroke 1981;12:454–9.

41 Gibbs JM, Wise RJS, Thomas DJ, Mansfield AO, Ross Russell RW. Cerebral haemodynamic changes after extracranial-intracranial bypass surgery. J Neurol Neurosurg Psychiatry 1987;50:140–50.

42 EC-IC bypass study group. Failure of extracranial-intracranial bypass to reduce the risk of ischaemic stroke: results of an international randomised trial. N Engl J Med 1985; 313:1191–200.

43 Humphrey P. Stroke and transient ischaemic attacks. J Neurol Neurosurg Psychiatry 1994; 57:534–43.

44 Frackowiak RSJ, Pozzilli C, Legg NJ, et al. Regional cerebral oxygen supply and utilization in dementia. A clinical and physiological study with oxygen-15 and positron tomography. Brain 1981;104:753–78.

45 Foster NL, Chase TN, Fedio P, Patronas NJ, Brooks RA, DiChiro G. Alzheimer's disease: focal cortical changes shown by positron emission tomography. Neurology 1983; 33:961–5.

46 Herholz K, Adams R, Kessler J, Szelies B, Grond M, Heiss W-D. Criteria for the diagnosis of Alzheimer's disease with positron emission tomography. Dementia 1990; 1:156–64.

47 Kumar A, Schapiro M, Grady C, et al. High-resolution PET studies in Alzheimer's disease. Neuropsychopharmacology 1991;4:35–46.

48 Haxby JV, Grady CL, Koss E, et al. Heterogeneous anterior-posterior metabolic patterns in dementia of the Alzheimer-type. Neurology 1988;38:1853–63.

49 Foster NL, Chase TN, Patronas NJ, Gillespie MM, Fedio P. Cerebral mapping of apraxia in Alzheimer's disease by positron emission tomography. Ann Neurol 1986;19:139–43.

50 Kuhl DE, Small GW, Reige WH. Cerebral metabolic patterns before the diagnosis of probable Alzheimer's disease. J Cereb Blood Flow Metab 1987;7:S406.

51 Montaldi D, Brooks DN, McColl JH, et al. Measurements of regional cerebral blood flow and cognitive performance in Alzheimer's disease. J Neurol Neurosurg Psychiatry 1990; 53:33–8.

52 Burns A, Philpot MP, Costa DC, Ell PJ, Levy R. The investigation of Alzheimer's disease with single photon emission tomography. J Neurol Neurosurg Psychiatry 1989;52:248–53.

53 Waldemar G, Bruhn P, Kristensen M, Johnsen A, Paulson OB, Lassen NA. Heterogeneity of neocortical cerebral blood flow deficits in dementia of the Alzheimer type: a [^{99m}Tc]-d,l-HMPAO SPECT study. J Neurol Neurosurg Psychiatry 1994; 57:285–95.

54 Kennedy AM, Frackowiak RSJ, Newman S, Roques P, Rossor MN. Presymptomatic deficits in individuals at risk of familial Alzheimer's disease: a PET study. Ann Neurol 1996 (in press).

55 Kamo H, McGeer PL, Harrop R, et al. Positron emission tomography and histopathology in Pick's disease. Neurology 1987;37:439–45.

56 Salmon E, Franck G. Positron emission tomographic study in Alzheimer's disease and Pick's disease. Archives of Gerontology and Geriatrics 1989;8:241–7.

57 Leenders KL, Frackowiak RSJ, Lees AJ. Steele-Richardson-Olszewski syndrome. Brain energy metabolism, blood flow and fluorodopa uptake measured by positron emission tomography. Brain 1988;111:615–30.

58 Karbe H, Grond M, Huber M, Herholz K, Kessler J, Heiss W-D. Subcortical damage and cortical dysfunction in progressive supranuclear palsy demonstrated by positron emission tomography. J Neurol 1992;239:98–102.

59 Foster NL, Gilman S, Berent S, Morin EM, Brown MB, Koeppe RA. Cerebral hypometabolism in progressive supranuclear palsy studied with positron emission tomography. Ann Neurol 1988;24:399–406.

60 Neary D, Snowden JS, Shields RA, et al. Single photon emission tomography using ^{99m}Tc-

HM-PAO in the investigation of dementia. *J Neurol Neurosurg Psychiatry* 1987;**50**: 1101–9.

61 Tyrrell PJ, Warrington EK, Frackowiak RSJ, Rossor MN. Progressive degeneration of the right temporal lobe studied with positron emission tomography. *J Neurol Neurosurg Psychiatry* 1990;**53**:1046–50.

62 Tyrrell PJ, Warrington EK, Frackowiak RSJ, Rossor MN. Heterogeneity in progressive aphasia due to focal cortical atrophy: A clinical and PET scan study. *Brain* 1990; **113**:1321–36.

63 Kuhl DE, Phelps ME, Markham CH, Metter EJ, Riege WH, Winter EJ. Cerebral metabolism and atrophy in Huntington's disease determined by [18]FDG and computed tomographic scans. *Ann Neurol* 1982;**12**:425–34.

64 Hayden MR, Martin WRW, Stoessl AJ, *et al.* Positron emission tomography in the early diagnosis of Huntington's disease. *Neurology* 1986;**36**:888–94.

65 Grafton ST, Mazziotta JC, Pahl JJ, *et al.* A comparison of neurological, metabolic, structural, and genetic evaluations in persons at risk for Huntington's disease. *Ann Neurol* 1990;**28**:614–21.

66 Mazziotta JC, Phelps ME, Pahl JJ, *et al.* Reduced glucose metabolism in asymptomatic subjects at risk for Huntington's disease. *N Engl J Med* 1987;**316**:357–62.

67 The Huntington's disease collaborative research group. A novel gene containing a trinucleotide repeat that is expanded and unstable in Huntington's disease chromosomes. *Cell* 1993;**72**:971–83.

68 MacMillan JC, Snell RG, Tyler A, *et al.* Molecular analysis and clinical correlations of the Huntington's disease mutation. *Lancet* 1993;**342**:954–8.

69 Aylward EH, Brandt J, Codori AM, Mangus RS, Barta PE, Harris GJ. Reduced basal ganglia volume associated with the gene for Huntington's disease in asymptomatic at-risk persons. *Neurology* 1994;**44**:823–8.

70 Kuhl DE, Metter EJ, Riege WH. Patterns of local cerebral glucose utilisation determined in Parkinson's disease by the ^{18}F-fluorodeoxyglucose method. *Ann Neurol* 1984;**15**: 419–24.

71 Raichle ME, Perlmutter JS, Fox PT. Parkinson's disease: metabolic and pharmacological approaches with positron emission tomography [abstract]. *Ann Neurol* 1984;**15**:S131–2.

72 Martin WRW, Beckman JH, Calne CB, *et al.* Cerebral glucose metabolism in Parkinson's disease. *Can J Neurol Sci* 1984;**11**:169–73.

73 Leenders KL, Palmer AJ, Quinn N, *et al.* Brain dopamine metabolism in patients with Parkinson's disease measured with positron emission tomography. *J Neurol Neurosurg Psychiatry* 1986;**49**:853–60.

74 Sawle GV, Colebatch JG, Shah A, Brooks DJ, Marsden CD, Frackowiak RSJ. Striatal function in normal aging: implications for Parkinson's disease. *Ann Neurol* 1990; **28**:799–804.

75 Eidelberg D, Takikawa S, Dhawan V, *et al.* Striatal ^{18}F-DOPA uptake: absence of an aging effect. *J Cereb Blood Flow Metab* 1993;**13**:881–8.

76 Martin WRW, Palmer MR, Patlak CS, Calne DB. Nigrostriatal function in humans studied with positron emission tomography. *Ann Neurol* 1989;**26**:535–42.

77 Sawle GV, Wroe SJ, Lees AJ, Brooks DJ, Frackowiak RSJ. The identification of presymptomatic parkinsonism: clinical and [^{18}F]Dopa PET studies in an Irish kindred. *Ann Neurol* 1992;**32**:609–17.

78 Sawle GV, Turjanski N, Brooks DJ. The rate of progression of clinical and subclinical Parkinson's disease. *J Neurol Neurosurg Psychiatry* 1992;**55**:1215.

79 Bhatt MH, Snow BJ, Martin WRW, Pate BD, Ruth TJ, Calne DB. Positron emission tomography suggests that the rate of progression of idiopathic parkinsonism is slow. *Ann Neurol* 1991;**29**:673–7.

80 Sawle GV. The rate of progression of Parkinson's disease. *Ann Neurol* 1992;**31**:229.

81 Sawle GV, Myers R. The role of positron emission tomography in the assessment of human neurotransplantation. *Trends Neurosci* 1993;**16**:172–6.

82 Widner H, Tetrud J, Rehncrona S, *et al.* Bilateral fetral mesencephalic grafting in two patients with parkinsonism induced by 1-methyl-4-phenyl-1,2,3,6-tetrahydropyridine (MPTP). *N Engl J Med* 1992;**327**:1556–63.

83 Brooks DJ, Salmon EP, Mathias CJ, *et al.* The relationship between locomotor disability, autonomic dysfunction, and the integrity of the striatal dopaminergic system in patients with multiple system atrophy, pure autonomic failure, and Parkinson's disease, studied with PET. *Brain* 1990;**113**:1539–52.

84 Brooks DJ, Ibañez V, Sawle GV, et al. Differing patterns of striatal ¹⁸F-dopa uptake in Parkinson's disease, multiple system atrophy and progressive supranuclear palsy. Ann Neurol 1990;28:547–55.

85 Bhatt MH, Snow BJ, Martin WRW, Cooper S, Calne DB. Positron emission tomography in Shy-Drager syndrome. Ann Neurol 1990;28:101–3.

86 Sawle GV, Brooks DJ, Marsden CD, Frackowiak RSJ. Corticobasal degeneration: a unique pattern of regional cortical oxygen metabolism and striatal fluorodopa uptake demonstrated by positron emission tomography. Brain 1991;114:541–56.

87 Brooks DJ, Ibanez V, Playford ED, et al. Presynaptic and postsynaptic striatal dopaminergic function in neuroacanthocytosis: a positron emission tomographic study. Ann Neurol 1991;30:166–71.

88 Calne DB, Langston JW, Martin WRW, et al. Positron emission tomography after MPTP: observations relating to the cause of Parkinson's disease. Nature 1985;317:246–8.

89 Burn DJ, Sawle GV, Brooks DJ. Differential diagnosis of Parkinson's disease, multiple system atrophy, and Steele-Richardson-Olszewski syndrome: discriminant function analysis of striatal ¹⁸F-dopa PET data. J Neurol Neurosurg Psychiatry 1994;57:278–84.

90 Tyrrell PJ, Sawle GV, Bloomfield PM, et al. Clinical and PET studies in the extrapyramidal syndrome of dementia of the Alzheimer type. Arch Neurol 1990;47:1318–23.

91 Sawle GV, Hymas NF, Lees AJ, Frackowiak RSJ. Obsessional slowness: functional studies with positron emission tomography. Brain 1991;114:2191–202.

92 Wolters ECh, Huang C, Clark C, et al. Positron emission tomography in manganese intoxication. Ann Neurol 1989;26:647–51.

93 Rosenberg NL, Myers JA, Martin WR. Cyanide-induced parkinsonism: clinical, MRI, and 6-fluorodopa PET studies. Neurology 1989;39:142–4.

94 Burn DJ, Brooks DJ. Nigral dysfunction in drug-induced parkinsonism: an ¹⁸F-dopa PET study. Neurology 1993;43:552–6.

95 Tedroff J, Aquilonius S-M, Laihinen A, et al. Striatal kinetics of [¹¹C]-(+)-nomifensine and 6-[¹⁸F]fluoro-L-dopa in Parkinson's disease measured with positron emission tomography. Acta Neurol Scand 1990;81:24–30.

96 Hantraye P, Brownell AL, Elmaleh D, et al. Dopamine fiber detection by [¹¹C]-CFT and PET in a primate model of parkinsonism. NeuroReport 1992;3:265–8.

97 Marek KL, Seibyl JP, Sandridge B, et al. SPECT imaging with [I-123]β-CIT demonstrates striatal dopamine transporter loss in parkinsonism. Neurology 1994;44 (suppl 2):A352.

98 Hagglund J, Aquilonius S-M, Eckernas S-A, et al. Dopamine receptor properties in Parkinson's disease and Huntington's chorea evaluated by positron emission tomography using ¹¹C-N-methyl-spiperone. Acta Neurol Scand 1987;75:87–94.

99 Wienhard K, Coenen HH, Pawlik G, et al. PET studies of dopamine receptor distribution using [(18)F]fluoroethylspiperone: findings in disorders related to the dopaminergic system. J Neural Transm 1990;81:195–213.

100 Rinne UK, Laihinen A, Rinne JO, Nagren K, Bergman J, Ruotsalainen U. Positron emission tomography demonstrates dopamine D-2 receptor supersensitivity in the striatum of patients with early Parkinson's disease. Mov Disord 1990;5:55–9.

101 Rinne JO, Laihinen A, Rinne UK, Någren K, Bergman J, Ruotsalainen U. PET study on striatal dopamine D₂ receptor changes during the progression of early Parkinson's disease. Mov Disord 1993;8:134–8.

102 Brücke T, Podreka I, Angelberger P, et al. Dopamine D2 receptor imaging with SPECT: studies in different neuropsychiatric disorders. J Cereb Blood Flow Metab 1991;11:220–8.

103 Tatsch K, Schwarz J, Oertel WH, Kirsch C-M. SPECT imaging of dopamine D2 receptors with ¹²³I-IBZM: initial experience in controls and patients with Parkinson's syndrome and Wilson's disease. Nucl Med Commun 1991;12:699–707.

104 Pizzolato G, Rosatto A, Briani C, et al. Alterations of striatal D2 receptors contribute to deteriorated response to L-dopa in Parkinson's disease (PD): a ¹²³I-IBZM study. Neurology 1993;43(suppl):A271.

105 Schwarz J, Tatsch K, Arnold G, et al. ¹²³I-iodobenzamide-SPECT predicts dopaminergic responsiveness in patients with de novo parkinsonism. Neurology 1992;42:556–61.

106 Burn DJ, Mathias CJ, Quinn N, Marsden CD, Brooks DJ. Striatal opiate receptor binding in Parkinson's disease and multiple system atrophy: ¹¹C-diprenorphine study. Neurology 1993;43(suppl):A270.

107 Gilman S, Koeppe RA, Junck L, Kluin KJ, Lohman M, St Laurent RT. PET studies of cerebellar bensodiazepine receptors with [¹¹C]flumazenil show increased binding in MSA

and decreased binding in OPCA. *Neurology* 1994;44:(suppl 6):A353.

108 Mayberg HS, Starkstein SE, Sadzot B, *et al.* Selective hypometabolism in the inferior frontal lobe in depressed patients with Parkinson's disease. *Ann Neurol* 1990;28:57–64.

109 Eidelberg D, Moeller JR, Dhawan V, *et al.* The metabolic anatomy of Parkinson's disease: Complementary [(18)F]fluorodeoxyglucose and [(18)]fluorodopa positron emission tomographic studies. *Mov Disord* 1990;5:203–13.

110 Playford ED, Jenkins IH, Passingham RE, Nutt J, Frackowiak RSJ, Brooks DJ. Impaired mesial frontal and putamen activation in Parkinson's disease: a positron emission tomography study. *Ann Neurol* 1992; 32:151–61.

111 Jenkins IH, Fernandez W, Playford ED, *et al.* Impaired activation of the supplementary motor area in Parkinson's disease is reversed when akinesia is treated with apomorphine. *Ann Neurol* 1992;32:749–57.

112 Rascol O, Sabatini U, Chollett F, *et al.* Supplementary and primary sensory motor area activity in Parkinson's disease. *Arch Neurol* 1992;49:144–8.

113 Rao SM, Binder JR, Bandettini PA, *et al.* Functional magnetic resonance imaging of complex human movements. *Neurology* 1993;43:2311–8.

114 Rao SM, Binder JR, Bandettini PA, *et al.* Relationship between movement rate and functional magnetic resonance signal change in primary motor cortex. *Neurology* 1994; 44(suppl 2):A262.

115 Turjanski N, Burn DJ, Lammertsma AA, *et al.* PET studies on D1 and D2 receptor status in chorea. *Neurology* 1993;43:A333.

116 Nygaard TG, Marsden CD, Fahn S. Dopa-responsive dystonia: long term treatment, response and prognosis. *Neurology* 1991;41:174–81.

117 Quinn N, Critchley P, Marsden CD. Young onset Parkinson's disease. *Mov Disord* 1987;2:73–91.

118 Sawle GV, Leenders KL, Brooks DJ, *et al.* Dopa-responsive dystonia: [¹⁸F]dopa positron emission tomography. *Ann Neurol* 1991;30:24–30.

119 Snow BJ, Nygaard TG, Takahashi H, Calne DB. Positron emission tomographic studies of dopa-responsive dystonia and early-onset idiopathic parkinsonism. *Ann Neurol* 1993; 34:733–8.

120 Sawle GV, Morrish PK, Playford ED, Burn DJ, Brooks DJ. Young-onset parkinsonism: clues from [¹⁸F]dopa PET studies. *Neurology* 1994;44(suppl 2):A353–4.

121 Engel J, Kuhl DE, Phelps ME, Mazziotta JC. Interictal cerebral glucose metabolism in partial epilepsy: its relation to EEG changes. *Ann Neurol* 1982;12:510–7.

122 Theodore WH, Newmark ME, Sato S, *et al.* ¹⁸F-fluorodeoxyglucose positron emission computed tomography in refractory complex partial seizures. *Ann Neurol* 1983;14: 429–37.

123 Abou-Khalil BW, Siegel GJ, Sackellares JC, Gilman S, Hichwa RD, Marshall R. Positron emission tomography studies of cerebral glucose metabolism in chronic partial epilepsy. *Ann Neurol* 1987;22:480–6.

124 Theodore WH, Jabbari B, Leiderman D, McBurney J, Van Nostrand D. Positron emission tomography and single photon emission tomography in epilepsy: comparison on cerebral blood flow and glucose metabolism. *Ann Neurol* 1990;28:262–3.

125 Engel J, Kuhl DE, Phelps ME. Patterns of human local cerebral glucose metabolism during epileptic seizures. *Science* 1982;218:64–6.

126 Ryvlin P, Philippon B, Cinotti L, Froment JC, Le Bars D, Mauguière F. Functional neuroimaging strategy in temporal lobe epilepsy: a comparative study of ¹⁸FDG-PET and ⁹⁹ᵐTc-HMPAO-SPECT. *Ann Neurol* 1992;31:650–6.

127 Sadzot B, Debets R, Maquet P, Comar C, Franck G. PET studies of patients with partial epilepsy: visual interpretation vs. semi-quantitation/quantitation. *Acta Neurol Scand Suppl* 1994;152:175–8.

128 Duncan R, Patterson J, Hadley DM, *et al.* CT, MR and SPECT imaging in temporal lobe epilepsy. *J Neurol Neurosurg Psychiatry* 1990;53:11–5.

129 Jackson GD, Connelly A, Cross JH, Gordon I, Gadian DG. Functional magnetic resonance imaging of focal seizures. *Neurology* 1994;44:850–6.

130 Di Chiro G, DeLaPaz RL, Brooks RA, *et al.* Glucose utilization of cerebral gliomas measured by [¹⁸F]fluorodeoxyglucose and positron emission tomography. *Neurology* 1982; 32:1323–9.

131 Patronas NJ, Di Chiro G, Kufta C, *et al.* Prediction of survival in glioma patients by PET. *J Neurosurg* 1985;62:816–22.

132 Sasaki M, Ichiya Y, Kuwabara Y, *et al.* Ringlike uptake of [(18)F]FDG in brain abscess:

a PET study. *J Comput Assist Tomog* 1990;**14**:486–7.

133 Kim KT, Black KL, Marciano D, *et al.* Thalium-201 SPECT imaging of brain tumours. *J Nucl Med* 1990;**31**:965–9.

134 Mazziotta JC. The continuing challenge of primary brain tumour management: the contribution of positron emission tomography. *Ann Neurol* 1991;**29**:345–6.

135 Glantz MJ, Hoffman JM, Coleman RE, *et al.* Identification of early recurrence of primary central nervous system tumours by [^{18}F]fluorodeoxyglucose positron emission tomography. *Ann Neurol* 1991;**29**:347–55.

136 Hatazawa J, Ishiwata K, Itoh M, *et al.* Quantitative evaluation of L-[methyl-C-11]methionine uptake in tumor using positron emission tomography. *J Nucl Med* 1989; **30**: 1809–13.

137 Bustany P, Chatel M, Derlon M, *et al.* Brain tumour protein synthesis and histological grades: a study by positron emission tomography (PET) and C-11-L-methionine. *J Neurooncol* 1986;**3**:397–404.

138 Tsurumi Y, Kameyama M, Ishiwata K, *et al.* (18)F-fluoro-2'-deoxyuridine as a tracer of nucleic acid metabolism in brain tumors. *J Neurosurg* 1990;**72**:110–3.

4 Imaging blood vessels of the head and neck

R J SELLAR

The modern era of blood vessel imaging began in 1929 when Forssmann injected himself with contrast medium through a large bore catheter.[1] Although recognised to be a hazardous procedure the diagnostic ability of angiography was quickly appreciated and a whole new field of neurosurgery rapidly emerged. Dott in Edinburgh wrapped a cerebral aneurysm in 1932[2] and Eastcott in London performed the first carotid endarterectomy in 1954.[3]

While angiographic techniques have continued to improve, so has the appreciation of the risks; when the benefits of treatment are minimal, such as in patients with low grade carotid stenosis, the risks of angiography can outweigh its benefits. This has led to the search for less invasive modalities to image the blood vessels. This chapter reviews these new methods, particularly Doppler ultrasonography (DUS), magnetic resonance angiography (MRA), and CT. It also discusses what is the role for angiography other than its accepted use for vascular lesions in the head such as aneurysms and arteriovenous malformations. The remaining role of angiography in imaging the carotid bifurcation is the current subject of heated debate.

The intensity of this debate was recently increased by the North American Symptomatic Carotid Endarterectomy Trial (NASCET)[4] and the European Carotid Surgery Trial (ECST)[5] both of which showed that 70% stenosis, when measured from an angiogram, could select a group of patients that benefited from carotid surgery but that non-invasive measurement, when performed as in NASCET, did not satisfactorily select these patients.[6]

Measurements on the carotid arteries

Methodological problems

Before reviewing the various methods of imaging the cerebral blood vessels it is important to understand that much of the controversy surrounding the investigation of patients, particularly those with arteriosclerotic disease, relates to the different methods of measuring the disease that are used. Measurement of angiographic carotid stenosis can be performed in at least three different ways and further methods still are used to measure stenosis detected by other modalities.

In the first place it is unlikely that good correlation will exist between two methods based on different physical principles. Angiographic measurements are of the anatomical transverse diameter of the lumen of the artery. Doppler flow measurements are physiological and relate to the state of the circulation. The Doppler signal at one point in time depends not only on the vessel's cross sectional area (not merely its diameter), but also on cardiac output and peripheral resistance.

Secondly, the probable discrepancy between such differing methods of measurement becomes far greater when the stenosis is asymmetric. The peak velocity produced by a given diameter stenosis can differ by 30% depending on whether the stenosis is concentric or asymmetric.[7]

The third point relates to angiography; many studies, including NASCET, require two views for measurement of carotid stenosis. Often on one view (usually the anteroposterior) the stenosis is obscured due to overlap from the external carotid vessel. If this is the case there is a potential for considerable error in measuring percentage stenosis and even if three views are taken large errors may still occur. Figure 4.1 shows that even if oblique and lateral projectives are available there can still be considerable error in estimating percentage stenosis. The variability of angiography between observers has not been fully tested.[8] There have been studies of error in measurement of carotid stenosis between observers but unfortunately it is unethical to repeat the entire procedure. This is a pity because it would have highlighted the problem of limited views and almost certainly helped to standardise angiographic procedures.

Perhaps more surprising is that even within each imaging modality there is little standardisation of the methods of measure-

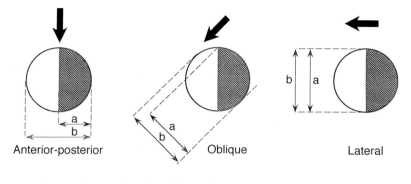

Anterior-posterior   Oblique   Lateral

➡ indicates direction of *x* ray beam

Figure 4.1   *Effect of different views on degree of apparent carotid stenosis*

ment. This is particularly true of measurement of angiographic stenosis. This has important consequences; the method used by NASCET[4] was significantly different from that used by ECST.[5] The denominator chosen by ECST was an imaginary diameter of the carotid bulb before it was diseased, whereas in NASCET it was the distal internal carotid artery at the point when the walls become parallel.

The difference in mensuration has recently been shown to result in an ECST measurement of 70% representing the same degree of stenosis as a NASCET measurement of 50%.[9] Because ECST produced a significant result for 70% and greater stenosis (these patients benefiting from surgery), it could be argued that the continuing NASCET trial may now be randomising the wrong group of patients in that the critical degree of stenosis is likely to be less than 50% NASCET stenosis rather than 70%.

Finally DUS, MRA, and angiography are often compared from correlation coefficients but the use of coefficient statistics is totally inappropriate when comparing two measures that are not calibrated against a true value.[10] There is a high correlation between foot size and height but this does not mean that the measurement of a neurosurgeon's foot will give you an accurate measure of his height. It is possible to obtain a high degree of correlation although one of the methods used is highly inaccurate due to bias. Doppler ultrasonography machines vary considerably[11 12] and it is probable that lack of calibration contributed significantly to the poor DUS results in multicentre trials.

105

In summary, unless the theoretical problems related to measurement are clearly understood, it is likely that the problems that non-invasive methods of investigating carotid disease have had in gaining credibility will continue.

Carotid Doppler ultrasound (DUS)

This review considers the non-invasive imaging techniques before the invasive ones. It is the safety of DUS that is one of its great advantages and it is a technique that has achieved widespread use as a screening test for carotid atherosclerosis. Carotid ultrasound was initially performed with continuous wave Doppler. Two separate transducers were used, one to transmit, the other to receive ultrasound signals. Doppler images were obtained, from which peak flow velocities could be calculated with the Doppler shift principle.[13] Pulsed wave Doppler uses the same transducer to transmit and receive waves; discrete volumes can be sampled with this technique, and this improves depth resolution. The next major advance was the elegant combination of real time imaging with Doppler information called duplex ultrasonography.[14] The stenosis could be measured from an image with calipers as well as assessed physiologically with Doppler.

The most recent development has been colour flow DUS, whereby flow information is colour coded and superimposed on the grey scale images (figure 4.2). This reduces the time of the examination by rapidly pinpointing the pathological regions. The angle of insonation can now be electronically set to keep the Doppler measurements accurate.

DUS criteria for significant carotid disease

Various Doppler measures have been proposed in addition to the real time image measures for detecting significant stenosis. Peak systolic and peak diastolic velocity can be measured both in the common carotid artery, at, or just distal to the stenosis and in the distal internal carotid artery well beyond the stenotic area. These measures can be used on their own or expressed as ratios. Peak systolic flow velocity adjacent to the stenosis has been found to correlate well with angiographic stenosis in two studies.[15 16] Examination of various diagnostic criteria showed peak systolic flow velocity to be the most straightforward measure with a

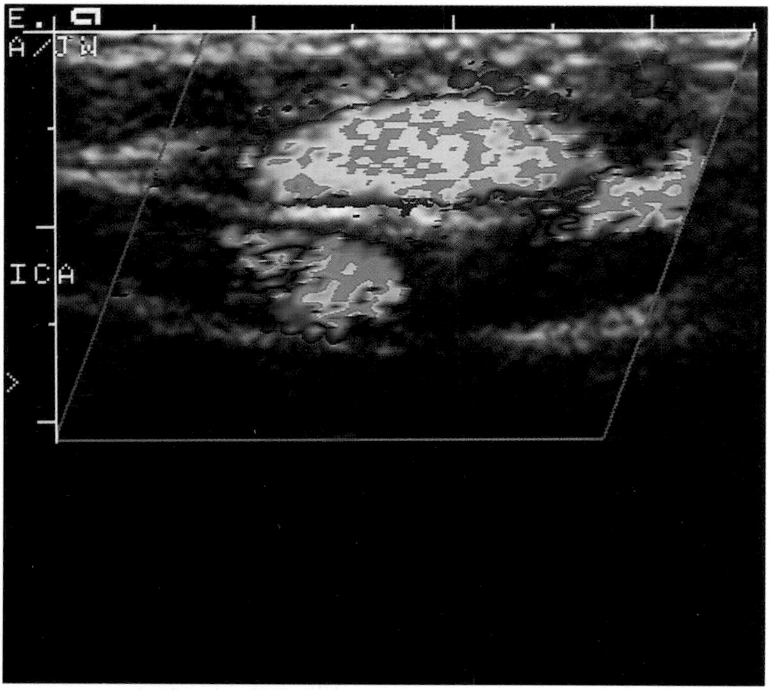

Figure 4.2   *Carotid ultrasonography with colour flow. High velocity signal is seen at the site of narrowing*

2·25–2·3 m/s threshold being used to predict 70% angiographic stenosis.

Both these studies generated receiver operator characteristic curves, which are useful as they allow the clinician to decide what sensitivity and specificity are required for a particular clinical situation and to choose a threshold that is appropriate. (For screening purposes a peak systolic flow velocity of about 1·25 m/s is typically used to select patients with 50% carotid stenosis.)

Other authors have found that in very severe stenosis the peak systolic flow velocity Doppler signal can decline and that peak diastolic flow is a more accurate method of detecting these patients.[17] The diagnosis of carotid occlusion can be made by the absence of pulsation from the internal carotid artery, and the pres-

107

ence of echogenic material filling the lumen. Doppler signals will be absent and the distal artery may be reduced in diameter.[14]

What is the role of DUS ?

Can DUS be relied on not only as a screening test but as the only and definitive diagnostic test before surgery? This is a question that has caused much heated debate.[8 12] It is easiest to approach this subject historically.

Many authors in the early 1980s found that there was high sensitivity, specificity, and accuracy in DUS as a technique for detecting carotid stenosis. A review by Cardullo *et al* of 16 studies concluded that DUS was 96% sensitive, 86% specific, and 91% accurate at detecting angiographic carotid stenosis greater than 50%.[18] The enthusiasm for DUS grew during the 1980s so that by 1987 Goodison *et al*[19] were claiming that the accuracy of DUS exceeded that of angiography; Hartnell,[20] although conceding that it was difficult for clinicians to change old habits, said it was time that surgeons used only DUS preoperatively because it was better than angiography for detecting severe stenosis. This momentum came to an abrupt halt when the NASCET results were published.[4] It was clear that 70% angiographic stenosis selected a group of patients that benefited from surgery but no equivalent Doppler measurements could satisfactorily select this group. Later the sonographic data was presented and the sensitivity for detecting 70% angiographic stenosis was only 59%.[6] These data have subsequently been criticised on account of poor quality control. There were, however, other causes of failure of ultrasound to pass the acid test of a randomised prospective multicentre trial.

Firstly there has been a tendency to rewrite the early ultrasound data. Zweibel, in his excellent review of DUS of the cerebral arteries in 1992,[14] states that the accuracy of carotid artery measurements is high. He quotes five papers to support this, all surprisingly published around eight years before his review.[21-25] The sensitivities range from 91–94% with equally impressive specificity and accuracies quoted (87–99%) for detecting significant carotid stenosis. By far the largest series is his own with 393 vessels insonated.[21] Because the common and external carotid arteries were assessed as well, in reality this means that 131 bifurcations in 78 patients were evaluated.

It is rewarding to look at this early paper in more detail and to quote the author's original comments: "the sensitivity level of HRS (high resolution sonography), CWD (continuous wave Doppler), and the combined procedures all were suboptimal for a screening study (72% CWD, 72% HRS, and 82% combined). If 50% decrease in diameter is considered to be the level at which carotid stenosis becomes haemodynamically significant, then these results cast doubt on the case of ultrasound as a screening procedure".

It is only if the studies that were of poor quality or in which the artery was wrongly localised are removed from the results that the sensitivities improve to acceptable levels. Ten years later, the same data were claimed by the author to show that DUS has a 94% sensitivity and 99% specificity for detecting 50% and greater stenosis and others went on to claim that DUS is so accurate that surgical decisions should be based on it.

More recent researchers have consistently achieved high sensitivities of 81% to 85% for DUS in detecting 50% stenosis but these are results achieved by specialised units on small numbers of patients.[15][26][27] Hunting et al have stated that if verification bias is taken into account sensitivities of greater than 70% will be difficult to achieve by DUS.[15]

Secondly, ultrasound is both highly operator and machine dependent; although colour flow has reduced the pitfalls for the operator, it still remains a highly skilled investigation. On account of the variability of results from different centres, doubt has been cast on its use for multicentre trials without proper calibration of the ultrasound equipment and certification of laboratories.[11]

Thirdly, there is no agreement as to which measurements should be used and considerable debate as to whether a battery of DUS tests including orbital plethysmography is required[28] or whether a single measure—for example, peak systolic flow velocity—is sufficient.

Finally the need for angiography before surgery has been underlined by two further studies. The first was from the NASCET Group describing an association between angiographic ulceration and increased risk of stroke, particularly in patients with very severe degrees of stenosis.[29] The second was a recent study by Griffiths et al,[32] which found concurrent intracranial disease in 26 out of a 100 consecutive patients referred for investigation of cerebrovascular disease. Eleven had aneurysms or arteriovenous malformations and 15 had tandem stenoses. There has been extensive debate on the subject of patients who have a second carotid stenosis typically situated in the carotid syphon.

Polak has stated that such tandem stenoses are rare, pointing out that they were present in only 2% of cases in NASCET and that in any case the decision regarding surgery or not is unaffected.[8] The studies he quotes in support of his case are, however, totally inappropriate. Firstly, the presence of tandem lesions was a specific exclusion criteria of NASCET,[4] so the incidence is likely to be low in this study! With respect to the second issue he cites Little et al[33]; this paper is concerned with the distinction of distal stenosis from flow artifacts rather than with the effect of tandem lesions on surgical decisions. Polak's defence of ultrasound in general is curious and is partly based on the argument that it must be good because its use is widespread. "Was it not performed in all ECST patients?" he asks.[8] In fact, no ultrasound data at all were collected for the ECST trial. In summary, DUS has only replaced angiography in a few centres where it is believed that the risks of angiography outweigh the benefits of accurate classification and knowledge of the intracranial circulation.

On the other hand the value of ultrasound as a screening test is established; using it in this way O'Leary and Polak were able to increase the incidence of haemodynamically significant stenosis in patients going on to angiography from 50% to 80%.[30] There are practical reasons why DUS is a good screening test for mild and moderate stenosis but less accurate in cases of severe stenosis. As the artery becomes progressively stenosed, the impedance of the plaque increases and this tends to cause blurring of the interfaces and reverberation artifact. Measurement of the stenosis with calipers is often difficult and ultrasound diagnosis is then dependent on the physiological data, typically the peak systolic velocity.[30] When complete occlusion occurs the distinction from very tight stenosis has always been a problem for ultrasonographers and the external carotid may be mistaken for the internal carotid artery (figure 4.3).[31]

A recent prospective study comparing DUS and MRA with conventional angiography by Houston et al[27] showed that DUS correctly identified all of the angiographic stenoses of greater than 50% but misclassified 60% of patients with angiographic moderate stenosis (50–80% in this series) as having severe stenosis and 37% of patients with angiographic occlusion were thought to have

110

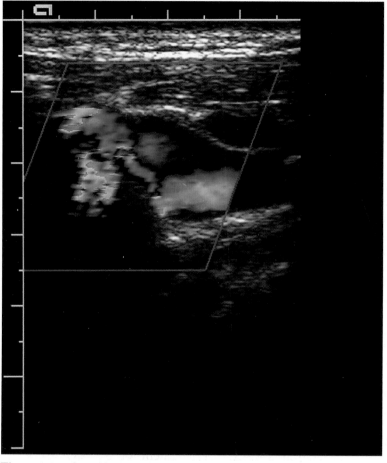

Figure 4.3   *Carotid ultrasonography. The tortuosity of the bifurcation and carotid vessels, as shown in this image, shows the difficulty in correct identification of vessels*

stenosed but patent carotid arteries. These findings confirm that DUS is an excellent screening test for 50% stenosis but has problems in classifying the more severe degrees and that angiography is required in patients for accurate classification of the severity of the stenosis.

111

Imaging of plaque with ultrasound

Ultrasound is the first of the imaging techniques to focus on other characteristics of plaque apart from its shape and size. Heavily calcified plaque is strongly echogenic. Fibrogenic plaque is also echogenic but relatively homogeneous whereas intraplaque haemorrhage results in heterogeneity within the plaque and areas that are anechoic. Some studies comparing the DUS detection of haemorrhage with surgical histology have been encouraging with sensitivities ranging from 72% to 74% and specificities of 79% to 80%.[14][34] Other studies showed no correlation, however, between DUS and histology.[35] The hypothesis that intraplaque haemorrhage leads to intimal inflammation and secondary mural thrombus is supported by several studies reporting an increased risk of transient ischaemic attacks and infarction in patients with DUS plaque haemorrhage. Conversely, postmortem studies of asymptomatic subjects have shown a high incidence of ultraplaque haemorrhage.[36] Hopefully, a larger prospective trial will show whether plaque morphology, particularly intraplaque haemorrhage, is indeed a risk factor.

Transcranial Doppler (TCD)

This technique uses the thin temporal bone above the zygoma as a window to image the middle cerebral artery and the other vessels close to the circle of Willis.[37]

Now that colour flow information has been added, it has become an increasingly valuable technique for studying the intracranial circulation in a non-invasive manner. Applications include following subarachnoid haemorrhage when TCD can detect spasm before clinical deterioration. We have found a 20% increase in peak systolic flow velocity of 120 cm/s to be an accurate predictor of clinically significant spasm. Transcranial Doppler has also been used to monitor hazardous procedures such as carotid endarterectomy giving warning of both hypoperfusion and hyperperfusion. Hypoperfusion may occur due to the effects of anaesthetic agents on the heart and on the autoregulation mechanism of the cerebral vessels. Hyperfusion is an unusual complication of endarterectomy but is thought to be due to a reduction in peripheral resistance of the cerebral circulation. Recently TCD has shown that emboli from the heart occur asymptomatically in patients with cerebrovascular disease.[38]

We have used TCD to monitor the progress of acute stroke and found that spontaneous reperfusion during the first week after a stroke does not result in the predicted oedema or an obviously increased tendency to haemorrhagic transformation, but leads to the converse and a reduced infarct size.[39]

Research with primate models in the 1970s indicated that middle cerebral artery reperfusion after 90 minutes resulted in profound reperfusion oedema and haemorrhage.[40] But our own results indicate that reperfusion in patients leads to less oedema and smaller infarct size suggesting that the animal model, which involved ligation of the middle cerebral artery, does not correspond to the effect of thrombus lodging in the middle cerebral artery. (There is some evidence that build up of toxins such as nitrous oxide causes vasodilatation and hence some reperfusion on a cyclical basis.) As thrombolysis becomes a more widespread treatment in stroke, TCD should be a valuable tool with which to monitor the success of treatment.

DUS in other vascular disease

Ultrasound has only a few "windows" in the skull to interrogate the cerebral arteries and visualisation of walls of small arteries is difficult.

It is not therefore an ideal method for studying diffuse disease such as vasculitis or fibromuscular hyperplasia, although the increased peripheral resistance will be reflected in the Doppler wave form. Arterial dissections are said to cause a backward and forward motion of blood in the internal carotid artery but we have found this sign unreliable; occurring also in acute middle cerebral artery occlusion.

Magnetic resonance angiography (MRA)

Few techniques have developed as quickly as MRA.[41] The first description of flow imaging was in 1985 by Wedeen et al.[42] The details of time of flight (TOF) angiography[43] and phase contrast MRA followed soon afterwards.[44]

Technique

Blood can be imaged in two different ways by MRI; either as a negative signal (black blood) or as a positive signal (white blood).[45]

113

Black blood

In conventional spin echo MRI, the pulse sequence consists of a 90° radiofrequency pulse to magnetise the slice and a 180° pulse, which rephases the exited protons before read out.

If blood flows out of the section being imaged in the time between these two radiofrequency pulses then a signal void occurs as there are no protons remaining for read out which then appears black on MRI. This phenomenon of a "flow void" can be magnified by using a presaturation band just outside the plane of interest. This reduces the alignment of protons along the Z axis (the direction of the main magnetic field) and thus reduces the availability of inflowing protons to produce a signal in response to the radiofrequency pulse. Clearly, using a thin section technique and long repetition time will increase the likelihood of blood protons leaving the slice before refocusing,[45] increasing the black blood effect. A long repetition time also increases the effect by increasing the signal from stationary tissues.

White blood

For positive signal imaging of the extracranial vessels the reverse principle is applied. The protons within the stationary tissues are saturated and the strong signal (white) comes from inflowing blood. For imaging white blood, two techniques have evolved—namely, TOF and phase contrast MRA.

Time of flight angiography

Time of flight angiography relies on rapid pulse sequences being applied to the area of interest so that the stationary tissues become saturated and only a few protons remain aligned along the main magnetic field and thus available to emit a signal.

Gradient echo pulse sequences are used that have a short repetition time (30–60 ms) and a small flip angle (30–60°).[46] If the repetition time becomes too short or if the flip angle is too large inflowing blood will also become saturated. A balance obviously has to be achieved because if the repetition time is increased too much not only will the saturation of blood be reduced but also that of the stationary tissues. The precise values used will depend on whether the blood is flowing across or in the plane of imaging. If the blood is flowing in plane the repetition time can be longer and the flip angle smaller. Imaging by TOF can be performed as a three dimensional volume slab or as a two dimensional technique whereby multiple thin sections are acquired; the second is more suitable for slow flow situations as blood is less likely to become saturated as it travels through a thin slice. These MRA techniques have recently been reviewed by Edelman.[46]

Phase contrast angiography

Phase contrast relies on the principle that inflowing blood causes a shift in phase of the MR signal.

Two images have to be acquired; the first uses a positive gradient to induce positive flow related phase shifts whereas the second image has a negative gradient applied. The two images are then subtracted to remove the signal from background tissue.[45] For coding in three directions at least six images are required.[44]

Saturation of inflowing blood does not occur and hence this technique is particularly suitable for slow flow situations such as that in veins, but it is time consuming.

Maximum intensity projection (MIP)

Raw data from these studies are projected into a three dimensional format by an elegant technique that stores the brightest signals from the data, which are then back projected as a two dimensional image. This maximum intensity projection can be tailored to the anatomy of interest, excluding veins and unwanted arteries.[47] The data can then be rotated in three dimensions to obtain the optimal view of the pathology (figure 4.4).

Recent developments

Magnetic resonance angiography has been steadily refined and some of the recent developments include using magnetisation transfer to increase the saturation of the stationary tissue.[48 49] Magnetic resonance angiography involves the mobile protons; the restricted protons held by large molecules such as proteins are usually not visible, on account of their ultrashort T2 relaxation time. But these restricted protons can be energised by a powerful off resonance radiofrequency pulse as they have a wide range of resonant frequencies.

The magnetisation imparted to this restricted pool of protons will then be transferred to the mobile protons in the stationary tissue helping to cancel out its signal. Flowing blood has very few

115

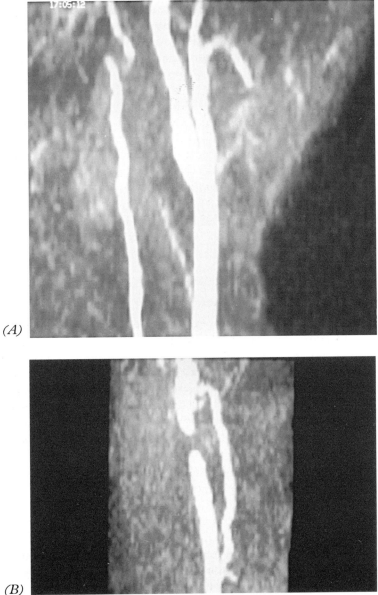

(A)

(B)

Figure 4.4 *(A) Time of flight magnetic resonance angiogram. Normal appearances of the carotid and vertebral arteries. (B) 2D time of flight magnetic resonance angiogram. The flow void in the internal carotid artery indicates tight carotid stenosis*

restricted protons and hence overall flow contrast is enhanced. Other techniques have evolved to improve the signal and reduce the saturation effects that occur in three dimensional TOF. These include tilted optimised non-saturating excitation (TONE), a technique that increases the flip angle as blood passes through the slice. This increases the signal from the flowing blood at a time when it is losing signal from saturation effects.

Travelling saturation bands may also be used; these are excited just before the arrival of blood and help to suppress the background signal. Sharper images have also been obtained by diastolic acquisition of images.[50] Cerebral blood flow can now be quantified by exciting a bolus that is then tracked along the blood vessels.[51] A similar technique of presaturation of the flow in a blood vessel can be employed for assessment of the collateral circulation to the territory supplied by the suppressed vessel.[52]

Uses of magnetic resonance angiography

Arteriosclerotic disease: technique

Some centres use a three dimensional TOF technique for imaging carotid arteries that is less affected by turbulence and in which diameter measurements correlate better with conventional angiography. When there is a very tight stenosis, however, flow rates through the stenosis start to fall and occlusions may be falsely diagnosed. On account of this we have used both a three dimensional and a two dimensional technique. The thin slices of two dimensional TOF are much less likely to result in saturation than the thicker slabs of the volume three dimensional TOF method.[53-56] The additional inspection of the individual images further reduces the chance of calling a tight stenosis an occlusion.[46 54]

Results

Several centres have already produced encouraging results using MRA as a screening test for carotid arteriosclerosis. Masaryk et al obtained an R value of 0·94 when correlating a three dimensional TOF technique with conventional x ray angiography.[54] For a screening test high sensitivity is important, particularly if the consequences of missing the diagnosis can be devastating for the patient.

Sensitivities higher than colour flow DUS have been obtained in some hands[57 58 60 61] although this experience is not universal.[59] A recent prospective blinded trial of a few patients found that the accuracy of MRA equalled that of DUS.[27] The most encouraging aspect of this series was that MRA correctly identified all the angiographic occlusions. Severe stenosis will cause variable lengths of complete loss of signal due to phase dispersal within the repetition time. This flow void has been found to be a sensitive (0·85) indicator of severe (70%) stenosis.[26] Ackerman and Candia[28] have pointed out, however, that others have found a 25% false positive rate for this sign and that flow voids have been seen with stenoses of only 55%.[26] They argue against the increasing practice of using an MRA flow void as an indication for surgery with no x ray angiographic confirmation. This leads us back to the question of measurement. If it is a 55% NASCET measurement—that is, the least stenosis that leads to a flow void—then ECST has shown that it is logical to offer surgery to these patients in any case.

The use of MRA in the diagnosis of carotid stenosis has many traps for the unwary; MRA may overestimate the length of stenosis.[62] If blood forms pools in an ulcer saturation effects can occur.[63] There are also artefacts from the maximum intensity projection algorithm, the background signal from the stationary tissue may become indistinguishable from the saturated slow flow that occurs along the arterial wall.[62] Then there are the potential problems for MRA from intraplaque haemorrhage[64] or intraplaque lipid which may give rise to bright signal despite the short repetition time. This causes T1 breakthrough from the background as this bright signal may prove indistinguishable from inflowing blood for the algorithm. It is important therefore to check the individual thin slices when assessing a stenosis as well as in suspected occlusion.[64]

In an experimental situation Podolak *et al*[65] have shown that especially in two dimensional angiography there are not only phase encoding errors but, on account of the time delay between the radiofrequency pulse and frequency encoding, the flow can displace the signal leading to exaggeration of the stenosis. This has led researchers to try to find a conversion factor, but unfortunately the overestimation of stenosis is a non-linear function.[66]

Magnetic resonance angiography has the same problem as DUS in that it uses flow data to infer an anatomical abnormality. But the similarity of the images with angiography is deceptive and has lured some surgeons into operating without further studies.

Masaryk and Obuchawski have emphasised that current announcements concerning the demise of angiography were somewhat premature.[12]

Aneurysms and arteriovenous malformations

Magnetic resonance angiography has become increasingly useful for detecting aneurysms. Ross et al[67] reported a 95% accuracy for MRA when compared with conventional angiography. Only aneurysms of 5 mm diameter or less were missed and it has been claimed that the complication rate for these aneurysms is small; this seems to be the case with unruptured aneurysms,[68] but it is not everyone's experience with aneurysms that have previously ruptured.[69] Although not yet suitable for routine use in patients with subarachnoid haemorrhage there is possibly a role for MRA in those patients with negative x ray angiography. Aneurysms may not be recognised on conventional angiography because of overlapping, tortuous vessels, or if they contain thromboses at the time of angiography. It is also suggested that spasm surrounding vessels may render aneurysms difficult to see, but this is debatable. Magnetic resonance angiography has been reported as positive after conventional angiography failed to show an aneurysm.[70]

There is certainly a role for MRA in elderly patients presenting with 3rd nerve palsy. These aneurysms are nearly always larger than 5 mm. Computed tomography has also been successfully used for this purpose and the choice of technique will depend on local availability.[71] We also currently use it as a screening test for aneurysms in patients with a strong family history of subarachnoid haemorrhage, while explaining to these patients the limitations of this technique to detect small aneurysms. Finally, MRA may find a role in following up aneurysms that have been treated by platinum coiling in which a residual neck is suspected.

It should be stressed that MRA is not suitable for following up aneurysms that have been surgically clipped. Not only are there large artefacts from the metals used in patients who have had an aneurysm clipped but a death has occurred because of magnetic deflection of an aneurysm clip. Unfortunately the information available at the time of scanning concerning the clip was incorrect. If a patient with aneurysm clips has to be scanned, it has been recommended that the operation note is checked to make sure that the clip is of a type which is not ferromagnetic. Clips can even vary from batch to batch and the most recent recommendation is that all clips should be magnet tested before use. Arteriovenous malformations are clearly seen on MRI as well as MRA.[72] The size of the nidus can be assessed and used to follow up the effect of radiosurgery or embolisation treatment; MRA does not, however, give sufficient data on feeding vessels and venous drainage for treatment decisions to be made (figure 4.5).[73 74]

Other vascular lesions: vasculitis, dissection, and fibromuscular hyperplasia

Magnetic resonance angiography is not an ideal technique for imaging vasculitis. A recent study[75] of a few cases with MRI showed a reasonable correlation with angiography, but MRA was not used in this study; MRA is not the modality of choice because not only is there the potential pitfall of false positive diagnosis (the distal arteries may appear beaded due to slow flow from

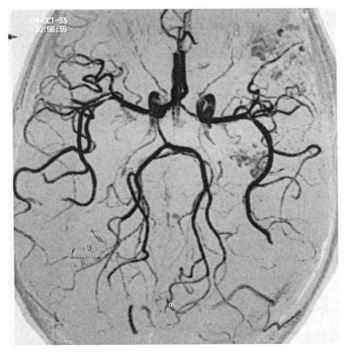

Figure 4.5   *3D time of flight magnetic resonance angiogram. The circle of Willis and larger cerebral arteries are well demonstrated. A diffuse arteriovenous malformation is seen in the right temporal area*

120

other causes such as venous thrombosis), but also vasculitis may involve arteries smaller than the current resolution of MRA. Arterial dissection is better shown on angiography although successful diagnosis has been made by MRI.[76 77] The associated thrombus may have a brighter signal than the adjacent flowing blood[64] confusing the maximum intensity projection algorithm. Fibromuscular hyperplasia is more likely to be a false positive diagnosis with MRA than a true one; the use of multiple thin slabs in two dimensional techniques[78 79] does not always align due to movement and gives rise to a "venetian blind" artefact not unlike fibromuscular dysplasia. As this condition is also associated with cerebral aneurysms, angiography is the more suitable technique.

Magnetic resonance venography

Some tests do not have to go through the full validation process; their clinical value is immediately recognised.[80] Magnetic resonance venography, particularly if venous sinus thrombosis is suspected, falls into this category and in our department has already supplanted conventional venography (figure 4.6). The same principles as those for MRA are used except that the saturation band is now placed to nullify inflowing arterial blood. A full understanding of MRA techniques is required as flow voids will occur when the slow venous flow remains in plane for any length of time, this commonly occurs in the transverse sinus near the torcular.[81 82] Reference to the individual T1 images is useful as thrombus will often give rise to a very bright signal and will confirm that a flow void is due to a clot.[83 84] Venous thrombosis may also give rise to parenchymal haemorrhage, infarcts, hydrocephalus, and dilatation of the deep periventricular veins. Some tumours, particularly meningiomas, encroach on the deep veins. This information is valuable to the surgeon as complete occlusion of the vein allows it to be sacrificed without danger.

The smaller veins may be better visualised by introduction of gadolinium which will also allow the circulation of some tumours to be seen on MRA.[85]

Combined DUS and MRA for screening the carotid

Recently several authors have suggested that a combination of these two tests may replace angiography for arteriosclerotic dis-

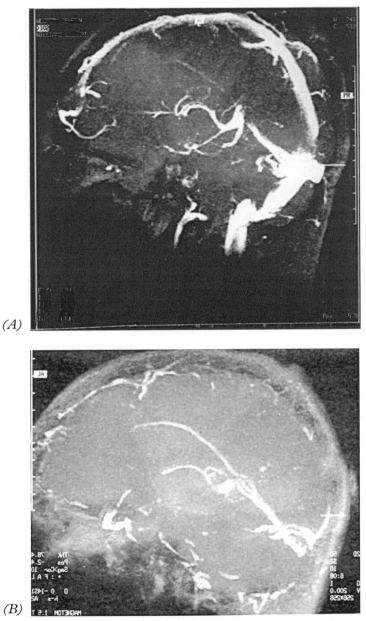

(A)

(B)

Figure 4.6   (A) 2D time of flight magnetic resonance venogram. Normal
appearance of the venous sinuses. (B) 2D time of flight magnetic resonance
venogram. Thrombosis of the superior sagittal sinus

ease.[27 29 62 86 87] This combination of tests is attractive as DUS is very sensitive for detecting stenoses up to 50% and MRA, and, particularly if a technique sensitive to low flow is selected, can often be used to distinguish between complete occlusion and very tight stenoses. The published data are as yet few, but Polak has already claimed that this combination of tests would result in a 99% sensitivity for detecting surgical cases. This claim is made on the basis that both tests have about 90% sensitivity; therefore, theoretically both tests combined will produce only one false positive result in 100.[8] This, however, makes the large assumption that the tests are completely independent, whereas we know that both tests have difficulties in the same pathological situations—for example, patients with complete or near complete occlusion and those with tortuous arteries. Masaryk and Obuchawski have criticised Polak's data on several counts, but mainly on the lack of any independent reference investigation—for example, x ray angiography—for some of the patients included in their paper.[12]

A recent study from Liverpool[87] overcomes many of the methodological objectives that have been made to the studies already mentioned. These workers compared prospectively DUS and MRA with x ray angiography (DSA). They avoided the error of using correlation coefficients in the analysis of their results and report the agreement of their tests at every degree of percentage stenosis (0–100%). This is valuable for the future as we are still uncertain at what percentage stenosis surgery becomes the appropriate treatment. In their hands, if DUS and MRA agreed then 6% of patients were misclassified when compared with DSA and they make the reasonable point that this degree of inaccuracy is offset by the absence of risk of DUS and MRA when compared with invasive radiology. Unfortunately there are few hospitals with such an experienced ultrasonographer. So, although early results are encouraging, the jury is still out.

Computed tomography

The advent of spiral CT[88] has meant that the cervical carotid artery can be scanned in under 30 seconds. Scan data are acquired continually as the patient moves through the scanner during an infusion of contrast medium.[89] Data processing currently takes longer, up to 10 minutes, and uses either the same image projection (maximum intensity projection) methods as in MRA or one of the other three dimensional display techniques that have been

123

developed specifically for CT. Early results have been impressive. A study by Marks *et al* of a group of 28 patients found a good correlation when CT was compared blind with angiography, with 89% of cases falling into the same three categories (0–30, 30–70, 70–100%) of narrowing.[61] Computed tomography has a very high sensitivity to contrast and both cases of occlusion were correctly identified. This may turn out to be one of the major advantages of the technique.

There are, however, also problems related to CT; scanning protocols typically include only a small segment, usually 6 cm, of the cervical carotid artery and lesions outside this small window will be missed.

Calcified lesions, if dense, will cause beam hardening and increase the apparent narrowing of the vessel lumen, particularly if the calcification is circumferential. Conversely, if the calcification is faint there is potential for a partial volume artefact and part of the density of the vessel wall being falsely interpreted as contrast medium. (The ability to show the degree of calcification may also be helpful in the selection of patients for angioplasty.) There are other advantages over MRA as currently performed in that the superior resolution of the CT images allows for cross sectional measurements to be made. The physiological effect of circumferential and asymmetric lesions is very different. Finally, angiographic ulceration has been shown to be an important risk factor in severe stenosis[29] but MRA is a relatively poor technique for demonstrating ulceration; CT may prove to be more sensitive for detecting ulcers.

In summary, CT has potential advantages as a technique for assessing carotid stenosis. It has the advantage over DUS and MRA that it can give a diameter measurement of carotid stenosis and does not rely on a physiological measurement. It is therefore more likely on theoretical grounds to be able to select patients that will benefit from surgery. But until these advantages become clear cut with larger series it is unlikely to win widespread acceptance on account of the high x ray dose and the requirement for an intravenous contrast agent.

Angiography

The modern era of angiography started with Seldinger[90] who in 1953 described his percutaneous technique with admirable brevity as "needle in, wire in, needle out, catheter over wire, wire out,

124

that is all". Since that time, developments in technology have resulted in smaller softer tipped catheters that cause less trauma to the arterial wall, contrast agents that are less toxic, and improved *x* ray equipment, particularly of high resolution digital substraction angiography (DSA) which has meant that carotid angiography can be performed very quickly (15–20 minutes).

Angiography for arteriosclerotic disease: technique

Angiographic techniques must be meticulous and not left in the unsupervised hands of junior staff, when the risks can be three times as high.[91]

Short examination times, small soft catheters, the use of safety J guidewires that are kept below the carotid bifurcation, non-ionic contrast agents, and DSA all probably reduce the risks.

We routinely perform a lateral and two oblique views as it has been shown that if two views only are used 40% of lesions are missed.[92] Some modern angiographic equipment can "spin" through 90° or 180° during a single slow injection and thus the projection revealing maximum stenosis can be selected for measurement. It is possible to include the carotid siphon and intracranial carotid vessels on a single image with even small image intensification systems (9 inches) reducing examination time.

Advantages of angiography

The advantages of angiography are that it is an established technique with proved ability to select patients who will benefit from carotid endarterectomy. It is a high resolution technique with high agreement between observers (figure 4.7).[93] It can demonstrate not only the carotid bifurcation region but also the carotid origin, carotid siphon, and distal branches. Proximal stenosis at the origin of the common carotid artery is rare (1·5%–5%),[94] so that many centres do not routinely perform arch aortography, particularly as proximal stenosis is seldom sufficiently severe to influence surgical decisions. Moseley has claimed that a case in which the common carotid artery was occluded would be the "case of the year" in his department.[95] Distal internal carotid disease, particularly involving the carotid siphon, may have a more sinister implication[96 97] and the incidence of "tandem stenosis" has probably been underestimated and 15% of those carefully investigated by angiography in a recent trial had significant intracranial carotid artery stenosis.[32] The plaque itself can be assessed not only in

125

terms of width and length but also for ulceration, which has recently been shown to be a risk factor for stroke.[29]

Risks of angiography

Before subjecting any patient to angiography it is important to try to ensure that the benefits outweigh the risks. Studies showing that the risks of angiography are markedly increased in the hands of the inexperienced support the view that most of the complications result from trauma to the wall of the vessel and clots forming either on the vessel wall or on the catheter during the procedure. Transcranial Doppler has recently been used to show that multiple emboli pass into the middle cerebral artery during angiography.[98] We reviewed the results of eight retrospective and seven prospective trials that assessed angiographic complications in patients with mild cerebrovascular disease and concluded that the overall permanent neurological complication rate was 1% in patients with symptomatic cerebrovascular disease.[91] Since these studies were performed, new catheter designs and DSA have led to reports of much lower complication rates. Grzyska *et al* reviewed the complications of angiography in 1095 patients and established a permanent complication rate of 0·09%,[99] but these patients were not preselected by ultrasound and only 30% of the angiograms were performed for cerebrovascular disease. Waugh and Sacharias reported even better results with only 0·03% of patients having permanent neurological disability.[100] Very low complication rates of angiography in patients with symptomatic cerebrovascular disease should be regarded with suspicion. The natural history of patients with transient ischaemic attacks is a 4·4% (or higher) risk of a stroke in the first month after the presenting event.[107] This means that the expected stroke rate in these patients during the 72 hours after angiography will be at least 0·5% and if preselected by carotid ultrasound, possibly as high as 1%. The effect of screening patients with DUS has resulted in only patients with more severe degrees of atheromatous disease having angiography and thus in some other centres increasing risks of angiography have been reported. A recent prospective study found a 4% permanent neurological complication rate from angiography.[101] These complications were during a 72 hour period after angiography and some are likely to be unrelated to the procedure in these patients at risk.[102] Unfortunately there is likely to be publication bias in these studies. Centres with a high complication rate are unlikely to publish their results in a competitive market unless they are keen to abandon angiography! I suspect that the complication rate remains at around 1% in most centres with the advantages of improved technology being cancelled out by preselection of more severely diseased patients by DUS.

The neurological complications of angiography may be reduced by using intravenous DSA. Good results in some hands have been achieved with acceptable images in 80% of patients.[103 104] Inadequate contrast due to poor left ventricular function, or artefact from patient swallowing during the procedure combined with poor overall resolution of the images have, however, prevented its widespread acceptance. The reasons for this failure have been reviewed by Cebul and Paulus.[105] There has been a surprisingly high systemic complication rate reported by some authors. Turner *et al* found a 9·1% incidence of myocardial ischaemia and pulmonary oedema.[106] The improving technology of DSA has resulted in intravenous DSA achieving more acceptable, higher resolution images, and of a resurgence of interest in the technique.

Aneurysms

Angiography is the investigation of choice in acute subarachnoid haemorrhage. Routinely, we perform angiography of both carotid arteries and the dominant vertebral artery.

Three views are taken of each carotid: anteroposterior, lateral, and oblique. If no aneurysm is demonstrated then further views may be indicated with the purpose of opening out vessel loops.[108] These further views are focused by the apparent source of bleeding shown by CT. If a single vertebral artery injection does not opacify both posterior inferior cerebellar arteries, bilateral vertebral angiography is performed. Occasionally a more limited protocol is used—for example, in elderly patients in whom a posterior circulation aneurysm would be treated conservatively the vertebral angiogram may not be performed, or in patients who have large deep hemispheric bleeds in whom the purpose of angiography is to exclude an underlying vascular abnormality on the side of the bleed. In such circumstances a single carotid angiogram is often obtained.

Information on the patency of the circle of Willis can be important to the surgeon. The anterior communicating artery may need to be preserved if both anterior cerebral arteries fill from one

127

carotid artery and the other anterior cerebral artery is hypoplastic. Cross compression studies are sometimes performed to distinguish between hypoplastic and absent A1 segments.

In 75%–85% of patients with acute subarachnoid haemorrhage, an underlying aneurysm or vascular malformation will be shown. The cause of failure of initial angiography is often uncertain but may be due to thrombosis, spasm, misinterpretation of tortuous vessel loops, or a perimesencephalic bleed that may not be aneursymal in origin.[70] Repeat angiography is of debatable value with some series having only a 2% detection rate of aneurysms and Moseley has argued that the risks of repeat angiography often outweigh the benefits.[110] Our own experience is of a higher incidence of detecting aneurysms by repeating angiography. This is possibly due to a policy of performing angiography early on often uncooperative patients, but Wolpert and Caplan have reported results similar to our own, finding aneurysms in 5% of repeated studies.[111]

Because the risks of angiography in this group of patients is small,[112] we do perform repeat angiograms at four weeks or when the spasm has resolved (on transcranial Doppler) on all patients unless the quantity of blood on CT is small and restricted to the perimesencephalic cisterns, the proximal interhemispheric, or sylvian fissures. Such a distribution indicates a perimesencephalic bleed and the yield of repeat angiograms on such patients with perimesencephalic blood is low.[110]

Multiple aneurysms are present in 10%–30% of patients.[111 113] The correct management of the unruptured aneurysms is the subject of a current multicentre trial. At present our current policy is to operate on or coil unruptured aneurysms in young patients with aneurysms that are greater than 5 mm. We are currently following small aneurysms with MRA, as the available evidence suggests that rupture of these aneurysms is rare.[68]

Angiography is an integral part of the treatment of aneurysms as well as diagnosis. Aneurysms can be treated angiographically in several ways.

All methods rely on preliminary angiography to assess the anatomy of the aneurysm, in particular the size, shape, and neck size. Subsequent treatment depends on the site and size. "Berry" aneurysms found around the Circle of Willis and at the bifurcations of the main cerebral arteries can be treated by introducing platinium coils into the lumen or by balloons positioned either in the neck or within the sac of the aneurysm.[114] The most recent development is to use coils, the detachment of which can be controlled. These coils, developed by Guglielmi et al,[115] are released by passing a small current down the mandril to the coil. This causes thrombosis within the aneurysm and then releases the coil by electrolysis of the solder between the coil and its steel mandril wire (figures 4.7 and 4.8). Balloon placement within aneurysms is now less common and in many centres is restricted to parent vessel occlusion in the treatment of carotid aneurysms. Modern DSA equipment contributes significantly to the speed and safety with which these procedures can be carried out. The position of the embolic material can be rapidly assessed and any prolapse into the feeding arterial systems rectified. The road map facility enables the radiologist to visualise the arteries during superselective catheterisation and prevents the guide wires from passing through the aneurysm wall.

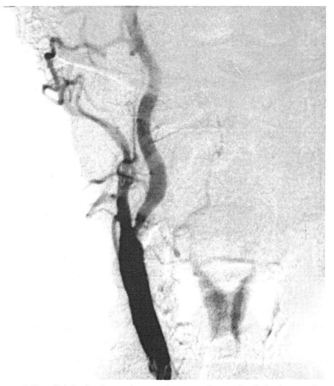

Figure 4.7   *Digital subtraction angiogram. Stenosis of the internal carotid artery; degree of stenosis depends on method of measurements*

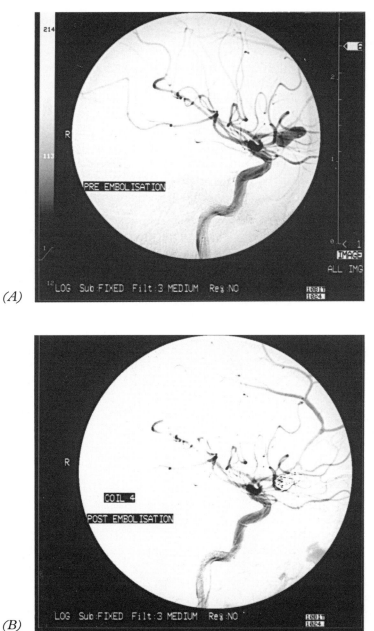

(A)

(B)

Figure 4.8   *Digital subtraction angiogram. An anterior communicating artery aneurysm is shown before (A) and after (B) coiling with platinum coils*

Arteriovenous malformations

Angiography is the only modality that demonstrates fully the vessel architecture of arteriovenous malformations. This information is essential for planning treatment, either by surgery, intra-arterial embolisation, or radiosurgery, each or all of which may have a role. The risks of surgery have been graded by Spetzler and Martin.[116] Grading depends on the location, the size of the nidus, and whether the venous drainage is to the superficial or deep veins. Pre-embolisation assessment includes identification of the number of feeders, the venous drainage, any external carotid supply, and an estimate of the rate of flow.[117] Lesions with multiple small tortuous feeders are usually difficult to embolise fully. Stereotactic radiosurgery on the other hand is most suited to lesions that are less than 3 cm, with deep lesions typically responding better than peripheral lesions. No prospective trial has yet shown the superiority of any particular treatment and this will be difficult to design because a combined approach using two of these treatments is often required. Occasionally, thrombosis of an arteriovenous malformation will cause it to be missed on angiography but the presence of methaemoglobin and haemosiderin often enable visualisation by MRI. These thrombosed malformations do not require treatment. Small arteriovenous malformations that are compressed by a large haematoma in the acute phase can also be missed if angiography is performed early. In young non-hypertensive patients or with peripherally situated haematomas we repeat angiography when the mass effect has resolved, usually after two to four weeks.

Other vascular lesions

Cranial arteritis may be restricted to the cranial circulation or may be part of a collagen vascular disease such as systemic lupus erythematosus. Rarer causes include drug misuse, particularly with amphetamines, heroin and cocaine, and radiation.[110] Arteries show evidence of narrowing and dilatation or "beading", which may be focal or widespread. Cranial arteritis involves the proximal vessels as do most of the drug induced vasculitides.

Systemic lupus erythematosus and polyarteritis attack the medium and small vessels, occasionally with the formation of small aneurysms.[118] Radiation affects the very small arteries so that often no changes are noted on angiography, although in rare cases a

131

larger vessel is involved.[119] The contraceptive pill has been reported to result in not only venous but also arterial occlusions.[111]

Fibromuscular dysplasia is best recognised on angiography.[120] The classic irregular narrowing of the carotid artery (figure 4.9) can be mimicked by pressure waves induced at the time of intraarterial contrast injection but these waves can be distinguished by their regularity. This disease, which is commoner in females, can be associated with intracranial aneurysms.

Dissection of the carotid or vertebral arteries often follows direct neck trauma. In the absence of trauma, the patients sometimes give a history of sudden neck pain. The typical appearance is of a carotid artery which tapers gradually like a "rat's tail" (figure 4.10).[121]

It is rare to see an intimal flap or false lumen except when induced by angioplasty.

Marfan's disease and Ehlers-Danlos syndrome, in which the elastic fibres of the arterial media are inherently weak, are diseases associated with dissections and caroticocavernous fistulae. These

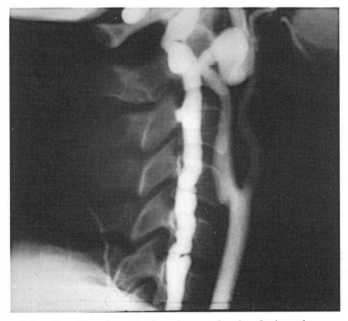

Figure 4.9 *Carotid and vertebral angiogram showing the irregular narrowing and dilatations of fibromuscular hyperplasia*

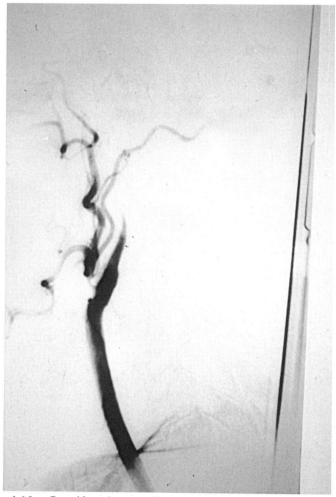

Figure 4.10   *Carotid angiogram. The internal carotid artery tapers giving a "rat's tail" appearance typical of dissection*

are difficult to treat conventionally as the arteries are often further traumatised by balloon placement.

Venography

The main indication for venography is suspected venous obstruction due either to thrombosis or tumour. Venous throm-

133

bosis can be due to otitis media or mastoiditis, pregnancy or the pill, malignancy, and trauma.

Magnetic resonance venography (MRV) has to a large extent replaced conventional venography but when not available or if the MRV result is unsatisfactory, conventional venography is still performed. Meticulous technique is again required; bilateral catheterisation of the carotid arteries with simultaneous injection is recommended by Newton and Potts,[122] but even then interpretation can be difficult. Abnormalities such as tumours adjacent to the sinuses can cause sufficient narrowing to mimic complete obstruction.

The central lumen of the vein may not opacify due to streaming of contrast along the vessel walls. Secondary features such as reversal of flow in the cortical veins and drainage into collateral pathways are useful signs to confirm the presence of obstruction.

Costs

The cost and the charge of examinations differs considerably around the world and even local costs are difficult to assess in the National Health Service (NHS) of the United Kingdom.[123] The costs of an individual examination will depend on patient throughput in a unit, over how long a period equipment is written off and replaced, salary costs, etc. Our own costs are based on using modern equipment with a moderately high throughput of patients and writing off the equipment over an eight year period. The charges to patients referred from other centres are as follows:

	Cost/ exam	Equipment	Exams/ year
Angiography	£350	GE DX Highline	1000
MR including angiography	£167	Siemens 1·5T 63SP	5000
Colour flow ultrasound	£95	Acuson XP/10 + ART	2000

In the new climate NHS these charges should approximate to costs (apart from an additional 10% administration fee). Angiography will often involve overnight hospital accommodation with a charge of £200 a night to be added to the costs. If patients can be spared angiography by using a screening test such as DUS, considerable cost savings can be made.[123]

Summary

Atherosclerotic disease

Patients with transient ischaemic attacks or a non-disabling stroke who are surgical candidates should be screened with Doppler ultrasound, or MRA/CT, or both. The choice will depend on local expertise and availability. If DUS is used it is recommended that the equipment is regularly calibrated and a prospective audit of results, particularly of those patients that go on to angiography, is maintained locally. Those patients found to have the DUS equivalent of a 50% stenosis should have angiography only if surgical or balloon angioplasty treatment is contemplated. Angiography should be performed with meticulous technique to minimise risks.

Aneurysm and arteriovenous malformations

Angiography remains the investigation of choice for patients with subarachnoid haemorrhage. Magnetic resonance angiography and CT can demonstrate the larger aneurysm but because even small aneurysms can rupture with devastating effects, these techniques are not the examination of first choice. Angiography is also the only technique that adequately defines the neck of an aneurysm.

This information is becoming increasingly important in management decisions—for instance, whether to clip or use a coil. Likewise angiography is the only technique to fully define the vascular anatomy of arteriovenous malformations although the size of the nidus can be monitored by MRA and this is a useful method of follow up after stereotactic radiosurgery, embolisation, or surgery. There are specific uses for MRA such as in patients presenting with a painful 3rd nerve palsy and as a screening test for those patients with a strong family history of aneurysms.

Vasculitis, fibromuscular hyperplasia, and dissection

These rare arterial diseases are best detected by angiography, although there are increasing reports of successful diagnosis by MRA. There are traps for the many unwary and MRA does not give an anatomical depiction of the arteries but a flow map. Slow flow may lead to signal loss and a false positive diagnosis of vasculitis.

135

Conclusion

Imaging techniques for the cerebral blood vessels develop so rapidly that it is difficult to say with confidence what the status is at any one time. The pace of new developments leads to its own problems. When has a technique improved to the point that a proper prospective randomised controlled trial is indicated? Clinical outcome should be the gold standard against which tests should be measured. But studies using clinical outcome as the endpoint, such as NASCET, take 10 years to complete and by that time the technique has been superseded. Thus clinicians must often make do with small trials that may be retrospective and use a gold standard such as angiography, which itself has many disadvantages as a test. The analysis of such data to develop a sensible local policy will always remain a challenge.

"Errors in judgement must occur in the practice of an art which consists largely in balancing probabilities"

Sir William Osler

I thank Dr J Wardlaw and Dr I Marshall for their help with the manuscript.

1 Geddes LA, Geddes LE. *The catheter introducers*. Chicago: The Mobium Press, 1993:15.
2 Todd NV, Howie JE, Miller JD. Norman Dott's contribution to aneurysm surgery. *J Neurol Neurosurg Psychiatry* 1990;**53**:455–8.
3 Eastcott HHG, Pickering GW, Robb C. Reconstruction of internal carotid artery in a patient with intermittent attacks of hemiplegia. *Lancet* 1954;ii:994–6.
4 North American Symptomatic Carotid Endarterectomy Trial Collaborators. Beneficial effect of carotid endarterectomy in symptomatic patients with high grade carotid stenosis. *N Engl J Med* 1991;**325**:445–53.
5 European Carotid Surgery Trialists Collaborative Group. MRC European Carotid Surgery Trial: interim results for symptomatic patients with severe (70–99%) or with mild (0–29%) carotid stenosis. *Lancet* 1991;**337**:1235–43.
6 Rankin RN, Fox AJ, Thorpe K, *et al* for NASCET collaborators. *Carotid ultrasound: correlation with angiography in a multicentre trial*. Presented to the American Society of Neuroradiology, St Louis: 31 May–5 June, 1992.
7 Spencer MP, Reid JM. Quantification of carotid stenosis with continuous wave Doppler ultrasound. *Stroke* 1979;**10**:226–330.
8 Polak JF. Noninvasive carotid evaluation. *Carpe Diem Radiology* 1993;**186**:329–31.
9 Rothwell PM, Gibson RT, Slattery J, Sellar RJ, Warlow CP. Equivalence of measurement in carotid stenosis. A comparison of three methods on 101 angiograms. *Stroke* 1994; **25**:2435–9.
10 Bland M, Altman DEG. Statistical methods for assessing agreement between two methods of clinical measurement. *Lancet* 1986;i:307–10.
11 Howard G, Chambless LE, Baker WH, *et al*. A multicentre validation study of Doppler ultrasound versus angiography. *J Stroke Cerebrovasc Dis* 1991;**1**:166–73.
12 Masaryk TJ, Obuchowski NA. Noninvasive carotid imaging caveat emptor. *Radiology* 1993;**186**:325–8.
13 Carroll BA. Carotid sonography. *Radiology* 1991;**178**:303–13.
14 Zweibel WJ. Duplex sonography of cerebral arteries: efficacy limitations and indications. *AJR Am J Roentgenol* 1992;**158**:29–36.
15 Huning MGM. Polak JF, Barlaw MM, O'Leary DH. Detection and quantification of carotid artery stenosis. Efficiency of various Doppler velocity parameters. *AJR Am J*

Roentgenol 1993;**160**:619–25.

16 Robinson ML, Sacks D, Perlmutter GS, Merinelli DC. Diagnostic criteria for carotid duplex—sonography. *AJR Am J Roentgenol* 1988;**151**:1045–9.

17 Roederer GO, Langlois YE, Jager KA. A simple spectral parameter for accurate classification of severe carotid disease. *Bruit* 1984;**8**:174–8.

18 Cardullo PA, Cutler BS, Brownwell-Wheeler L. Detection of carotid artery disease by duplex scanning. *J Diag Med Sanogr* 1986;**7**:63–73.

19 Goodison SF, Flanigan P, Bishara P, Schuler JJ, Kikta MJ, Meyer JP. Can duplex scanning supplant arteriography in patients with focal carotid territory symptoms? *J Vasc Surg* 1987;**5**:551–7.

20 Hartwell GG. Controversies in radiology: Doppler of the carotid artery. *Clin Radiol* 1989;**40**:177–88.

21 Zweibel WJ, Austin CW, Sackett JF, Strother CM. Correlation of high-resolution, B-mode and continuous wave Doppler sonography with arteriography in the diagnosis of carotid stenosis. *Radiology* 1983;**149**: 523–32.

22 Clark WM, Hatten HP. Non-invasive screening of extracranial carotid disease: duplex sonography with angiographic correlation. *AJNR Am J Neuroradiol* 1981;**2**:443–7.

23 Benedict PJ, Jackson WP, Becker GJ. Comparison of ultrasound scanning/Doppler with digital subtraction angiography in evaluating carotid arterial disease. *Medical Instruments* 1983;**3**:220–2.

24 Cardullo PA, Cuttler BS, Wheeler AB, Arous EJ, Hapmann JB. Accuracy of duplex sonographic scanning in the detection of carotid arterial disease. *Bruit* 1984;**8**:181–6.

25 Wetzner SM, Tutunjian J, Marich KW. Focus on duplex sonographic scanning: a vascular diagnostic technology. *American Review of Diagnostics* 1983;**1**:31–6.

26 Mittl RLJ, Broderick M, Carpenter JP, *et al*. Blinded-reader comparison of magnetic resonance angiography and duplex ultrasonography for carotid artery bifurcation stenosis. *Stroke* 1994;**25**:4–10.

27 Houston J III, Lewis BD, Weibers DO, Meyer FB, Reiderer SJ, Weaver AL. Carotid artery: prospective blinded comparison of two dimensional time of flight MR angiography with conventional angiography and duplex US. *Radiology* 1993;**186**:339–44.

28 Ackerman RH, Candia MR. Identifying clinically relevant carotid disease. *Stroke* 1994;**25**:1–3.

29 Eliasziw M, Streiflet JY, Fox AJ, Hachinski VC, Ferguson GG, Barnett JHM. Significance of plaque ulceration in symptomatic patients with high grade carotid stenosis. *Stroke* 1994;**25**:304–8.

30 O'Leary DH, Polak JF. High resolution carotid sonography; past present and future. *AJR Am J Roentgenol* 1989;**153**:699–704.

31 Zweibel WJ, Crummy AB. Sources of error in Doppler diagnosis of carotid occlusive disease. *AJR Am J Roentgenol* 1981;**2**:231–42.

32 Griffiths PD, Worthy S, Gholkar A. Incidence of vascular pathology in patients investigated for carotid stenosis. *Neuroradiology* 1995 (in press).

33 Little JR, Sawhny B, Weinstein M. Pseudo tandem lesions of the internal carotid artery. *Neurosurgery* 1980; **15**:574–77.

34 Stepetti AV, Schultz D, Feldhans RT, *et al*. Ultrasonographic features of carotid plaque and risks of subsequent neurological deficits [abstract]. *Radiology* 1989;**171**:883.

35 Wolverson MF, Bashiti HM, Peterson GJ. Ultrasonic classification of alteromatous plaques using a high resolution real time scanner. *Ultrasound Med Biol* 1983; **6**:669–709.

36 Imparto AM, Riles TS, Mintzer K, *et al*. The importance of haemorrhage in the relationship between gross morphologic characteristics and cerebral symptoms in 376 carotid artery plaques. *Ann Surg* 1983;**197**:195–8.

37 Norris JW. Does transcranial doppler have any clinical value? *Neurology* 1990;**40**:329–31.

38 Grosset PG, Georgiaris MD, Abdullah MD, Lees KR. Doppler emboli signals vary according to stroke subtype. *Stroke* 1994;**25**:382–4.

39 Wardlaw JM, Dennis MS, Lindley RI, Warlow CP, Sandercock PAG, Sellar RJ. Does early reperfusion of a cerebral infarct influence cerebral infarct swelling in the acute stage or the final clinical outcome? *Cerebrovascular Diseases* 1993;**3**:86–93.

40 Symon L. *Experimental cerebral infarction. Progress in stroke research*. Bath: Pitman Medical, 1979:79–93.

41 Crosby DC, Turski PA, Davis WC. Magnetic resonance angiography and stroke; techniques, applications and limitations. *Neuroimaging Clinics of North America* 1992;**2**: 509–31.

42 Wedeen V, Meuci R, Edelman RR, et al. Projective imaging of pulsatile flow with magnetic resonance. Science 1985;230:946–8.
43 Haase A, Frahm J, Matthaei D, Hanicke W, Merbolt KD. FLASH imaging: rapid NMR imaging using low flip angle pulses. J Magn Reson Imaging 1986;67:256–66.
44 Dumoulin C, Souza S, Walker M, Wagle W. Three-dimensional phase contrast angiography. Magn Reson Med 1989;9:139–49.
45 Edelman RR, Mattle HP, Wallner B, et al. Extracranial arteries; evaluation with "black blood" MR angiography. Radiology 1990;177:45–50.
46 Edelman RR. MR angiography: present and future. AJR Am J Roentgenol 1993;161:1–11.
47 Baker MC, Kucharczyk J, Sevick RJ, Mintorovitch J, Moseley ME. Recent advances in the MR imaging/spectroscopy of cerebral ischemia. AJR Am J Roentgenol 1991;156: 1133–44.
48 Wolff SC, Balaban RS. Magnetisation transfer contrast (MTC) and tissue water proton relaxation in vivo. Magn Reson Med 1988;10:135–44.
49 Edelman RR, Ahn S, Chien D, et al. Improved time of flight MR angiography of the brain using magnetisation transfer contrast. Radiology 1992;184:395–9.
50 Saloner D, Salby K, Anderson CM. MRA Studies of arterial stenosis. Improvements by diastolic acquisition. Magn Reson Med 1994;31:196–203.
51 Edelman RR, Mattle HP, Kleefield J, Silver MS. Quantification of blood flow with dynamic MR imaging and presaturation bolus tracking. Radiology 1989;171:551–6.
52 Edelman RR, Mattle HP, O'Reilly GV, Wentz KV, Liv C, Zhao B. Magnetic resonance imaging of flow dynamics of the circle of Willis. Stroke 1990;21:56–65.
53 Lasster RE Jnr, Acker JD, Halford HH, II, Nauert TC. Assessment of MR angiography versus arteriography for evaluation of cervical carotid bifuracation disease. AJNR Am J Neuroradiol 1993;14:681–8.
54 Masaryk AM, Ross JS, DiCello MC, Modic MT, Paranadi L, Masaryk TJ. 3DFT MR angiography of the carotid bifurcation. Potential and limitations as a screening examination. Radiology 1991;179:797–804.
55 Lewin JS, Laub G. Intracranial MR angiography: a direct comparison of 3 time of flight techniques. AJNR Am J Neuroradiol 1991;12:1133–9.
56 Keller PJ, Drayer BP, Fram EK, Williams KD, Dimoulin CC, Souza SR. MR angiography with two-dimensional acquisition and three dimensional display. Radiology 1989;173:527–32.
57 Anderson CM, Saloner D. Leere, et al. Assessment of carotid artery stenosis by MR angiography; comparison with X-ray angiography and colour-coded Doppler ultra-sound. AJNR Am J Neuroradiol 1992;13: 989–1003.
58 Mattle HP, Kent KC, Edelman RR, Atkinson DJ, Skillman JJ. Evaluation of the extracranial carotid: correlation of magnetic resonance angiography, duplex ultra sonography and conventional angiography. J Vasc Surg 1991;13:838–45.
59 Polak JF, Bajakian RC, O'Leary DH, Anderson MR, Donaldson MC, Jolesz FA. Detection of internal carotid stenosis: comparison of MR angiography, colour Doppler sonography and arteriography. Radiology 1992;182:35–40.
60 Heirserman JE, Draper BP, Fram EK, et al. Carotid artery stenosis: clinical efficacy of two dimensional time of flight MR angiography. Radiology 1992;182:761–8.
61 Marks MP, Napel S, Jordan TE, Enzmann DR. Diagnosis of carotid artery disease: preliminary experience with maximum-intensity projection spiral CT angiography. AJR Am J Roentgenol 1993;160:1267–71.
62 Laub G. Displays for MR angiography. Magn Reson Med 1990;14:222–9.
63 Anderson CM, Saloner D, Tsuruda JA, Shapeero LG, Lee RE. Artifacts in maximum-intensity projection display of MR angiograms. AJR Am J Roentgenol 1990;154:623–9.
64 Yousem DM, Balakrishnan, Debrun GM, Bryan RN. Hyperintense thrombus on GRASS MR images: potential pitfall in flow evaluation. AJNR Am J Neuroradiol 1990;11:51–8.
65 Podolak MJ, Hedlund LW, Evans AJ, Herfkens RJ. Evaluation of flow through simulated vascular stenosis with gradient echo magnetic resonance imaging. Invest Radiol 1989;24:184–9.
66 Sitzer M, Furst G, Fischer H, Siebler M, Fehlings T, Kleinschmidt A, et al. Between-method correlation in quantifying internal carotid stenosis. Stroke 1993;24:1513–8.
67 Ross JS, Masaryk TJ, Modic MT, Ruggier PM, Haacke EM, Selman WK. Intra cranial aneurysms: evaluation by MR angiography. AJR Am J Roentgenol 1990;155: 159–65.
68 Wiebers DO, Whisnant JP, Sundt TM, O'Fallon WM. The significance of unruptured intracranial saccular aneursysms. J Neurosurg 1987;66:23–9.

69 Weir B. *Aneurysms affecting the nervous system*. Baltimore: Williams and Williams, 1987: 303–63.
70 Curness T, Shogry ME, Clark DC, Elsner JH. MR Angiographic demonstration of intracranial aneurysm not seen on conventional angiography. *AJNR Am J Neuroradiol* 1993;14:974–7.
71 Teasdale E, Statham P, Straiton J, Macpherson P. Non-invasive radiological investigation for oculo motor palsy. *J Neurol Neurosurg Psychiatry* 1990;53: 549–53.
72 Potchen ET, Haacke EM, Siebert JE, Cottschalk A. *Magnetic resonance angiography: concepts and applications*. St Louis: Mosby, 1993:394.
73 Houston J, III, Rufenacht DA, Ehman RL, Weibers DO. Intracranial aneurysms and vascular malformations: comparison of time of flight and phase contrast MR angiography. *Radiology* 1991;181:721–30.
74 Marchal G, Bosmans H, Van Fraeyenhoven L, *et al.* Intracranial vascular lesions: optimation and clinical evaluation of three-dimensional time of flight angiography. *Radiology* 1990;175:443–8.
75 Greenan TJ, Grossman RI, Goldberg HI. Cerebral vasculitis: MR imaging and angiographic correlation. *Radiology* 1992;182:65–72.
76 Goldbert HI, Grossman RI, Comori JM, Ashburh AK, Bilaniuk LT, Zimmerman KA. Cervical internal carotid artery dissecting haemorrhage: diagnosis using MR. *Radiology* 1986;158:157–61.
77 Quint D, Spickler E. Magnetic resonance demonstration of vertebral artery dissection; report of two cases. *J Neurosurg* 1990;72:964–7.
78 Heiserman JE, Drayer BP, Fram EK, Keller PJ. MR angiography of cervical fibromuscular hyperplasia. *AJNR Am J Neuroradiol* 1992;13:1454–7.
79 Blatter DD, Parker DC, Robinson RO. Cerebral MR angiography with multiple overlapping thin slab acquisition: Part II Early clinical experience. *Radiology* 1992; **183**:379–89.
80 Perlmutter JS. New techniques in neuroimaging: When are pretty pictures useful? *Current Opinion in Neurology* 1993;6:889–90.
81 Rippe DJ, Boyko OB, Spritzer LE, *et al.* Demonstration of dural sinus occlusion by use of MR angiography. *AJNR Am J Neuroradiol* 1990;11:199–201.
82 Mattle HP, Wentz KV, Edelman RR, Wallner B, Finn JP, Barnes P, *et al.* Cerebral venography with MR. *Radiology* 1991; **178**:453–8.
83 Isewsee CH, Reul J, Throw A. Magnetic resonance imaging of thrombosed dural sinuses. *Stroke* 1994;**25**:29–34.
84 Padayachee TS, Bingham JB, Craves MT, Colchester AC, Cox TC. Dural sinus thrombosis: diagnosis and follow up by magnetic angiography and imaging. *Neuroradiology* 1991;33:165–7.
85 Creasy JL, Price RR, Presbery T, Goins D, Partain CL, Kessler RM. Gadolinium enhanced MR angiography. *Radiology* 1990;175:280–3.
86 Polak JF, Kalina P, Donaldson MC, O'Leary DH, Whittemore AD, Mannick JA. Carotid endarterectomy: pre-operative evaluation of candidates with combined Doppler sonography and MR angiography. Work in progress. *Radiology* 1993;186:333–8.
87 Young GR, Humphrey PRD, Shaw MDM, Nixon TE, Smith ETS. Comparison of magnetic resonance angiography, duplex ultrasound, and digital subtraction angiography in assessment of extracranial internal carotid artery stenosis. *J Neurol Neurosurg Psychiatry* 1995;57:1466–78.
88 Schwartz RB, Towes KM, Chernoff DM, *et al.* Common carotid bifurcation: evaluation with spiral CT. *Radiology* 1992;185:513–9.
89 Kallender WA, Polakin A. Physical performance characteristics of spiral CT scanning. *Med Phys* 1991;18:910–5.
90 Seldinger SI. Catheter replacement of the needle in percutaneous arteriography. *Acta Radiol* 1953;39:368–76.
91 Hankey GT, Warlow CP, Sellar RJ. Cerebral angiographic risk in mild cerebro-vascular disease. *Stroke* 1990;21:209-22.
92 Jeans WD, Mackenzie S, Baird RN. Angiography in transient cerebral ischaemia using three views of the carotid bifurcation. *Br J Radiol* 1986;59:135–42.
93 Chikos PM, Fisher CD, Hirsch JH, Harley TD, Thiele BC, Strandness DE Jr. Observer variability in evaluating extra cranial carotid artery stenosis. *Stroke* 1983;14:885–92.
94 Goldstein ST, Fried AM, Young B, Tibbs PA. Limited usefulness of aortic arch angiography in the evaluation of carotid occlusive disease. *AJR Am J Roentgenol* 1982;**138**: 103–8.

95 Moseley I. *Diagnostic imaging in neurological disease*. Edinburgh: Churchill Livingston, 1986:125.
96 Schuler TJ, Flanigan P, Lim CT, Keifer T, Williams LR, Behrend AJ. The affect of carotid syphon stenosis on stroke rate death and relief of symptoms following elective carotid endorterectomy. *Surgery* 1982;**92**:1058–67.
97 Mastos MA, Van Bemmelen PS, Hodgson KJ, Berkmeter CD, Ramsay DE, Sumner DS. The influence of carotid siphon stenosis on short and long term outcome after carotid endartectomy: fact or fiction [abstract]. *J Vasc Surg* 1992;**16**:475.
98 Markus H. Transcranial Doppler detection of circulating cerebral emboli. *Stroke* 1993;**24**:1246–50.
99 Grzyska V, Freitag J, Zeumer H. Selective cerebral inter-arterial DSA. Complication rate and control of risk factors. *Neuroradiology* 1990;**32**:296–9.
100 Waugh JR, Sacharias N. Arteriographic complications in the DSA era. *Radiology* 1992;**182**:293–246.
101 Davies KN, Humphrey PR. Complications of cerebral angiography in patients with symptomatic carotid territory ischaemia. *J Neurol Neurosurg Psychiatry* 1993;**56**:967–72.
102 Baum S, Stein G, Kuroda KK. Complications of 'no arteriography'. *Radiology* 1966;**86**:835–8.
103 Wood GW, Lukin RR, Tomsick TA, Chambers AA. Digital subtraction angiography with intravenous injection; assessment of 1000 carotid bifurcations. *AJR Am J Roentgenol* 1983;**140**:855–9.
104 Ducos de Lahitte M, Marc-Vergnes JP, Rascol A, Guiraud B, Manelfe C. Intravenous angiography of the extracranial cerebral arteries. *Radiology* 1980;**137**:705–11.
105 Cebul RD, Paulus RA. The failure of intravenous digital subtraction angiography in replacing carotid angiography. *Ann Intern Med* 1986;**104**:572–4.
106 Turner WH, Murie JA. Intravenous digital subtraction angiography for extra cranial carotid artery disease. *Br J Surg* 1989;**76**:1247–50.
107 Hankey GJ, Warlow CP. *Transient ischaemic attacks of the brain and eye*. London: WB Saunders, 1994:269.
108 Kricheff I. Angiographic investigation of cerebral aneurysms. *Neuroradiology* 1972;**105**:72–5.
109 Forster DMC, Steiner L, Hakanson S, Bergvall U. The value of repeat pan angiography in cases of unexplained subarachnoid haemorrhage. *J Neurosurg* 1978;**48**:712–6.
110 Moseley I. *Diagnostic imaging in neurological disease*. Edinburgh: Churchill Livingstone, 1986:104.
111 Wolpert SM, Caplan LR. Current role of cerebral angiography in the diagnosis of cerebrovascular disease. *AJR Am J Roentgenol* 1992;**159**:191–7.
112 Heiserman JE, Dean BC, Hodak JA, *et al*. Neurologic complications of cerebral angiography. *AJNR Am J Neuroradiol* 1994;**15**:1401–7.
113 Maurice William RS. *Subarachnoid haemorrhage*. Bristol: Wright; 1987:135.
114 Higashida R, Halback V, Hieshena GB, *Endovascular therapy of aneurysms. Interventional neuroradiology*. New York: Raven Press, 1992:51–72.
115 Guglielmi G, Vinveza F, Sepetka I, *et al*, Electrothrombosis of saccular aneurysms via endo vascular approach Part 1: electrochemical basis, technique, and experimental results. *J Neurosurg* 1991;**75**:1–7.
116 Spetzler RF, Martin NA. A proposed grading system for arteriovenous malformation. *J Neurosurg* 1986;**65**:476–89.
117 Berenstein A, Lasjaunias P. *Surgical neuro angiography. 4. Endovascular treatment of cerebral lesions*. Berlin: Springer Verlag, 1992:27;25–80.
118 Burrows EH, Leeds NE. *Vascular abnormalities in neuroradiology*. New York: Churchill Livingstone 1981:75–117.
119 Brandt-Zawadzki M, Anderson M, De Armour SJ, *et al*. Radiation-induced large intra cranial vessel occlusive vasculopathy. *AJR Am J Roentgenol* 1980;**134**:51–5.
120 Newton TH, Potts DF. *Radiology of the skull and brain angiography*. Saint Louis; CV Mosby 1974, P 1707.
121 Anson J, Crowell RM. Cerviocranial arterial dissection. *Neurosurgery* 1991;**29**:89–96.
122 Newton TH, Potts DF. *Radiology of the skull and brain angiography*. St Louis: CV Mosby, 1974:939–45.
123 Hankey GJ, Warlow CP. Cost effective investigation of patients with suspected transient ischaemic attacks. *J Neurol Neurosurg Psychiatry* 1992;**55**:171–6.

5 Imaging of the spinal cord

JOHN M STEVENS

Methods of investigation

Historical perspective

Air myelography

The first contrast medium used to show the spinal cord was air. The first reports of its use to localise intraspinal tumours came from Jacobeus in 1921 and Dandy in 1925.[1] The technique was later refined to show the entire spinal canal; this involved complete replacement of the CSF by air and distension of the spinal subarachnoid space.[2] Adequate visualisation of the spinal cord usually required tomography. Spinal roots were not shown, and many types of pathology such as vascular malformations or arachnoiditis were either not shown or easily misinterpreted. However, despite the fact that the technique was difficult to achieve and very hard on the patient, it remained the preferred method for visualising the spinal cord in many centres until the advent of non-toxic water soluble contrast only just over 10 years ago.

Oil myelopathy

At the time that air myelography was being developed, it was found accidentally that iodised oils could be moved through the spinal subarachnoid space under the influence of gravity. They proved easier to use than air, and quickly established oil myelography as the technique of choice especially in the lumbar spinal canal. It received even greater impetus from the appearance in 1940, of iophendylate (Myodil; Pantopaque), a preparation that

141

was less viscous than the earlier Lipiodol and better for demonstrating the spinal cord. Myodil was very opaque to x rays and special techniques such as tomography were not required. It was very slowly absorbed and could be left in the canal and rerun postoperatively to check the adequacy of decompression. Its main disadvantage was its immiscibility with CSF; it tended to break up into globules, forming a layer in the spinal canal, which made it difficult to demonstrate both anterior and posterior surfaces of the spinal cord unless large amounts were used. For nearly 40 years, Myodil was generally the agent of choice, with air being reserved for special situations, such as spinal dysraphism and syringomyelia. As late as 1989, eminent names in spinal surgery were still declaring their preference for Myodil, mainly because of experiences with non-diagnostic water soluble myelograms in which the contrast medium had become too dilute. Myodil is now no longer manufactured, and existing stocks have been withdrawn because of the frequency with which it caused chronic adhesive arachnoiditis.[3 4]

Water soluble myelography

The advantages of water soluble over oily contrast media were established by use of a substance called Abrodil in Scandinavian countries, which provided superior images of the cauda equina and root sheaths. Other ionic water soluble media such as Conray and Dimer-X enjoyed limited use, but all were too toxic to use other than to show the lower lumbar thecal sac, and therefore are irrelevant to the present review. However, a revolution in myelography occurred when the new non-ionic water soluble medium metrizamide (Amipaque) appeared. This was far less neurotoxic than previous ones. It could be used safely around the spinal cord. However, inadvertent deposition in the head when running the contrast medium into the cervical region often caused generalised seizures, a risk minimised by introducing it by lateral C1–2 puncture.[5]

By 1983, similar and even less toxic media had been developed and metrizamide was quickly withdrawn. These agents, such as iohexol, do not cause arachnoiditis in the concentrations used in clinical practice, and by 1989, Skalpe and Sortland were able to state that "Epileptic seizures have not been reported following myelography with Omnipaque [iohexol], so it seems that fear of this complication can be virtually disregarded."[6]

These media are still not perfect: most patients experience post-myelography headache, and about 5% become confused or develop symptoms such as radicular pain or meningism.[7] Further agents have been developed, but clinical trials now are difficult to mount because myelography is so little used. Iohexol should be injected by lumbar puncture wherever possible to reduce the risk of injury to the spinal cord or vertebral artery in lateral cervical puncture.[8] Myelography may cause neurological deterioration due to: *the spinal puncture*, causing injury to the spinal cord or intraspinal bleeding; *the disease*, resulting in increased cord compression during the positioning required for radiography; *the procedure*, causing raised intraspinal pressure below a subarachnoid block.[7 8]

x Ray computed tomography (CT) of the spine

Soon after its introduction for cranial imaging CT was used in the spine. It provided the valuable cross sectional perspective of the spinal canal, formerly very difficult to achieve with conventional radiography. Artefacts caused by bone degrade intraspinal contrast in spinal CT. *Intravenous* contrast media increase contrast between extradural tissues and CSF, and *intrathecal* contrast media provide excellent visualisation of the spinal cord and other intradural structures. Patients requiring myelography usually are booked for CT as well, the findings on the myelogram or the clinical features serving to direct the CT examinations to specific levels. Computed tomography is almost exclusively a cross sectional technique; sagittal and coronal projections require reformatting from stacks of axial slices, and resolution in reformatted planes is not as good as in the plane of data acquisition. Radiation dose can be very considerable, and new guidelines for the use of CT in Britain have been published recently.[9]

Magnetic resonance imaging (MRI)

During the period when myelography was being greatly improved, MRI appeared, and within just a few years myelography was pushed almost into obsolescence. With modern high resolution MRI, almost all intradural features demonstrable by myelography can be shown, usually better, by MRI. Myelography is now indicated only when satisfactory MRI cannot be obtained because it is contraindicated (pacemakers, mechanical heart

143

valves, aneurysm clips); it cannot be done (claustrophobia and anaesthesia refused or unsafe, patient cannot fit into the magnet due to obesity, scoliosis, or limb contractures); or it is not available quickly enough, due to lack of on call service or other logistical problems.

Several recent developments have had a special impact on MRI of the spinal cord.

Volumetric (3-D) acquisitions

The deployment of fast image techniques has permitted three dimensional spatial encoding within a few minutes. This results in multiple contiguous images, no interslice gaps, and section thicknesses down to 1 or 2 mm. However, the best images of the spinal cord structure are still usually obtained from thicker slices. The best results from volumetric MRI acquisitions are usually obtained on high-field machines.

Fast spin echo (FSE)

Several phase encoding steps are made at each excitation instead of just one, which greatly reduces acquisition times, and permits use of much larger matrices. This results in twice the resolution in even shorter data acquisition periods. The penalty is slight loss of contrast and increased sensitivity to physiological motion, for which it is more difficult to compensate than when single phase encoding steps are used.

Phased array coils

Spinal imaging requires surface coils, and the phased array configuration enables data to be acquired simultaneously from two or even more surface coils. This permits imaging of the entire spinal cord over one acquisition period and greatly reduces imaging time. Vertebral level counting, sometimes difficult or impossible from single coils, especially in the thoracic region, also becomes easy.

A wide variety of postprocessing options are available on most imagers, or can be purchased separately. These permit multiplanar reformatting in real time, three dimensional surface rendering, colour coding, and many other modifications. The ability to reconstruct in a curved plane is potentially useful in scoliosis, but we have found this of only limited value because most major curvatures are in more than one plane.

Artefacts

These are important to consider because they can closely simulate intraspinal disease. *Phase dispersion* across the image, due to magnetic susceptibility variation and chemical shift effects, reduces sensitivity to biological signal differences, and reduces boundary definition. The *truncation artefact*, generated at boundaries by image processing, is particularly significant at the CSF-spinal cord interface, and is one possible cause of the band of high or low signal seen in the centre of the cord in midsagittal images. It also causes difficulty in defining the position of the cord-CSF boundary where the problem is compounded by susceptibility effects. Phantom studies have shown that both electronic and caliper measurements of the spinal cord, especially in the phase-encoding direction, can be artificially reduced by over 2 mm and may create a spurious impression of spinal cord flattening.[10]

Motion artefacts

Motion artefacts are generated by cardiosynchronous and oscillatory motion of CSF. This motion has been documented and roughly quantified by MRI. At C2/3, movement is estimated at about 0·65 ml per cardiac cycle, downwards on systole and upwards on diastole.[11] New data confirm older work indicating that the primary driving force behind intracranial and spinal canal CSF flow is expansion of the brain during vascular systole. The spinal cord and brain stem also descend very slightly on systole and oscillate anteroposteriorly with CSF flow.[12] In classic studies, Rubin *et al*[13] showed how the oscillatory motions generate linear artefacts parallel to the cord-CSF interface at roughly harmonic intervals across the images in the phase encoding direction, producing signal variation in the spinal cord image which could be easily misinterpreted as intramedullary pathology.[12] Areas of turbulent CSF flow in regions where subarachnoid septa exist, particularly in the thoracic spine, can result in signal variations simulating intradural masses or enlarged vessels. Many strategies have been developed to minimise these problems, but results can be less consistent than is desirable.

The thoracic cord in particular is difficult to image well, especially in cross section, where cardiac motion and the proximity of the aorta add to the motion generated artefacts.

145

Metallic artefacts

Metallic artefacts can be particularly destructive of image quality. Many spinal operations utilise metal stabilisation devices, such as plates, rods, screws, and loops, and patients often require postoperative imaging at some stage. Ferromagnetic substances such as stainless steel generate major local artefacts and usually render spinal imaging useless. Tiny fragments from drills and punches, invisible on plain radiographs, may also result in devastating artefacts.[14][15] Design of implants can also be important such as the avoidance of conductive loops.[16] Using titanium for manufacture may have advantages.[17] A wide range of titanium devices has become available only recently, however, and the long term stability and biological effects of these new materials remain under evaluation.[18]

Special techniques

New methods of brain imaging are usually eventually applied to the spine. Many are being evaluated and only some will be given passing reference here.

Phase contrast imaging utilises bipolar phase encoding gradients; the first brings all spins into phase, the second records reduced signal from moving spins as they dephase relative to stationary spins, due to their motion. This can be used to demonstrate molecular diffusion. One method displays apparent diffusion coefficients across the image and fluid filled cavities appear much brighter than solid areas.[19] Phase contrast imaging can also be used to demonstrate coherent CSF flow and movement of the neural axis. *Phase contrast cine MR* produces images that represent velocity as a function of time throughout the cardiac cycle, and by the direction of the phase shift indicate flow direction.[20] *Spatial modulation* of *magnetism* (SPAMM), also referred to as *presaturation bolus tracking,* is a method whereby regions are tagged by applying a narrow band of saturation before the pulse sequence. This produces a dark stripe across the image which bends in the direction of movement. Multiple presaturation bands can be used to produce a "zebra stripe" pattern, and coupling with a cine loop increases sensitivity in detecting minimal movement.[21] This has been used extensively to study syringomyelia. *Susceptibility contrast weighted dynamic MRI* has been used to study blood flow in spinal tumours and arteriovenous malformations.[22][23] A susceptibility weighted dynamic gradient recalled echo sequence is used to

146

detect the large, transient signal reduction that occurs on the first pass of a bolus dose of intravenous gadolinium through the lesion. *Fluid attenuated inversion recovery (FLAIR)* sequences are said to offer improved lesion detectability by permitting heavily T2 weighted acquisition to be accomplished with suppression of all signal from CSF. This removes motion artefact from CSF, which appears paradoxically as signal void on heavily T2 weighted images. However, cysts and cystic lesions within the cord also appear as signal void. Most other pathology appears as hyperintensity. At present, imaging with FLAIR is slow and of low resolution,[24] and like most of the functional imaging methods listed, it has found little general clinical application to the present.

Spinal sonography

Intraoperative spinal sonography has been used widely in some centres. A minimum of a two or three level laminectomy wound is required, filled with water or saline to act as an acoustic window.[25][26] Although considerable utility has been achieved,[25] experience has shown that it may not distinguish tumour from cord tissue, may incorrectly identify cysts as solid masses due to unusual echogenicity of some cyst fluids, and cannot reliably distinguish tumorous from non-tumorous cysts.[26] Surprisingly large transverse excursion of the spinal cord and roots is observed normally, lagging slightly behind the cardiac cycle, and breathing and the Valsalva manoeuvre produce additional abrupt movement. *Percutaneous spinal sonography* is possible in infants.[27][28] The spinal canal can also be imaged in adults by angling the probe parallel to an intervertebral disc space. *Transoesophageal* transducers have been used with some success to image the thoracic cord, but clinical utility is virtually non-existent with the availability of MRI. *Transuterine sonography* has been used to identify dysraphic states in the fetus,[29] but MRI may also be employed for this purpose.

Plain radiographs of the spine

Plain films have little part to play in the investigation of spinal cord disease. Inferences can be made about possible sites of spinal cord compression in conditions such as spondylotic myelopathy and trauma, and they may suggest the site and type of cord involvement in dysraphic states. The role of plain films in the preliminary investigation of patients with intraspinal lesions was reviewed by Naidich *et al* as late as 1986.[30] The spinal canal is usually enlarged in children with intramedullary tumours. Greatest sensitivity is achieved by graphing the interpediculate distances and comparing them with normal values, but even then the false positive rate is at least 11%. Therefore, plain radiographs have only a very limited screening value even in children.

Spinal angiography

The technique of spinal angiography was developed over 30 years ago by Djindjian and Doppman. Today it is indicated only for localisation of the major radiculomedullary arteries before operations on the spine, or to study vascular malformations associated with arteriovenous shunts, and before endovascular treatment of various spinal lesions. To demonstrate all the spinal cord arteries, selective injections into the intercostal, lumbar, lumbosacral, vertebral, deep, and ascending cervical arteries is required. Searches for dural fistulae may also require selective injections into branches of the external carotid artery. General anaesthesia is desirable although not essential. Moderate, usually transient, neurological deterioration occurs not uncommonly after extensive spinal angiography,[31] but paraplegia is rare.[32] Thus spinal angiography can be a very laborious undertaking; short cuts have been devised using other imaging modalities and these will be discussed with vascular malformations.

Imaging methods in present use in modern units

● Spinal MRI	By far the most efficacious and utilitarian
● Myelography and CT (computed myelography)	For use mainly when spinal MRI is not available, contraindicated, or unsatisfactory
● Spinal angiography	In specific conditions
● Spinal sonography	In very limited situations
● Plain x ray films	Mainly to evaluate subluxation and fractures

Shape, internal structure, and biomechanics of the spinal cord

Size and shape

Spondylotic flattening of the formalin fixed spinal cord is commonly found at necropsy, and was often considered to be a fixation artefact. Modern imaging has made it abundantly clear that this is not so. Good qualitative agreement is found between the appearance of the spinal cord on cross sectional imaging in living subjects and formalin fixed cords at necropsy,[33 34] but clinical measurement is problematic. The most robust measure of *size* is cross sectional area. Area measurements could theoretically be accurate within about ±5%,[35] but on clinical images it is clear that nothing like this is actually achieved. Electronic window settings profoundly influence all measurements of the cord on computed myelography[36] and on MRI many other factors are also involved. This is shown by the mean values derived by various workers for their control populations. To give three examples: mean normal cord cross sectional areas at C2 (where spondylosis is not expected) of 62 mm²,[37] 86·6 mm²,[35] and 110 mm²[2 38] have been reported. Close correlations between area measurements made by computed myelography and MRI were reported by Fukushima *et al* ($r = 0·901$)[34]; but the mean values were very different—namely, 0·38 (SD 0·14) cm² on computed myelography and 0·50 (SD 0·16) cm² on MRI. Yu and his colleagues concluded that each department needed to define its own normal range.[39] It is hardly surprising that no workers have shown a stable relation between cord size, patient age, or body size. Few measurements have been published for the thoracic cord, but we can console ourselves that medical science is not too much the poorer for that.

Two simple measurements of cord shape have been used: circularity (4π area/circumference²),[35] and the compression ratio (ratio of the anteroposterior to transverse diameters)[35 40 41] Abnormal shapes have also been classified qualitatively in specific types of cord compression, especially cervical spondylosis and its variants, the most comprehensive being by Yu *et al.*[39]

Internal structure

The internal structure of the spinal cord on MRI seems remarkably similar to an anatomical preparation stained with myelin. More myelinated regions generally yield a lower signal than less

149

myelinated ones. Magnetic resonance imaging has consistently shown variations in texture in histologically uniform regions, such as the anterior horns in the sacral area, Clarke's column, and the dorsal horn complex; the gracile fascicles yield a slightly higher signal than the cuneate.[42 43] In some types of image, the subpial zone has yielded a high signal,[44] and it is uncertain if this represents an MR artefact or the narrow band of subpial degeneration commonly seen in the cords of aging subjects. It is notable that some authors have forgotten the T1 shortening that occurs with formalin fixation, making it difficult to obtain images with T1 weighted contrast.

Biomechanical properties

Deformation of the cord by transverse compression of up to about 20% requires minimal force, whereas deformation in excess of 50% requires forces exceeding capillary perfusion pressure and begins to disrupt both transverse and longitudinal axons.[45 46] Moreover, spinal cord substance has only a limited capacity for elastic recoil. It has been shown by measurements of cord deformation between flexion and extension on computed myelograms that only about 20% of a deformation recovers elastically.[47] This has an important implication for interpreting CT and MRI images, which are generally performed in positions where the available space for the spinal cord is maximised. Because of its lack of elasticity, it is safe to conclude that if the spinal cord is normal in cross sectional shape, it is not being significantly compressed in any situation occurring in the patient during normal daily activities; and when deformity is present, it is safe to conclude that the deformity shown reasonably represents the magnitude of intermittent compression. We developed the simple concept of congruous cord deformity, to help distinguish deformation due to intermittent compression from that due to atrophy. When the available subarachnoid space appears capacious on cross sectional images, compression is suggested, nevertheless, if the deformity of the spinal cord is reciprocally congruous with the visible (disc/osteophyte), or expected (reducible subluxation) deformity of the spinal canal; in cord atrophy the deformation is incongruous.[48]

The compressed spinal cord usually increases in size after operative decompression. Fukushima et al[34] measured a mean postoperative increase in size of the compressed spinal cord of 13%, varying between 5% and 20% in different patient subgroups, which is of the order expected from cord elasticity studies. The cord also often changes shape after decompression, becoming less flattened or altered in some other way, because it is very easily deformed by varying conditions.

Cord motion

The cord lies about 2 mm more posteriorly in the supine than in the prone position, and the cord and vertebral midlines differ by up to 2 mm in over 40% of non-scoliotic subjects.[49]

On phase contrast MRI the range of normal cardiosynchronous oscillatory longitudinal movement of the upper cord has been measured to be only 0·4–0·5 mm.[12] Initial studies caused excitement because they suggested that assessment of tethering could be made without objective influence of morphological appearances. Reduced oscillatory motion has been seen in the presence of cord tethering, and increased oscillatory motion in Chiari associated syringomyelia.[21] However, the actual relevance of any of these findings in the absence of morphological changes, such as a low lying conus medullaris, has, in my opinion, yet to be demonstrated.

Pathological states in cord substance

Necrosis

Water soluble contrast medium in the subarachnoid space diffuses freely into neural tissue, and x ray attenuation of spinal cord substance measured on CT equilibrates dynamically at about 20% of that in the subarachnoid space, being removed by the capillary-venous system.[50] When necrosis occurs, hydrophobic lipid is broken down and the capillary bed destroyed. Contrast medium continues to accumulate in the necrotic region until the CSF concentration falls, and passive diffusion out of the area takes several hours. Necrotic areas thus appear as circumscribed areas of contrast enhancement on computed myelograms, often most conspicuous after six to 12 hours.[51]

On MRI, colliquative necrosis appears as a circumscribed area of signal change. Necrosis, from whatever cause, most often involves mainly the central parts of the spinal cord, in particular the grey matter and ventral parts of the posterior columns. Involvement is usually bilateral, producing either a localised con-

151

fluent lesion or, more often, bilateral lesions resulting in an appearance likened to snakes' eyes on cross sectional images.[52]

Wallerian degeneneration

Antegrade degeneration in the long tracts of the spinal cord is seen with pathological states that cause axonal damage. Typically it appears as descending degeneration in the anterior part of the lateral column and ascending degeneration in the posterior columns, which, in diseases of the cervical spine, is often most severe in the fasciculus cuneatus.[33 41 44 53]

Wallerian degeneration is shown only by MRI. Its appearances have been studied mostly in the brain stem, and only recently in the spinal cord. Four stages are distinguishable on imaging, which evolve over about 14 weeks.[54] For up to four weeks, MRI is normal and the chronic stage, characterised by volume loss and increased MR signal, persists indefinitely. Enhancement with intravenous contrast agents does not occur at any stage. In the spinal cord only the chronic stage has been described,[44 55] but recent experimental studies with magnetisation transfer imaging have demonstrated abnormalities in the earliest stage.[56]

Cystic degeneration and syringomyelia

Syringomyelia may result from any pathological process that is liable to cause spinal cord necrosis. It represents an end stage which itself may be progressive and promote further cord damage. The cavities are usually located dorsal to the central canal, with which they may or may not communicate. They may be single or multiple. Only about 15% extend beyond C2, and those that do so usually bifurcate around the decussations in the medulla oblongata and come to lie ventral to the floor of the fourth ventricle. Hydromyelia is a cavity consisting mainly of a dilated central canal and communicating with the fourth ventricle. It is closely associated with hydrocephalus, and is collapsed by ventricular shunting.[57]

Chiari I associated syringomyelia

In the currently most widely accepted hydromechanical theory of causation, this begins as a hydromyelia which subsequently loses communication with the fourth ventricle early in life, resulting in the condition often being referred to as syringohydromyelia.

Obstruction of the foramen magnum or the outlets of the fourth ventricle by the descended cerebellar tonsils is central to most hydromechanical theories. In support, phase contrast cine MRI has demonstrated absence of CSF in the cisterna magna due to the abnormal cerebellar tonsils, and restoration of CSF flow after foramen magnum decompression, accompanied by collapse of the syrinx. Also, two groups have recently separately reported a new observation on dynamic MRI: accentuated caudal displacement of the cerebellar tonsils and spinal cord with cardiac systole, which was restored to the normal range, or obliterated altogether, by decompression of the foramen magnum.[21 58] Oldfield et al[58] proposed intermittent piston like obstruction of the foramen magnum by the tonsils.

Although these mechanisms may operate in patients in whom the cerebellar tonsils do obstruct the foramen magnum, other workers have shown that the foramen magnum is not obstructed by the abnormal cerebellar tonsils in at least 20% of patients, and the cerebellum would need to move more than 10 times as far as has been recorded to cause intermittent obstruction.[59 60] Furthermore, no association exists between the distension or cranial extent of the syrinx and the presence or absence of foramen magnum obstruction, or degree of tonsillar descent[59]; indeed, syringomyelia occurs significantly more frequently with mild rather than with severe tonsillar descent.[60 61]

Additional complications have arisen with respect to the nature of the Chiari I malformation itself. Firstly, assessment of the level of the cerebellar tonsils on midline sagittal MR images has greatly overestimated the prevalence of tonsillar descent below the foramen magnum. Indeed, a prevalence of between 15% and 20% is still generally accepted[61] despite the previous assessments on myelography and computed cisternography indicating a prevalence of less than 1%. However, the recent volumetric MBI study of Savy et al has confirmed the second figure to be correct.[62] Although the apparent prevalence of tonsillar ectopia on sagittal MRI in the study was 20%, it was explained by partial volume averaging and was therefore spurious. Secondly, in over 50% of patients with true cerebellar ectopia, the medulla oblongata is also elongated. Indeed, a linear relation has been shown between the presence of medullary elongation and severity of the descent of the cerebellar tonsils,[63] which results in the obex often lying in the cervical canal, not the cranial cavity, and actually lying *below* the tonsils in about half of such cases.[59 60 63] These anatomical facts are usually ignored in hydromechanical explanations of syringomyelia and pose appreciable difficulties. Finally, it now seems certain that the Chiari I lesion is an acquired deformation of the rhombencephalon, and not a congenital malformation at all. Serial MRI examinations have clearly shown the development of typical Chiari I deformities postnatally,[64 65] the cause apparently being a lower rate of growth of the basicranium relative to the cerebellum in the first two years of life (figure 5.1).

Dynamics and clinical aspects

On air myelography, an important diagnostic finding was whether an enlarged cervical cord collapsed in the head up position. Syringomyelia was collapsing, cord tumours or non-fluctuant cysts were not. Similar observations could be made on water soluble myelography, but the change in cord size was smaller and in the opposite direction, opacified CSF being denser than cyst fluid.[51] However, serial MRI has sometimes disclosed large fluctuations in cord size with no intervention whatsoever, and not associated with any change in clinical status.[59 60 66]

There are numerous surgical strategies for collapsing a distended syrinx,[67] the commonest being foramen magnum decompression and syringoperitoneal shunting, either of which will collapse 70%–80%. The hypothesis of Williams holds that CSF enters the cord from above, due to intermittent pathological raising of intracranial over intraspinal pressure.[68] This has been challenged by new intraoperative measurements indicating higher intraspinal pressures,[69] lending support to the alternative hypotheses, which propose that raised intraspinal CSF pressure forces CSF into the cord via the dorsal root entry zone, or Virchow-Robin spaces. Park et al[69] treated a small series of patients with Chiari-associated syringomyelia by lumboperitoneal shunting, and found that this also collapsed the syrinx in about 80% of cases. This approach has been used in different types of syringomyelia, with similar success[70–72]; the obvious advantage over syringoperitoneal shunting is that it does not interfere with the spinal cord, and it is much less painful and hazardous than foramen magnum decompression.

No correlation can be shown between the degree of distension, or indeed the extent, of a syrinx and severity of clinical features.[51 73–75] Vaquero et al studied 30 patients clinically and with

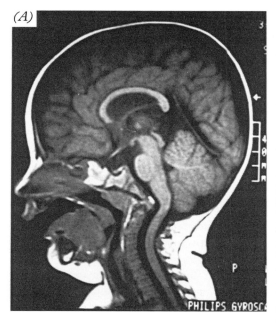

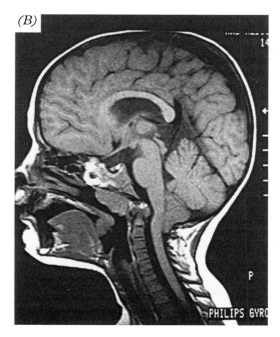

Figure 5.1 *Two approximately midsagittal T1 weighted MR images, the image (A) being made when the child was aged 1 year, and (B) three years later. The child was mildly hypotonic from birth but otherwise developmentally normal. No new symptoms accompanied the cerebellar descent into the spinal canal shown on the second MRI and no operative intervention of any kind had taken place. A mildly exaggerated kyphosis of the craniovertebral junction was shown on the initial MRI, but was probably within the range of normal variation. The second MRI shows thickening of the periodontal soft tissues, enough to mildly compress the anterior aspect of the neural axis; this thickening is sometimes noted as an incidental finding in young children who have no evidence of a connective tissue disorder, and in whom the odontoid process is ossifying normally as in this case*

MRI, both preoperatively and postoperatively, and showed that collapse of the syrinx was achieved in 29, but only 46% improved clinically, and 27% continued to deteriorate despite MRI showing persistent collapse of the syrinx.[75] Furthermore, Sherman et al used serial MRI to show that Chiari associated and post-traumatic syringomyelia successfully collapsed by surgical intervention may still continue to propagate through the cord.[73] Assessment of CSF dynamics by MRI has been just as disappointing in predicting clinical progression or outcome,[73] despite several claims to the contrary based on isolated cases and no follow up data.

Spinal cord compression and injury

In 25% of their control population Yu et al found the spinal cord to be at least moderately compressed by osteophytes at C5/6 or C6/7.[35]

Some workers have found an apparently linear correlation between numerical evaluation of cord compression (cord cross sectional area or compression ratio) and clinical disability,[34 40 41 53] whereas others have not.[37 76 77] However, all studies indicate that when cord compression is sufficient to reduce cord cross sectional area by more than 60%, clinical dysfunction is usually present. Canine models have suggested that lower limb paralysis appears only when gradually applied cord compression exceeds 50%, and that the relation between compression and clinical dysfunction is non-linear, following a catastrophe model rather than a linear one.[47] However, more is involved than mere static compression.

In a canine model of chronic spinal cord compression at C5, Al-Mefty et al showed that progressive paraplegia developed in most animals at a mean of seven months after only 30% compression of the cord.[78] In a series of patients with chronic malunited fracture of the dens, Crockard et al showed a log linear relation between reduction in cord cross sectional area, as measured on computed myelograms, and time in years since injury.[79] In another canine model, Anderson showed that a rapidly applied deformation of the cord of only 20%–30% produced much greater damage than slow compression of up to 50%–60%, and that this consisted mainly of haemorrhagic damage to the grey matter in the first, and mainly white matter change in the second.[80] In chronic compression, although blood flow reduction is maximal in the anterior columns in contact with the compressive agent, paradoxically it is the lateral and the anterior parts of the posterior columns that show pathological change.[47] In the brain, diffuse axonal injury is the result of shearing forces generated by rotatory acceleration. Similar forces are generated in the spinal cord, where the pia mater is restrained more than the rest of the cord structure by the dentate ligaments and spinal roots, generating shearing forces maximal in the lateral and dorsal columns.[33] In the brain, very severe rotatory acceleration causes diffuse vascular injury, which is characterised by haemorrhagic damage in the basal ganglia, similar to the grey matter damage seen in the spinal cord. However, because the changes in white matter generally seem more suggestive of vascular insufficiency than diffuse axonal injury, most workers currently believe that progressive cord damage is due to repeated episodes of momentary arrest of the microcirculation. The resulting changes are maximal in the vascular watershed area, and tend to lead to cavitation, especially in the ventral parts of the posterior columns; this is readily shown by MRI.[78]

Imaging

Only MRI consistently shows the changes in the spinal cord that result from compression. They are best shown on T2 weighted images. The distribution is usually characteristic, consisting of diffuse signal change at the site of maximal compression, with variable extension to the *central* part of the cord, often bilateral, and resulting in an appearance reminiscent of snakes' eyes.[44 52 78 80] These changes are shown on T1 weighted images only when damage is particularly severe, and consist of low signal; when present they are a sign of poor prognosis. This is not so for signal changes on T2 weighted images, which often disappear completely after operative decompression, but persist when operative outcome is poor.[52 82] The pathological substrate for reversible MRI changes is not known, but it is often assumed to be oedema. The size of the spinal cord at the site of compression is also of prognostic importance. Several studies have shown that when the cord is reduced in size by more than about 50%–60%, operative outcome is poor.[34 37 76] However, this applies only to compression in cervical spondylosis and subluxation. The cord tolerates far greater compression from benign tumours such as meningiomas and schwannomas and functional recovery remains likely after decompression even when the cord is severely compressed.

157

In a recent computed myelographic study of 56 patients with spondylotic myelopathy who had a poor operative outcome,[83] an alternative cause for the myelopathy (usually multiple sclerosis) was established in only 14·3%. The spinal cord was reduced in size by 60% or more at the site of previous compression in only 26·8%, and only 15·6% had evidence of cord necrosis. In 57·1%, operation failed to decompress the spinal canal. Another study by the same workers has put paid to the idea that osteophytes usually regress or disappear after interbody fusion: some osteophytes were as large as they had been up to eight years after the preoperative computed myelogram, and in no case did any measurable regression occur.[84]

Clinicoradiological approach to cord compression in spondylosis and subluxations in the cervical spine

In patients with suspected compressive myelopathy, osteophytes, disc protrusions, or subluxation are irrelevant when the spinal cord is normal or only mildly flattened. Cord deformation of up to about 40% is also most likely to be irrelevant, unless appropriate signal change is present in the cord on MRI at the site of compression. Usually, however, signal change is present only in severely compressed cords.

Cord deformation of over 50% is likely to be relevant, but this is also the point at which clinical recovery from decompression is becoming less likely. Therefore, it seems appropriate to consider surgery in asymptomatic or mildly affected subjects as a prophylactic measure when cord compression is approaching 50%, in children and young adults. However, in most patients with cervical spondylosis, such operations will be less appropriate because of age and low expectation of deterioration within the relevant time frame.[47]

Acute spinal cord injury

It is now established in animal models that the extent of signal change shown in the spinal cord on MRI is related to the severity of injury,[85 86] and clinical studies have also shown a general association between the extent of signal change on MRI and functional outcome.[87–89] Mild or transient loss of function after spinal injury is not usually accompanied by signal change in the cord on MRI.[87–89] In more severe injury, evidence of haematomyelia is present on MRI in only about 50%. Cord swelling is mild and not

158

always present even within seven days of injury, and ongoing cord compression is usually absent.[87]

Progression from an acute injury to localised cystic myelopathy has been followed by serial imaging, most cysts being asymptomatic.[82] There is good evidence that cysts result from colliquative necrosis, and extension of spindle shaped cores of ectopic necrotic tissue along the bases of the dorsal horns into adjacent uninjured parts of the spinal cord is observable on MRI.[84-86 89] These necrotic cores are likely to be the basis of the elongated cavities that may occur within a few weeks of injury,[82] some of which distend and propagate and become associated with a progressive ascending myelopathy.[51 82] Progressive post-traumatic myelopathy can also occur in the absence of cavitation,[51 90] and is associated with ascending central necrosis in the spinal cord, manifesting as signal changes on T2 and T1 weighted MR images[90] and abnormal contrast medium accumulation on computed myelography.[51] Other abnormalities such as adhesions, and occasionally cord compression, are found in some cases; some workers consider these to be the cause of progressive cord damage.

Spinal cord injuries in children differ in some ways from those in adults.[91] Children may have extensive cord contusion or infarction with minor, remote, or no spinal fracture. Any signal change found on MRI is usually followed by considerable persistent functional loss.

Vertebral artery injury has recently been reported as occurring in nearly 46% of cases of midcervical fracture dislocation.[92] However, it is notable that spinal cord infarction due to vascular injury from subluxation, trauma, or cervical spondylosis and related conditions is exceptionally rare, and its documentation is confined to only two or three case reports over the past 30 years. Extensive and severe adhesive arachnoiditis and superficial siderosis are also described as rare, late complications.[93]

Vascular lesions of the spinal cord

Anatomy and physiology

The blood supply of the spinal cord has recently been reviewed in detail by Lasjaunias and Berenstein.[94] The anterior spinal artery supplies a centrifugal arterial system and radial arteries from the vascular network on the surface of the cord form a centripetal system. A watershed zone between these systems has been defined consisting of the inner 25% of the white matter and the outer edge of the grey matter, excluding the posterior 50% or more of the posterior horns. Regional blood flow in cord white matter of primates has been estimated to be as low as 10 ml/100 g/min and in grey matter as 58 ml/100 g/min, which is only about half cerebral blood flow measured by similar techniques. The bases of the dorsal horns seem the most vulnerable regions within the cord to ischaemia or hypoxaemia.

Two main groups of veins drain the spinal cord. The central veins, collecting from both halves and central parts of the cord, and the radial veins from capillary plexuses at the periphery of both grey and white matter. A coronal plexus of veins on the surface of the spinal cord forms a longitudinal network which drains out of the spinal canal along the medullary veins which accompany the spinal roots at varying intervals. These veins are narrowed as they traverse the dura mater, the narrowings perhaps functioning as weak antireflux valves. Although gravity favours inferior venous drainage, in the cervical region cranial venous anastomoses seem of particular importance. High cervical obstruction has been shown to cause venous congestion and stagnant hypoxia in the central parts of the spinal cord in the cervical enlargement.

Spinal cord infarction

The MRI appearances have been described in many cases.[95-97] The commonest change has been diffuse signal increase on T2 weighted images, most often involving the lower thoracic region. Cord swelling has been mild or absent even in the acute phase. Central haemorrhage has been noted.[94] In some cases only the ventral part of the cord has been involved, either limited in extent, confined to grey matter, or more diffusely in both grey and white matter.[95] Diffuse contrast enhancement may be seen after intravenous gadolinium in patients examined 10–21 days after onset, but not earlier or later.[96] An association with infarction in adjacent vertebral bodies has been noted.[96]

Venous infarction of the cord has been reported less often, and in two recent cases the MRI abnormality consisted of unilateral signal change.[44 97] One was confirmed by necropsy to be thrombosis of the posterolateral pial vein complex,[44] and the other was speculated to be due to thrombosis in these veins induced by a YAG laser during removal of an intradural neurinoma at C2. Serial MRI in the second case disclosed diffuse cord swelling and signal change from C1 to C3, which reduced within one month to a circumscribed area of signal change involving nearly all the lateral half of the spinal cord, confined to the site of surgery.

Spinal vascular malformations

Dural arteriovenous fistulae

Spinal vascular malformations used to be classified according to the extent of the abnormal intradural vessels, which was a descriptive rather than a functional approach. In the early years of spinal angiography, surgeons believed that most of the vessels were arteries, as did many reputable neuropathologists until very recently. However, the careful observations of Kendall and Logue revolutionised thinking about these lesions and now form the basis of the modern functional classification. Most spinal arteriovenous malformations are dural arteriovenous fistulae, the enlarged intradural vessels being veins not arteries. The fistula is located in the dura mater close to the nerve roots, usually in the thoracic region in older patients,[98][99] but can occur in the lumbosacral theca or in the dura mater around the foramen magnum or the posterior cranial fossa.[100] Slow, aberrant venous drainage is an important feature, and is presumed to be due to thrombosis of radicular veins. Their precise anatomy requires spinal angiography for elucidation. Treatment is often straightforward, by operative or endovascular occlusion of the fistula. However, haemodynamic improvement does not always occur because the thrombotic aspect of the disease may remain, with impaired venous drainage of the spinal cord.[48] Complications of dural fistulae include intramedullary haemorrhage, cord atrophy, and cavitation in the cord, usually above the fistula.[98]

High resolution MRI should detect most clinically relevant arterialised veins, but overdiagnosis is possible. Conventional myelography probably remains the most sensitive and specific technique for their detection. However, enlarged or conspicuous intradural veins that drain normally, even if filled by a fistula, are not usually associated with clinical myelopathy.[99] Virtually all patients with clinical myelopathy have signal changes in the lower part of the spinal cord on MRI, usually surrounded by a small rim of apparently unaltered cord tissue. The signal change often disappears partially or completely when the fistula is successfully closed and symptoms remit, and may reappear if the fistula

161

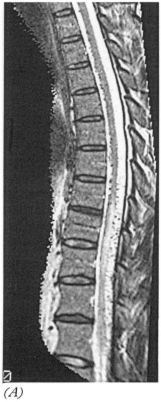

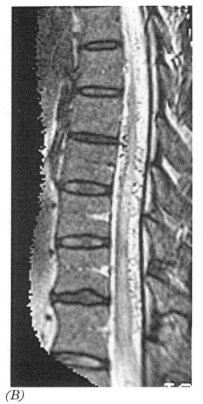

(A)

(B)

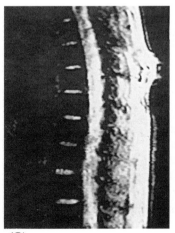

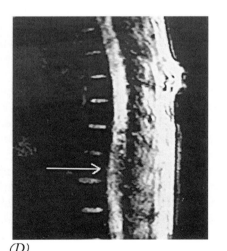

(C)

(D)

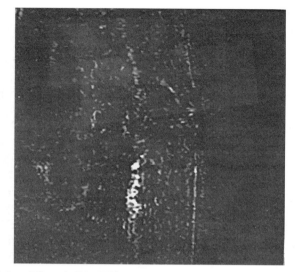

(E)

Figure 5.2   *(A) and (B). Midsagittal MR images of the thoracic spinal cord, made with phased array coils and using a T1 weighted, fast spin echo sequence. The lower half of the spinal cord shows extensive mainly central signal change, and multiple abnormal veins are clearly visible in the subarachnoid space: (C), (D) and (E). A series of midsagittal images of the thoracic spine from a dynamic susceptibility weighted MR study. Image C was immediately before the arrival of the bolus of Gd-DTPA, D immediately after and the veins across one level (T8) are filled with the contrast medium in this frame. Subtraction and contrast reversal (E) highlight the contrast filled veins, and combined with subsequent frames, provides a good indication of where they are filling from. The angiographer now knows to begin the search at the level of T8, or at levels immediately adjacent, with a high expectation of finding a dural fistula there (images kindly lent by Dr J W Thorpe, NMR Research Group, Institute of Neurology, London, UK; see Thorpe et al[23] for details)*

reopens. There may be patchy enhancement of spinal cord substance after intravenous gadolinium.[98 100]

The site of the fistula can be detected reliably by susceptibility contrast weighted dynamic MRI when the intradural veins are large enough to be shown easily. A series of heavily susceptibility weighted fast images is acquired in the midsagittal plane after an intravenous bolus of gadolinium, and the point at which signal nulling first appears in the intradural veins indicates the level of the fistula (figure 5.2).[23] Spinal angiography can then be directed at this level, greatly speeding up the diagnostic and therapeutic process.

Intramedullary arteriovenous malformations

These may be either a nidus, or a direct arteriovenous fistula, located within cord substance or on the pia mater. Fistulae are more common in children. The nidus is often visible on MRI as a focal expansion of the cord closely associated with serpiginous signal voids indicating the draining veins and sometimes enlarged arteries. Successful endovascular treatment may be feasible, even for intramedullary lesions, but multiple sessions may be required, obliteration is often incomplete, and the recurrence rate is high.[101]

Cavernomas and capillary angionmas

These are less common in the cord than in the brain. On MRI, they appear usually as localised expansions of the spinal cord, with sharply circumscribed signal change,[98 102] which cannot be distinguished from small intramedullary haemorrhages. Intravenous gadolinium enhancement may demonstrate otherwise invisible lesions in rare cases of multiple capillary haemangiomas.[103]

Neoplastic and inflammatory intramedullary processes

Neoplastic processes

Astrocytomas and *ependymomas* occur about equally in the spinal cord itself, but ependymomas are much more common in the filum terminale. Extramedullary ependymomas occur occasionally in the extradural part of the filum, involving the sacrum.[50] *Glioblastomas* are rare in all ages, as are *oligodendrogliomas*. Isolated reports are to be found of *subependymonas* of the cervical cord and *gangliogliomas* of cervicothoracic cord and filum terminale. *Metastases* are not uncommon. *Primary lymphoma* affecting only the spinal cord has now been reported several times. Reports of exceptionally rare neoplasms arising within or directly involving the cord have included *melanoma; intramedullary neurofibromas* arising from Schwann cells in nerves encasing blood vessels of the cord; intramedullary *teratoma,* associated with precocious puberty; *primitive neuroectodermal tumour; mesenchymal chondrosarcoma* without dural attachment, and *paraganglioma of the filum terminale.*

Finally, there is the relatively common spinal capillary *haemangioblastoma*, and its well known association with Von Hippel-Lindau disease. Screening of all family members with abdominal

164

CT and spinal MRI with gadolinium enhancement has been recommended by several workers because 40% of affected patients may be asymptomatic at the time of screening.

On clinical imaging, the hallmark of intramedullary neoplasms is expansion of the spinal cord, usually greater than in inflammatory conditions. Lobulation, or eccentric enlargement is extremely suggestive of this. Both astrocytomas and, especially, ependymomas can appear as very well circumscribed signal change on MRI. Sometimes circumscribed lesions appear etched out by a salient low signal pseudocapsule, around the entire circumference or capping the cranial and caudal extremities, consisting of dense gliosis or haemosiderin staining; this is more frequent with ependymomas.[50] Enhancement after intravenous gadolinium is usual, unlike benign intracranial gliomas which usually do not enhance. Enhancement is patchy, and does not reliably indicate all neoplastic areas.

Haemangioblastomas and metastases usually have a different appearance. They are well defined, and enhance strongly after intravenous gadolinium. About 50% of haemangioblastomas are associated with enlarged intrathecal veins, visible on all types of image including MRI. Spinal cord oedema is common with metastases and is well shown in white matter with MRI[44]; it may be difficult to distinguish from cavitation.

Three types of cyst occur in association with intramedullary neoplasms, and about 70% will have at least one type: *intratumoral cysts,* the walls containing or consisting of neoplastic tissue; *capping cysts,* cone shaped cavities extending for one or two spinal segments into uninfiltrated cord cranial and caudal to the tumour; and *syringomyelia,* undistinguishable from other causes remote from the tumour.[50] Even on MRI and intraoperative sonography, it can be difficult to distinguish some cystic from solid or necrotic tissue.

Inflammatory processes

Until the era of MRI, imaging was usually negative in these conditions, but virtually all inflammatory processes produce changes in cord substance detectable by MRI. Unfortunately, they all look alike and most have been confused with neoplasia. Diagnosis usually depends on clinical evolution, laboratory tests, or even cord biopsy, and in many cases the diagnosis remains uncertain.

Multiple sclerosis

The primary demyelinations, which include acute disseminated encephalomyelitis, present a range of stage dependent changes,[50] and the stages follow a roughly predictable time course that can be helpful in establishing a diagnosis.

Stage 1: perivenous inflammation and oedema—On MRI the cord may show mild fusiform enlargement if the lesion is large enough, with poorly defined signal change throughout the involved area, either diffuse or sparing the cord periphery. Clinical dysfunction is at its peak during this phase. Patchy or diffuse enhancement occurs after intravenous gadolinium within the area of signal change, but not coextensive with it. Similarity with cord glioma is particularly close at this stage, which lasts two to eight weeks.

Stage 2: demyelination and glial proliferation—Once MRI cord swelling has subsided, a smaller, more circumscribed area of signal change is evident, and enhancement no longer occurs after intravenous gadolinium. This is how most multiple sclerosis presents on MR images. Visualisation is considerably improved by the heavy T2 weighting provided by Spinal FLAIR MRI.[104] Lesions tend to involve sectors of the cord white matter, extending to the periphery of the cord, best shown on cross sectional T2 weighted images. The posterior columns and the posterior parts of the lateral columns are most commonly involved. The lesions are usually unilateral, or extend across the midline; they do not have the appearance of snakes' eyes. These features should distinguish plaques of demyelination arising in the cervical cord near sites of spondylotic compression, from cord damage due to the compression alone.

Stage 3: atrophy—the spinal cord is small or focally or diffusely flattened. In rare cases it becomes cavitated.

Nearly all multiple sclerosis lesions eventually progress to stage 3. Acute disseminated encephalomyelitis lesions usually arrest before this stage, often not progressing beyond stage 1, and most regress completely. The prognostic significance of brain lesions, which are found at presentation in about 60% of patients with clinically isolated cord syndromes, has been reviewed recently.[105]

166

Sarcoidosis

Involvement of the spinal cord is much less frequent than that of the brain or peripheral nerves in established cases. The appearances on myelography and MRI can be dramatic, although only a few cases have been fully described.[106][107] The cord may show pronounced and extensive fusiform or irregular expansion, with variable signal changes on T1 and poorly circumscribed high signal on T2 weighted images. Patchy, non-uniform enhancement usually occurs after intravenous gadolinium and may persist for months. The solid enhancing areas have been shown to consist of astrocytic gliosis in which are embedded typical sarcoid granulomas. One operated case was found also to have extensive cystic change involving almost the entire cord, the cyst containing xanthrochromic fluid. Milder forms, indistinguishable from focal multiple sclerosis, have also been documented.[50] The cord is usually involved along with the brain. Lexa and Grossman[106] described cord involvement in three of 24 established cases of neurosarcoidosis. The association of changes in periventricular or peripheral white matter in the brain and leptomeningeal enhancement after intravenous gadolinium is particularly suggestive of sarcoidosis. Intravenous gadolinium is definitely helpful in identifying meningeal disease and locating additional lesions, which may clinch a difficult diagnosis. Rapid reduction in contrast enhancement, accompanied by clinical improvement, was seen in 90% of patients in response to steroid treatment.[106]

Spinal tuberculosis

Spinal tuberculosis has a range of involvement similar to that of sarcoidosis. Meningeal fibrosis with chronic cavitatory myelopathy is more common, especially in countries where tuberculosis has a high prevalence, such as in India, and an MR appearance consisting of multiple superficial enhancing lesions after intravenous gadolinium is probably seen more often.[108] The diagnosis should be made from the CSF.[108] Response to antituberculous treatment is variable, as in the brain, and may be preceded by a period of apparent worsening of the appearances.

Intramedullary abscess (pyomyelia)

Pyomyelia may occur from haematogenous dissemination, but is exceptionally rare. More often there is an underlying abnormality, such as a dermal sinus.[109][110] A peripherally enhancing liquefying mass in a swollen oedematous cord is shown by MRI.

Acute varicella myelopathy

Herpes zoster can present with neurological disability before the onset of the cutaneous rash, consisting usually of unilateral limb weakness with or without long tract signs.[111] Magnetic resonance imaging has shown mild enlargement of the spinal cord, with diffuse signal change in the ipsilateral posterolateral portion and coextensive enhancement after intravenous gadolinium. Three or four segments are involved, a little more extensive than the dermatome distribution of the cutaneous rash when it appears. Only partial resolution may follow, with residual signal change in the cord and persistence of some dysfunction. The condition can occur in fit patients as well as the immunosuppressed. It is considered to be due to direct involvement of the spinal cord by the virus.

Tropical spastic paraparesis

This is a progressive vacuolar leukomyelopathy showing a strong association with human T cell lymphotrophic virus type 1 HTLV-1. The clinical course is relentlessly progressive. The thoracic region is usually involved. Extensive patchy signal change has been shown in the dorsolateral part of the spinal cord, with patchy, sometimes superficial, enhancement after intravenous gadolinium.

Listeria meningoencephalomyelitis

Listeria monocytogenes produces an encephalomyelitis characterised by multiple microabscesses. Mass lesions can form, simulating malignant tumours. Extensive brain stem and spinal cord involvement has been reported several times. A case presenting as an isolated abscess in the cervical spinal cord was described recently, showing the MRI features of an abscess.

Lyme disease

Lyme disease may cause an acute transverse myelitis with extensive cord involvement, often associated with involvement of the peripheral nerves. Damaerel et al [112] recently described a case involving just the spinal meninges, and we have encountered a similar case. In both, only postgadolinium MRI was abnormal, showing pronounced, diffuse enhancement of the pia mater of the brain stem and entire spinal cord. In our case, MRI of the head a few hours after the spinal examination showed that the gadolinium had diffused into the CSF producing a positive-contrast cisternogram (figure 5.3).

Granulomatous angiitis of the spinal cord

Granulomatous angiitis is a condition characterised by granulomata involving vascular walls, disseminated through the meninges and neural tissue, which only rarely involves the spinal cord. A case with extensive signal change throughout the spinal cord, showing no enhancement after intravenous gadolinium, has been

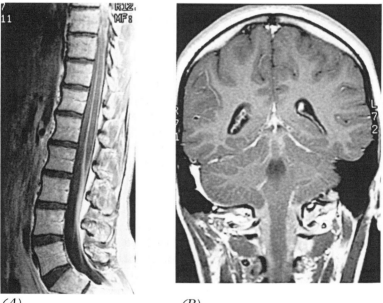

(A)   *(B)*

Figure 5.3   (A) *A midsagittal T1 weighted MRI of the thoracolumbar spine after intravenous Gd-TPA in a case of Lyme disease. The roots of the cauda equina and superficial layers of the spinal cord are enhanced with the contrast medium. The spinal cord appeared normal on unenhanced T1 and T2 weighted images. (B) Coronal T1 weighted MRI of the brain two hours after intravenous Gd-DTPA. All the CSF in the basal cisterns is enhanced by the contrast medium which has diffused into it from the diffusely enhancing meninges*

169

reported, and another otherwise similar case which showed extensive mainly superficial enhancement after gadolinium suggestive of metastatic disease ensheathing the cord.

Congenital abormalities of the spinal cord

These have been extensively reviewed by Naidich *et al*, to whom the interested reader is referrred for details.[113][114] Some represent disorders of neuralation of the neural plate and disjunction of the neuroectoderm from the ectoderm; and these include meningomyelocele and lipomas of the spinal cord. In the first, the unneurulated neural plate (placode) remains part of the integument. In the second, a localised region of the neural tube has failed to neurulate before disjunction occurred and mesenchyme contacting the exposed dorsal surface of the neural plate has differentiated into adipose tissue; disjunction usually is complete and the overlying dura mater is intact, to create an apparently intramedullary intradural lipoma. Spinal roots emerge from the ventral surface of the unnerurulated neural placode in both conditions.

The commonest malformations involve the more caudal part of the neural tube, most of which forms by canalisation of the caudal cell mass which develops in the tail fold of the embryo. When the tail fold disappears, this part of the cord normally undergoes retrogressive differentiation to form the filum terminale. A useful descriptive term for this group of conditions is lipomyelomeningodysplasia to emphasise the elements usually present to some degree in all. The spinal cord or thickened filum extend down, unusually to the sacral segments, and blend with a lipoma which extends through a dural defect and neural arch defect of variable size and and length to blend with subcutaneous fat. The site of blending with the dura mater and its extent, usually referred to as "tethering", is variable, as is the size and distribution of the lipoma and degree of meningeal ectasia. The spinal cord does not expand into a normal lumbar enlargement, and the conus medullaris usually lies at or below L3, its position sometimes being difficult to define.

Another group of conditions appears to be due to much more focal, even punctate failures of disjunction. A *dorsal dermal sinus* extends from skin dimple through or between neural arches to dura, and very occasionally intradurally; about 20% of spinal *dermoids* and *epidermoids* are connected to a dorsal dermal sinus. The neuroectoderm, and ectoderm normally are briefly connected in embryonic life, via the neurenteric canal or adhesion. Persistence of the normal adhesion, or aberrant adhesions at other levels, can result in a connection from foregut to spinal canal, along which neurenteric cysts may form. Intradural *spinal neurenteric cysts* were well reviewed recently by Brooks et al,[115] and present a reasonably characteristic appearance on MRI. Persistence of a communication with the skin of the back is a *dorsal enteric fistula*.

Diastematomyelia is a relatively common anomaly often considered also to be due to aberrant neuroentodermal adhesions. Over a variable number of segments the spinal cord develops as two, usually unequal hemicords, not duplications, although often there are two central canals, median sulci, and anterior spinal arteries. Sometimes this division takes the form only of a deep cleft, but usually the hemicords are entirely separate. In over 50% of cases, both are enclosed in a common dural tube; the rest are associated with splitting of the dura mater also, and a bony spur arising from malformed thickened laminae then often penetrates between the dural tubes. The spinal cord can be affected at any level, or rarely the filum terminale or medulla oblongata.

Finally, excessive retrogressive differentiation of the tail fold and caudal cell mass can lead to varying degrees of sacral and sacrolumbar agenesis, often referred to as the *caudal regression syndromes*. The spinal cord is abnormally short, the conus lying in the thoracic region at a variable level.

Many of these often dramatic anomalies are asymptomatic, and remain so throughout life. Much recent literature still is concerned with their diagnosis, which is now easy, and often seems to exaggerate the importance of timely surgical intervention. This is especially true in the concept of tethering. It has been documented recently that the filum terminale is thicker than 2 mm and filled with fat in 4% of normal patients, and that the conus medullaris lies at the level of the lower part of L2 in about 2% of the normal population. Some workers have indicated that the conus may be tethered, but normal in position, and others that functional MRI or sonography may demonstrate tethering in the absence of any morphological abnormalities. I remain aloof from such opinions at the present time. In cases with progressive disability due to the lesion, structural imaging can be important in demonstrating normal cord tissue giving rise to spinal nerves and in suggesting an operative goal such as debulking of a lipoma or the drainage of a cyst. High resolution MRI has replaced the need for myelography and CT in preoperative assessment of such cases.

Degenerative diseases

Although modern imaging is demonstrating abnormalities in many of these conditions, diagnosis remains clinical.

Subacute combined degeneration

Several reports have demonstrated *reversible* signal changes in the spinal cord on MRI.[116 117] Signal change is seen mainly or exclusively in the dorsal columns in the thoracic or cervical regions, extending over many segments, and presumably represents intramyelinic oedema. Therapy has resulted in complete resolution of the MR changes within six weeks.

Motor neuron disease

Changes have been noted on T2 weighted MRI in the corticospinal tracts (high signal) and motor cortex (low signal).[118 119] The low signal is considered to be due to mineral deposition in pigments which often form in association with neuronal degeneration, the main one being iron. Oba *et al*[119] studied 15 patients, and found reduced signal in the motor cortex of 14, and *increased* signal in the pyramidal tracts of only seven. Areas of the cortex other than the precentral gyrus were also involved in five. Two patients were negative on their first MRI, but became positive as the disease progressed. However, caution is required before accepting these findings because they are significantly different from those in large necropsy surveys, which the authors failed to discuss. Cord atrophy is also demonstrable in established cases, sometimes showing a rather characteristic anterolateral flattening on cross sectional images. Profound atophy of the lower cervical cord has been reported in the benign juvenile variant of motor neuron disease.

Friedreich's ataxia

Atrophy of the upper cervical spinal cord and medulla oblongata, and signal change posteriorly, were seen in 13 and nine patients respectively in a series of 14 patients with clinically established Friedreich's ataxia reported by Mascalchi *et al*.[120] The degree of atrophy and signal change showed no relation with chronicity or severity of the clinical features. Among the cerebellar ataxias, Friedreich's is the only one which is *usually* accompanied by involvement of the upper spinal cord on MRI.

Conclusion

Nowhere has MRI had greater impact than in the assessment of the spinal cord. To date some of the most interesting, and often unexpected observations include: (1) reversible changes in spinal cord substance in a variety of conditions, such as cervical spondylotic myelopathy and subacute combined degeneration; (2) changes in the substance of the spinal cord in radicular herpes zoster, some forms of sensory neuropathy; (3) degeneration in the cerebral cortex possibly occurring earlier and more often in motor neuron disease than formerly known; (4) many cord diseases such as multiple sclerosis and HTLV associated myelopathy often being accompanied by asymptomatic cerebral lesions; (5) Chiari type 1 malformations being a secondary deformation of the entire rhombencephalon, not just the cerebellum, and acquired in the first two years or so of life; (6) the progression of syringomyelia and its clinical manifestations apparently not being related to size of the cavity or the motility of the fluid within it. Syringomyelia is a disease which, despite interesting new dynamic observations never before possible, remains as obscure as ever.

1 Shapiro R. *Myelography*. 3rd ed. Chicago: Year Book Medical Publishers Inc, 1975.
2 Jirout J. Pneumographic examination of the cervical spine. *Acta Radiol* 1958;50:221–45.
3 Johnson AJ, Burrows E. Thecal deformity after lumbar myelography with iophendylate (Myodil) and meglumine iothalamate (Conray 280). *Br J Radiol* 1978;51:196–202.
4 Kendall BE, Stevens JM, Thomas D. Arachnoiditis. *Current imaging* 1991;2:113–9.
5 Sortland O, Skalpe IO. Cervical myelography by lateral cervical and lumbar injection of Metrizamide: a comparison. *Acta Radiol* 1977;355(suppl):154–63.
6 Skalpe IO, Sortland O. *Myelography*. 2nd ed. Oslo: Tano, 1989.
7 Shaw DD, Back-Gansmo T, Dahlstrom K. Iohexol: summary of North American and European clinical trials in adult lumbar, thoracic and cervical myelography, with a new non-issue contrast medium. *Invest Radiol* 1985;**suppl 20**:44–50.
8 Robertson HJ, Smith PD. Cervical myelography. Survey of modes of practice and major complications. *Radiology* 1990;**174**:79–83.
9 National Radiation Protection Board. *Protection of the patient in x-ray computed tomography*. Chiltern: NRPB, 1992.
10 Youser DM, Janick PA, Atlas SW, *et al.* Pseudo atrophy of the cervical portion of the spinal cord on MR images: a manifestation of the truncation artefact? *AJNR Am J Neuroradiol* 1990;**11**:373–7.
11 Enzmann DR, Pelc AJ. Cerebrospinal fluid-flow measured by phase contrast cine MR. *AJNR Am J Neuroradiol* 1993;**14**:1301–7.
12 Mikulis DJ, Wood ML, Zerdoner OAM, Poncelet BP. Oscillatory motion of the normal cervical spinal cord. *Radiology* 1994;**192**:117–21.
13 Rubin JB, Enzmann DR. Dyke Award. Harmonic modulation of proton MR precessional phase by pulsatile motion: origin of spinal CSF flow phenomenon. *AJR Am J Roentgenol* 1987;**148**:983–94.
14 Heindel W, Friedmann G, Bunke J, Thomas B, Firsching R, Ernestus RI. Artefacts in MR imaging after surgical intervention. *J Comput Assist Tomogr* 1986;**10**:596–9.

15 Yoshino MT, Temeltas OM, Carter LP, et al. Metallic postoperative artefacts on cervical MR. AJNR Am J Neuroradiol 1993;14:747–9.

16 Clagman DA, Murakami ME, Vines FS. Compatibility of the cervical braces with MR imaging: a study of nine non-ferrous devices. AJNR Am J Neuroradiol 1990;11:231–390.

17 Miruis SE, Gecsler F, Joslyn JN, Zrebeet H. Use of titanium wire in cervical spine fixation as a means to reduce artefacts. AJNR Am J Neuroradiol 1988;9:1229–31.

18 Williams DF. Editorial; titanium: epitome of biocompatibility or cause for concern? J Bone Joint Surg 1994;76B:348–9.

19 Berry I, Sigal R, Lebas J, Mark AS, Le Bihan D. Magnetic resonance imaging: principles, techniques and imaging protocols. In: Manelfe C, ed. Imaging of the spine and spinal cord. New York: Raven Press, 1992:157–94.

20 Enzmann DR, Pelc NJ. Normal flow patterns of intracranial and spinal cerebrospinal fluid defined with phase-contrast cine MR imaging. Radiology 1991;178:467–74.

21 Terae S, Miyasaka K, Abe S, et al. Increased pulsatile movement of the hindbrain in syringomyelia associated with Chiari malformation: cine MRI with presentation bolus tracking. Neuroradiology 1994;36:125–32.

22 Maeda M, Itoh S, Kimura H, et al. Vascularity of meningiomas and neuromas: assessment with dynamic susceptibility-contrast MR imaging. AJR Am J Roentgenol 1994;163:181–6.

23 Thorpe JW, Kendall BE, MacManus D, Miller DH. Dynamic gadolinium enhanced MRI with detection and localisation of spinal arterio-venous malformations. Neuroradiology 1994;36:522–9.

24 White SJ, Haginal JV, Young JR, Bydder GM. Use of fluid attenuated inversion recovery (FLAIR) pulse sequences for imaging the spinal cord. Magn Reson Med 1992;28:153–62.

25 Montalvo BM, Quencer RM. Intraoperative sonography in spinal surgery: state of the art. Neuroradiology 1986;28:551–90.

26 Plainfosse B, Brunon J, Nelson MD, David P, Hurth M. Intraoperative ultrasound. In: Manelfe C, ed. Imaging of the spine and spinal cord. New York: Raven Press, 1992:599–620.

27 Rowland Hill CA, Sibson PI, Britton JA, Hall DMB. Ultrasound of the neonatal conus medullaris: normal position and use in identification of occult spinal dysraphism. Neuroradiology 1994;36:165.

28 Di Pietro MA, Venes JL. Real time sonography of the pediatric spinal cord: horizons and limits. Concepts in Pediatric Neurosurgery 1988;8:120–32.

29 Winter RK, McKnight IL, Byrne RA, et al. Diastematomyelia: prenatal ultrasonic appearances. Clin Radiol 1989;40:291–4.

30 Naidich TP, Dopundoulakis SH, Poznanski AK. Intraspinal masses: effect of plain spine radiography. Paediatric Neuroscience 1986;12:10–17.

31 Kendall BE. Spinal angiography. In: Du Boulay GH, ed. A textbook of radiological diagnosis. 5th ed. Vol 1. The head and CNS. London: Lewis, 1982:563–80.

32 Moseley IF, Tress BM. Extravasation of contrast medium during spinal angiography, a cause of paraplegia. Neuroradiology 1977;13:55–7.

33 Hughes JT. Disorders of the spine and spinal cord. In: Hume Adams J, Duchen IW, eds. Greenfield's Neuropathology, London: Edward Arnold, 1992:1083–116.

34 Fukushima T, Takaaki I, Taoka Y, Takata S. Magnetic resonance imaging study of spinal cord plasticity in patients with cervical compression myelopathy. Spine 1991;16:534–8.

35 Yu YL, Jones SJ. Somatosensory evoked potentials in cervical spondylosis: correlation of median ulnar and posterior tibial nerve responses with radiological findings. Brain 1985;108:273–300.

36 Seibert CE, Barnes J, Dreisback JN, et al. Accurate CT measurement of the spinal cord using metrizamide: physical factors. AJNR Am J Neuroradiol 1981;2:75–8.

37 Fujiwara K, Yonenobu K, Ebara S, Yamashita K, Ono K. The prognosis of surgery for cervical compression in myelopathy. J Bone Joint Surg 1989;71B:393–8.

38 Sherman JL, Nassaux AB, Citrin CM. Measurements of the normal cervical spinal cord on MR imaging. AJNR Am J Neuroradiol 1990;11:369–72.

39 Yu YL, Du Boulay GH, Stevens JM, Kendall BE. Computer assisted myelography in cervical spondylotic myelopathy and radiculopathy. Brain 1986;109:259–78.

40 Fujiwara K, Yonenobu K, Hiroshima K, Ebara S, Yamashita K, Ono K. Morphometry in cases with compression myelopathy. Spine 1988;13:1212–6.

41 Ogino H, Tada K, Okada K, et al. Canal diameter, antero-posterior compression ratio, and spondylotic myelopathy of the cervical spine. Spine 1983;8:1–15.

42 Beuls E, Gelan J, Vandersteen M, et al. Microanatomy of the excised human spinal cord and the cervico-medullary junction examined with high resolution MR imaging at 9.4 Tesla. AJNR Am J Neuroradiol 1993;14:699–707.

43 Solsberg MD, Lemaire C, Resch L, Potts DS. High resolution MR imaging of the cadaveric human spinal cord: normal anatomy. AJNR Am J Neuroradiol 1990;11:3–7.

44 Ohshio I, Hatayama A, Kaneda K, et al. Correlation between histopathological features and magnetic resonance imaging of spinal cord lesions. Spine 1993;18:114–9.

45 Brieg A, Turnbull IM, Hasseter O. Effects of mechanical stresses on the cervical cord in cervical spondylosis: a study on fresh cadaver material. J Neurosurg 1966;25:45–66.

46 Stevens JM, O'Driscoll DM, Yu YL, et al. Some dynamic factors in compressive deformity of the cervical spinal cord. Neuroradiology 1987;29:136–42.

47 Stevens JM. The compressed spinal cord. Current medical literature. Medical Imaging 1993;5:3–8.

48 Stevens JM, Kendall BE, Crockard HA. The spinal cord in rheumatoid arthritis with clinical myelopathy: a computed myelographic study. J Neurol Neurosurg Psychiatry 1986;49:140–51.

49 Holsheimer J, Den Boer JA, Struijk JJ, Rozeboom AR. MR assessment of the normal position of the spinal cord in the spinal canal. AJNR Am J Neuroradiol 1994;15:951–9.

50 Balériaux D, Parizel P, Bank WD. Intraspinal and intramedullary pathology. In: Menelfe C, ed. Imaging of the spine and spinal cord. New York: Raven Press, 1992:832–90.

51 Stevens JM, Olney JS, Kendall BE. Post-traumatic cystic and non-cystic myelopathy. Neuroradiology 1985;27:48–56.

52 Mehali TF, Pezzuti RT, Applebaum BI. Magnetic resonance imaging and cervical spondylotic myelopathy. Neurosurgery 1990;26:217–27.

53 Ono K, Ota H, Tada K, Yamomoto T. Cervical myelopathy secondary to multiple spondylotic protrusions—a clinicopathological study. Spine 1977;2:109–25.

54 Kuhn MJ, Mikulis JJ, Ayoub DM, et al. Wallerian degeneration after cerebral infarction: evaluation with sequential imaging. Radiology 1989;172:179–82.

55 Terae S, Taneichi H, Aburni K. MRI of Wallerian degeneration of the injured spinal cord. J Comput Assist Tomogr 1993;17:700–3.

56 Lexa FJ, Grossman RI, Rosenquist AC. MR of Wallerian degeneration in the feline visual system: characterisation by magnetisation transfer rate with histopathological correlation. AJNR Am J Neuroradiol 1994;15:201–12.

57 Naidich TP, Zimmerman RA, McLone DG, et al. Congenital malformations of the spine and spinal cord. In: Manelfe C, ed. Imaging of the spine and spinal cord. New York: Raven Press, 1992:621–704.

58 Oldfield EH, Muraszko K, Shawker TH, Patronas NJ. Pathophysiology of syringomyelia associated with Chiari I malformation of the cerebellar tonsils: implications for diagnosis and treatment. J Neurosurg 1994;80:3–15.

59 Clifton A, Stevens JM, Kendall BE. Idiopathic and Chiari associated syringomyelia in adults: observation on the cerebrospinal fluid pathways at the foramen magnum. Neuroradiology 1991;33(suppl):167–9.

60 Stevens JM, Serva W, Kendall BE, et al. Chiari malformation in adults: relation to morphological aspects to clinical features and operative outcome. J Neurol Neurosurg Psychiatry 1993;56:1072–7.

61 Barkovich AJ, Wippold FJ, Sherman JJL, Citrin CM. Significance of cerebellar tonsillar position on MRI. AJNR Am J Neuroradiol 1986;7:795–9.

62 Savy L, Stevens JM, Taylor DJ. Apparent cerebellar ectopia: a reappraisal using volumetric MRI. Neuroradiology 1994;6:360–3.

63 Stevens JM, Clifton A, Kendall BE. Relationship between cerebellar tonsillar descent, medullary elongation and the basi cranium in hindbrain deformities of Chiari type. Neuroradiology 1994;36:163.

64 Payner TD, Prenger E, Berger TS, Crone KR. Acquired Chiari malformations: incidence, diagnosis and management. Neurosurgery 1994;34:429–34.

65 Huang PP, Constantine S. "Acquired" Chiari I malformations. J Neurosurg 1994;80:1099–102.

66 Birbamer G, Buchberger W, Felber S, et al. Spontaneous collapse of post-traumatic syringomyelia: serial magnetic resonance imaging. Eur Neurol 1993;33:378–81.

67 Milhorat TH, Johnson WD, Miller JI, et al. Surgical treatment of syringomyelia based on magnetic resonance imaging criteria. Neurosurgery 1992;31:231–42.

68 Williams B. Pathogenesis of syringomyelia. Lancet 1972;i:142–3.

69 Park TS, Cail WS, Broneldus WC, et al. Lumbo-peritoneal shunt combined with myelotomy for treatment of syringo-hydromyelia. *J Neurosurg* 1989;70:721–7.
70 Vissilouthis J, Panandreon A, Anagnostasas S. Thecoperitoneal shunt for post-traumatic syringomyelia. *J Neurol Neurosurg Psychiatry* 1994;57:755–6.
71 Vissilouthis J, Panadreon A, Anagnostasas S. Thecoperitoneal shunt for syringomyelia. Report of three cases. *Neurosurgery* 1993;33:324–8.
72 Vengsarkar VS, Panchal VS, Tripathis PB, et al. Percutaneous thecoperitoneal shunt for syringomyelia. Report of three cases. *J Neurosurg* 1991;74:827–31.
73 Sherman JL, Barkovich AJ, Citrin CM. The MR appearances in syringomyelia: new observations. *AJNR Am J Neuroradiol* 1986;7:985–95.
74 Grant R, Hadley DM, MacPherson P, et al. Syringomyelia—cyst measurement by magnetic-resonance imaging and comparison with symptoms, signs, and disability. *J Neurol Neurosurg Psychiatry* 1987;50:1008–14.
75 Vaquero J, Martinez R, Arias A. Syringomyelia-Chiari complex. Magnetic resonance imaging and clinical evaluation of surgical treatment. *J Neurosurg* 1990;73:14–68.
76 Hunter JV, Stevens JM, Kendall BE, et al. Radiological assessment of transoral surgery in rheumatoid arthritis using dynamic CT myelography. *Neuroradiology* 1991;33 (suppl):413–5.
77 Yu YL, Stevens JM, Kendall BE, de Boulay GH. Cord shape and measurement in cervical spondylotic myelopathy and radiculopathy. AJNR *Am J Neuroradiol* 1983;4:839–12.
78 Al-Mefty O, Harkey HL, Marawi I, et al. Experimental compressive cervical myelopathy. *J Neurosurg* 1993;79:550–61.
79 Crockard HA, Heileman AE, Stevens JM. Progressive myelopathy secondary to odontoid fractures: clinical, radiological and surgical features. *J Neurosurg* 1993;78:579–86.
80 Anderson TE. Spinal cord contusion injury. Experimental dislocation of haemorrhagic necrosis and subacute long axonal conduction loss. *J Neurosurg* 1985;62:115–9.
81 Schonman-Claeys E, Frija S, Caenol CA, et al. MR imaging of acute spinal cord injury: results of an experimental study in dogs. *AJNR Am J Neuroradiol* 1990;11:459–65.
82 Yamashita Y, Takahaiki M, Matsumoto Y, et al. Chronic injuries of the spinal cord: assessment with MR imaging. *Radiology* 1990;175:849–545.
83 Clifton AG, Stevens JM, Whitear PW, Kendall BE. Identifiable causes for poor outcome in surgery for cervical spondylosis. Post-operative computed myelography and MR imaging. *Neuroradiology* 1990;32:450–5.
84 Stevens JM, Clifton AG, Whitear P. Appearances of posterior osteophytes after sound anterior interbody fusion in the cervical spine: a high definition computed myelographic study. *Neuroradiology* 1993;35:227–8.
85 Hackney DB, Ford JC, Markowitz RS, et al. Experimeal spinal cord injury: MR correlations to intensity of injury. *J Comput Assist Tomogr*, 1994;18:357–62.
86 Fujii H, Yore K, Sakou I. Magnetic resonance imaging study of experimental acute spinal cord injury. *Spine* 1993;18:2030–4.
87 Kulkarni MR, McArdle CB, Kapanick D, et al. Acute spinal cord imaging: MR imaging at 1.5T. *Radiology* 1987;164:837–43.
88 Silberstein M, Hennessy O. Implications of focal spinal cord lesions following trauma—evaluation with magnetic resonance imaging. *Paraplegia* 1993;31:160–7.
89 Beers GJ, Rague GH, Wagner SG, et al. Magnetic resonance imaging of spinal trauma. *J Comput Assist Tomogr* 1988;12:755–61.
90 Falcone S, Quencer RM, Green BA, et al. Progressive post-traumatic myelomalacic myelopathy: imaging and clinical features. *AJNR Am J Neuroradiol* 1994;15:747–54.
91 Davies PC, Reisner A, Hudgins PA, et al. Spinal injuries in children: role of MR. *AJNR Am J Neuroradiol* 1993;14:607–17.
92 Willis BK, Greiner F, Orrison WW, Benzel EC. The incidence of vertebral artery injury after mid-cervical fracture or subluxation. *Neurosurgery* 1994;34:435–42.
93 Bonito V, Agostinis C, Ferraresi S, Defanti CA. Superficial siderosis of the central nervous system after brachial plexus injury with pseudo meningoceles. *J Neurosurg* 1994;80: 931–4.
94 Lasjaunias P, Berenstein A. *Surgical neuroangiography.* Vol 3. *Functional vascular anatomy of brain, spinal cord and spine.* New York: Springer Verlag, 1990:15–87.
95 Mawad ME, Rivera V, Crawford S, et al. Spinal cord ischaemia after resection of thoracoabdominal aortic aneurysms: MR findings in 24 patients. *AJNR Am J Neuroradiol* 1990;11:987–91.
96 Yuh WT, Marsh CY, Wang AK, et al. MR Imaging of spinal cord and vertebral body

infarction. *AJNR Am J Neuroradiol* 1992;13:145–54.

97 Henderson FC, Crockard HA, Stevens JM. Spinal cord oedema due to venous stasis. *Neuroradiology* 1993;35:312–5.

98 Rodesch G, Berenstein A, Lasjaunias P. Vasculature and vascular lesions of the spinal cord. In: Manelfe C, ed. *Imaging of the spine and spinal cord.* New York: Raven Press, 1992:565–98.

99 Willinsky R, Lasjaunias P, Terbrugge K, Hurth M. Spinal angiography in the investigation of spinal arteriovenous fistula. A protocol with application to the venous phase. *Neuroradiology* 1990;32:114–6.

100 Gaensler EHL, Jackson DE, Halbach VV. Arterio-venous fistulas of the cervicomedullary junctions as a cause of myelopathy: radiological findings in two cases. *AJNR Am J Neuroradiol* 1990;11:518–22.

101 Biondi A, Merland JJ, Reizine D, *et al.* Embolization with particles in thoracic intramedullary arterio-venous malformations: long term angiographic and clinical results. *Radiology* 1990;177:651–8.

102 Barnwell SL, Dowd CF, Davis RL, *et al.* Cryptic vascular malformations of the spinal cord: diagnosis by magnetic resonance imaging and outcome of surgery. *J Neurosurg* 1990;72:403–7.

103 Hida K, Tada M, Chandler WF, *et al.* Intramedullary disseminated capillary haemangioma with spinal cord swelling—case report. *Neurosurgery* 1993;33:1099–106.

104 Thomas DJ, Pennock JM, Hajnel A, *et al.* Magnetic resonance imaging of the spinal cord in multiple sclerosis by fluid attenuated invasion recovery (FLAIR). *Lancet* 1993;314:593–4.

105 Morrissey SP, Miller DH, Kendall BE, *et al.* The significance of brain magnetic resonance imaging abnormalities at presentation with clinically isolated syndromes suggestive of MS: a 5 year follow up study. *Brain* 1993;116:135–46.

106 Lexa FJ, Grossman RI. MR of sarcoidosis in the head and spine: spectrum of manifestations and radiographic response to steroid therapy. *AJNR Am J Neuroradiol* 1994;15: 973–82.

107 Stevens JM. Infections of the central nervous system. In: Butler P, ed. *Imaging of the nervous system.* London: Springer-Verlag, 1990:107–30.

108 Junger SS, Stem BJ, Levine SR, *et al.* Intramedullary sarcoidosis—clinical and magnetic imaging characteristics. *Neurology* 1993;43:333–7.

109 Rogg JM, Benzil DL, Haas RL, Knucky NW. Intramedullary abscess, an unusual manifestation of a dermal sinus. *AJNR Am J Neuroradiol* 1993;14:1393–5.

110 Hardwidge C, Palsingh J, Williams B. Pyomyelia: an intramedullary abscess complicating lumbar lipoma with spina bifida. *Br J Neurosurg* 1993;7:419–22.

111 Esposito MB, Arrington JA, Murtaugh FR, *et al.* MR of the spinal cord on a patient with herpes zoster. *AJNR Am J Neuroradiol* 1993;14:203–4.

112 Demaeral R, Wilms G, Van Lierde S, *et al.* Lyme disease in childhood presenting as primary leptomeningeal enhancement without parenchymal findings on MR. *AJNR Am J Neuroradiol* 1994;15:302–4.

113 Naidich TP, Zimmerman RA, McLone DG, *et al.* Congenial anomalies of the spine and spinal cord. In: *Magnetic resonance imaging of the brain and spine.* New York: Raven Press, 1991:865–920.

114 Naidich TP, McLone DG, Harwood-Nash D. Spinal dysraphism. In: Newton PH, Potts DG, eds. *Modern neuroradiology.* Vol 1. *Computed tomography of the spine and spinal cord.* San Anselmo, CA: Clavadel Press, 1983:299–354.

115 Brooks BS, Duval ER, El Gammal T, *et al.* Neuro-imaging features of neurenteric cysts: analysis of nine cases and review of the literature. *AJNR Am J Neuroradiol* 1993;14: 735–6.

116 Berger JR, Quencer R. Reversible myelopahy wih pernicious anaemia, clinical MR correlation. *Neurology* 1991;41:947–8.

117 Murata S, Naritomi H, Sawada T. MRI in subacute combined degeneration. *Neuroradiology* 1994;36:408–10.

118 Friedman DP, Tartaglino LM. Amyotrophic lateral sclerosis: hyperintensity of the corticospinal tracts on MR images of the spinal cord. *Am J Roentgenol* 1993;160:604–6.

119 Oba H, Araki T, Ohotomo K, *et al.* Amyotrophic lateral sclerosis: T2 shortening in motor cortex at MR imaging. *AJNR Am J Neuroradiol* 1993;189:843–6.

120 Mascalchi M, Salvi F, Piacentini S, Bartolozzi C. Friedreich's ataxia: MR findings involving the cervical portion of the spinal cord. *AJNR Am J Neuroradiol* 1994;163:187–91.

6 Neuropsychological assessment

LISA CIPOLOTTI, ELIZABETH K WARRINGTON

Patients with brain damage may present with impairments of memory, language, perception, thought, action, and other functions. These cognitive deficits can occur both in multiple domains or as highly selective impairments. In the 19th century and early 20th century, neurologists investigated cognitive impairments in patients with neurological disease by clinical and descriptive methods. These methods provided new insights and allowed the isolation of distinct syndromes—for example, aphasia,[1 2] alexia and agraphia,[3] acalculia,[4] visual agnosia,[5] and amnesia.[6] Indeed, these discoveries formed the basis for the development of a new discipline, "neuropsychology", devoted to the study of the relation between the brain and cognitive functions. The clinical and descriptive methods, however, provided a poor standard of description of the cognitive impairments in these syndromes. They were ". . . little more than the bald statement of the clinical opinion of the investigator. . .".[7]

To deal with this lack, neuropsychologists developed principled techniques for the measurement of cognitive functioning. In the early days, psychometric tests, originally developed for the measurement of either scholastic attainment or occupational guidance, were used. In particular, tests for the measurement of intellectual and memory functions became available to the clinician.[8-11] Gradually, over the past four decades an increasing number of measurement tools have been specifically designed for investigating the cognitive functions of patients with suspected or confirmed cerebral disease. Neuropsychological assessment

178

involves the use of a series of tests that are "reliable"—in the same circumstances they produce the same result—and "valid"—they measure what they are designed to measure.

The aim of this paper is to provide an overview of the main methods for the assessment of cognitive function and an outline of what may prompt a neuropsychological assessment (see also Lezak,[12] Crawford et al,[13] and Hodges[14]). Before approaching a neuropsychological assessment it is necessary to have a general theoretical structure on which to base and interpret the different levels of disturbance that can arise as a result of cerebral damage (for a similar view see Hodges[14]). In the next three sections we discuss our general theoretical schema; the methods of assessment of cognitive function; and the purposes of a neuropsychological examination.

General theoretical schema

Our approach makes the assumption that impairments in cognitive function can best be studied and understood by (a) assuming that there is a high degree of functional specialisation in the cerebral cortex; (b) by undertaking a modularity approach to the analysis of complex cognitive skills; and (c) by assuming that brain damage can selectively disrupt some components of a cognitive system.[15] The extent to which these assumptions have a direct anatomical substrate is less established.

The idea that the human brain is highly differentiated in terms of its functional organisation is not new. The phrenologists in the early 19th century were already speculating that the convoluted surface of the brain reflected the juxtaposition of a large number of discrete cerebral organs each subserving a particular psychological faculty.[16] Several years after these accounts, neurologists began to study and record impairments of the higher cortical functions and their accompanying cerebral lesions. Aphasic disorders were extensively studied and the specialised language functions of the left hemisphere were recognised.[1 2 17] Subsequently, after the pioneering work of Jackson,[18] the specialised visuoperceptual functions of the right hemisphere were also recognised. These early workers not only localised a number of specialised functions in the brain but they also discussed their findings within a theoretical framework. For example, Lichtheim[19] produced a complex diagram of the various subcomponents of the language system by

179

incorporating and expanding on Wernicke's[2] original scheme. In his diagram, the various subcomponents of the language functions are represented as a series of "centres" (for example, the concept centre, the centre of the motor images of the words, the centre of the auditory images of the words), each of which was thought to be located in a specific area of the brain. These different functional centres were thought to be connected with each other through sets of fibre tracts. This approach—those adopting it were termed the "diagram makers"—has some resemblance to that of modern cognitive neuropsychology theorists.

Despite this, the idea that cognitive skills such as language could consist of multicomponents and be localised in different, highly specialised areas of the brain came under attack from the "global theorists".[20-23] Of particular relevance here is the development of "mass action" theories. These theories proposed that there was no differentiation in the cortex for specific cognitive functions; rather, that it was equipotential with respect to cognitive abilities.[24] According to such a view, any form of neurological damage would deplete by a greater or lesser extent the available amount of some general cognitive resource and not specific cognitive functions. The amount of damage to the general cognitive resource, also termed intellect or abstract attitude, would depend on the extent of the brain damage and not on the site of the damage.

The notion that different brain regions are specialised for different cognitive functions regained popularity in the 1950s and the modern revolution in imaging techniques has made it possible to visualise these structures in the living human brain. The idea that there are cognitive processing systems that involve only specialised brain regions is now accepted ". . . as one of the cornerstones of modern brain science . . .".[25] For about 95% of right handers and 70% of left handers major language, literacy (reading, writing, and calculation), verbal short term memory, verbal long term memory, semantic memory, and praxis are represented in the left hemisphere. The right hemisphere is involved in non-verbal processing such as the analysis of perceptual and spatial stimuli, spatial short term memory, visual long term memory, spatially directed attention, face recognition, topographical knowledge, and in some prosodic components of language. For those few people who do not have normal lateralisation this pattern seems to be reversed, although a very small proportion of subjects may have bilateral organisation of some cognitive skills. The anterior parts of both hemispheres have been accepted as being implicated in problem solving processes that are required in a wide range of situations including practical routines and social interactions as well as abstract reasoning tasks.[7] The most posterior parts of both hemispheres are involved in early visual processing. Subcortical, as well as cortical, brain regions, are involved in attention and alertness. Subcortical brain regions are also involved in episodic memory, in some aspects of long term memory, and in the motor control of language.[12]

A modularity approach to the analysis of cognitive skills implies that each complex cognitive process can be thought of as consisting of a series of functionally independent specialised subprocesses.[7 26-29] The interaction of these subprocesses results in the complex cognitive skills. The way in which the cognitive processes are organised is often characterised, similarly to the "diagram maker" approach, in terms of flow diagrams that attempt to detail the way that the different subprocesses are brought together to perform a specific task. Empirical support for the modularity approach can be obtained at various levels including the neurophysiological, neuroanatomical, and neuropsychological.[30 31] For example, numeracy has been fractionated into several independent components: cognitive mechanisms for number comprehension, number production, arithmetical fact retrieval, and arithmetical procedures.[32]

The idea that complex cognitive skills are carried out by distinct subprocesses combined with the idea that there are highly specialised areas in the brain, has led many cognitive neuropsychologists to assume that a cerebral lesion can damage only some subprocesses within complex cognitive skills. Indeed, cognitive neuropsychologists have succeeded in showing many dissociations between the subcomponents of cognitive skills that allow valid conclusions about the nature and functions of the impaired processing components to be drawn.

Methods of assessment of cognitive functions

One of the fundamental principles underlying neuropsychological assessment is to establish whether the subject is still functioning at their premorbid optimal level or whether there has been a deterioration. Therefore, the methods used for assessing cognitive functioning in neuropsychology need to be able to provide: (*a*) an indirect measure of the premorbid skills of a person and (*b*) a measure of the present cognitive state of that person. Once the two types of measures are obtained they can be compared. This should indicate: firstly, whether the functioning has changed from the premorbid state; and secondly whether this reflects organic or functional impairment. If the results indicate organic impairment then an attempt will be made to establish the extent of the change. It is not only useful to know that a change in cognitive functioning has occurred; it is also useful to know whether the change can be characterised as global or focal. If the cognitive impairment is focal, neuropsychological measures can be used to specify more precisely the cognitive impairments: whether the impairment is indicative of lateralised dysfunction or confined to the anterior or posterior regions of the brain. In exceptional cases, it is possible to document highly selective cognitive impairments with a known and relatively precise anatomical localisation.

A comprehensive neuropsychological examination would include the assessment of: (*a*) premorbid ability; (*b*) general intellectual level; (*c*) memory; (*d*) language; (*e*) calculation; (*f*) problem solving; (*g*) alertness and attention; (*h*) visual and space perception. Ideally a cognitive profile would be constructed from performance on tests of proved validity and comparable difficulty. A long term aim for the neuropsychologist is to achieve a level of measurement for all cognitive skills that permit comparison across tasks and is sensitive to change. The method described by Newman *et al* in their study that monitored subjects at risk for Alzheimer's disease exploited this methodology (figure 6.1).[33]

In the next section we do not attempt to describe all the tests and techniques available to the neuropsychologists for investigation of all these different areas of cognition. Rather we focus on three main areas of cognitive function: intelligence, memory, and language functions. These serve to illustrate the range of techniques and procedures available for the investigation of cognitive impairments.[33]

Assessment of premorbid ability

Various procedures are adopted for obtaining an indirect measure of a subject's premorbid skills, which can then be compared with his current level of performance. These procedures can be divided into two main types: methods that use demographic data

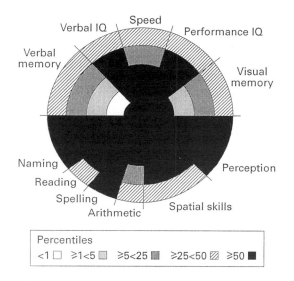

Percentiles
<1 □ ≥1<5 ▦ ≥5<25 ▨ ≥25<50 ▧ ≥50 ■

Figure 6.1 *Example of a circle diagram of cognitive skills. Sectors of the circle have been apportioned to each of the cognitive skills examined. The concentric circles represent the level of functioning in terms of percentile score. The levels of the subject's test performance are indicated by the degree of eccentricity within a sector. In this patient the most prominent feature was a global memory impairment more pronounced for verbal than visual material (diagram courtesy of Newman et al[33])*

such as age, sex, race, education, and occupation; and methods that use tests considered to be relatively resistant to neurological and psychiatric disorders. The first type of method is based on the known relation between a number of demographic variables and measured IQ*.[34] Not only may educational and occupational records be used as a rough estimate of a subject's optimal or premorbid level of functioning; they may also, through the use of various types of regression equations, provide a more precise and objective estimate.[35] One of the principle limitations of this type of technique, however, is that educational and occupational histories may not always be readily available and they may be incomplete, uninformative, or anomalous.

---

*The term IQ was first introduced by Stern[40] to describe a method of comparing one child's score on the Binet intelligence scale with the performance of average children of the same age. It is nowadays used to indicate intellectual level by comparing a subject's performance with the average scores attained by members of the same age group.

The second method involves the measurement of a cognitive skill that is known to be highly correlated with intellectual factors and resistant to brain damage. This method is obviously not reliant on pre-existing data. Some of the first methods of this type involved the use of vocabulary.[36] These methods were based on the finding that patients with brain disease retained old, well established verbal skills, such as those implicated in the verbal definition of words, long after other cognitive skills were impaired. The application of the same principle led to the development of various Wechsler deterioration indices.[12]

More recently, a measure of premorbid optimal level of functioning has been based on the overlearned skill of reading. Nelson and McKenna[37] first established that word reading skill, as measured by the Schonell graded word reading test[38] was highly correlated with general intelligence in a normal population. Nelson and O'Connell[39] then established that the reading of irregular words, such as "heir" or "chord", which cannot be pronounced correctly by applying the usual rules that map spelling on to phonology, were better indicators of premorbid intelligence (IQ) in demented subjects than estimates based on reading regular words. Nelson subsequently developed the National adult reading test (NART), which consists of 50 irregular words. Indeed, the NART has become one of the most commonly used measures of premorbid intelligence.[41] An American version of this test is also available.[42] One of the major limitations of the NART test is that it cannot be used with those who have poor literacy skills or in patients with obvious impairments of speech production or problems associated with dyslexia. In addition, there have been claims that patients with dementing disorders may not present with preserved irregular word reading.[43] Consequently these patients present with difficulties in reading the NART words, and this would result in erroneous low estimates of their premorbid IQ. In the cases of early dementia when language skills are relatively unimpaired, however, it has been shown that the NART remains stable over time and can be used as a predictor of the premorbid optimal level (Paque and Warrington, unpublished data).

Assessment of general intellectual level

Historically, intelligence has been defined in many different ways. For example, Spearman,[44] although he himself avoided the term intelligence, proposed the existence of a central intellectual ability, which he referred to as "g". Although he never actually defined what g was he thought that it involved "the eduction of relations and correlates".[44] In his formulation g referred to the determinant of shared variance among various tests of intellectual ability. An alternative view, associated with Thurstone[45] and Guilford,[46] involved the application of the term intelligence to a large set of diverse mental abilities (or factors). These included not only reasoning and problem solving on new data but also specialised knowledge derived from prior schooling or experience. In line with this, Cattell[47] distinguished between fluid intelligence, the ability to deal with novelty and to adapt one's thinking to a new cognitive problem, and crystallised intelligence, which reflects a knowledge base and skills that have been previously acquired through learning and experience.

The available measures of intelligence reflect these different formulations of the abilities underlying intelligence. For example, Raven's test, including the coloured progressive matrices,[11] the standard progressive matrices,[10] and the advanced progressive matrices (sets I and II),[48] are widely used for the clinical assessment of general intelligence. The various versions of this test are believed to weigh heavily on g and measure processes that are central to the definition of fluid intelligence (more recently also termed analytic intelligence[49]). Indeed, they require abstract reasoning, induction of relations, and eduction.[49] The test was developed as a "culture fair" measure of general intellectual ability and because of its non-verbal format, its ease of use, and its speed (especially the coloured progressive matrices), it has gained wide use in both clinical and research settings. This may be overoptimistic as educational level has subsequently been shown to have a major effect on the normal subject's performance.[50]

The Wechsler adult intelligence scale (WAIS)[51 52] is considered to be one of the core measures for evaluating general intellectual ability. It involves six verbal and five non-verbal subtests that sample various skills. These subtests are thought to measure various mental abilities as would follow from Thurstone's[45] and Guilford's[46] views, including both the explicit knowledge base derived from educational and previous experience and the ability to deal with and solve new cognitive problems. Verbal and performance IQs are determined from the use of the Wechsler scales. Much research has focused on discrepancies between verbal and performance IQ as a means of differentiating between left and

185

right hemisphere impairment[53] although this has not resulted in a general consensus.[12] Indeed, Warrington *et al*[54] suggested that such scales have little value as regards the localisation of a lesion or, for that matter, the identification of specific cognitive deficits. Nevertheless, the Wechsler adult intelligence scale-revised (WAIS-R), the successor of the WAIS, is the most often used psychological test of intellectual functioning and is a cornerstone for most neuropsychological test batteries. It is also widely used with geriatric patients, and recently, normative data for people who are 75 or older have become available.[55] Numerous studies are based on the WAIS-R.

Assessment of memory

Memory is not a unitary function but rather a collection of distinct and independent components, each of which is associated with different brain structures. A broad distinction is generally made between short and long term memory. Short term memory is considered to be responsible for the immediate retention of a limited amount of information; this information will decay in a matter of seconds if it is not refreshed. Long term memory retains larger amounts of information for longer periods—depending on the salience—which may be for minutes, days, and years. Short and long term memory functions can be further divided into verbal and visual memory according to whether they retain verbal or non-verbal information.[56] Long term memory is also subdivided into implicit (or procedural) and explicit (or declarative) memory.[57] Implicit memory retains information that affects behaviour but it is not available for conscious recollection (for example, motor skills, conditioned reflexes, priming). A further example is the three letter word stem completion task, which can be performed by guessing rather than by conscious recall.[58] In this task patients are presented with a list of words and their retention is tested either by standard recall and recognition techniques or by presenting the first three letters of the target item in a word completion task (for example, "cha"—chair). Explicit memory retains information that can be consciously accessed. It is subdivided into episodic and semantic memory.[59] Episodic memory contains information about temporally dated episodes or events and temporospatial relations among them (for instance, this can be for both autobiographical memories and memories of an artificial event such as a word list or short stories). Semantic memory contains our organised knowledge of concepts and facts as well as words and their meanings (for example, encyclopaedic memories). Most clinical assessments focus on three main types of memory functions: short term memory, episodic memory, and semantic memory.

Assessment of short term memory

The assessment of verbal short term memory usually requires the repetition of a progressively lengthening string of digits (digit span), letters, and words. The normal range of digits is five to nine. Spatial short term memory can be assessed with the Corsi block tapping test.[60] This requires the subject to tap a progressively lengthening sequence of blocks.

Assessment of episodic memory

Many tests and batteries are available for the assessment of episodic memory.[61] These use either a recall or recognition paradigm and typically assess the anterograde (the ability to acquire new information) rather than the retrograde component (the ability to recall previously learnt material). One of the oldest batteries used is the Wechsler memory scale (and the Wechsler memory scale-revised), which requires the recall of both complex verbal material (for example, short stories) and visual material (for example, reproduction of geometrical designs). Some of its sub-tests are not dependent on memory itself but rather on attentional processes (for example, mental control and orientation). Unfortunately all the subtests contribute to the final memory quotient. A more recently developed test for the assessment of long term verbal memory is the adult memory and information processing battery,[62] which has many similarities to the Wechsler memory scale. The Rivermead behavioural memory tests consist of a series of tests held to have ecological validity.[63] A task that is also very often used for assessing verbal anterograde recall is word list learning (for example, the auditory-verbal learning test[64]). For the assessment of non-verbal anterograde recall, the two most commonly used tests are the Rey-Osterreith complex figure test[65] and the Benton revised visual retention test.[66] Both require the recall of geometric figures.

Warrington[67] developed a test that used a recognition rather than a recall paradigm (the recognition memory test). The recognition paradigm was chosen because it is possible to have comparable tests of verbal and visual memory. This test incorporates the verbal and non-verbal dichotomy by having separate subtests with word and face stimuli. Age corrected percentile scores of a large standardisation sample are available. Validation of this test has shown that patients with right hemispheric lesions are impaired on the visual version and patients with left hemispheric lesions are impaired on the verbal version. It has also been shown that this test can detect minor degrees of memory deficit.[33] Clegg and Warrington[68] have also recently standardised and validated four "easy" memory tests (three recognition memory tests and a word paired associate learning test) for older adults (64 and older) that are recommended for patients in whom memory impairment is suspected but whose mental state (for example, poor attention, anxiety, or agitation) precludes longer or more demanding tests.

Most tests of retrograde verbal and visual recall have been devised for research rather than clinical purposes. They normally test recall and recognition of famous names and famous faces. Perhaps because they so quickly become dated their standardisation and validation are problematic. A relatively new test assessing autobiographical memory is an exception to this rule (autobiographical memory interview[69]). This test requires the recall of personal remote facts and incidents from three epochs: childhood, early adult life, and recent experience.

Assessment of semantic memory

Patients with a semantic memory disorder present a general loss of knowledge, including object and word meaning. This deficit can manifest itself as an inability to comprehend words and identify pictures and objects. The classic syndromes of transcortical sensory aphasia and visual associative agnosia have been identified with the impairment of semantic memory.[70] There are no standardised batteries for the assessment of semantic memory because, unlike episodic memory, it has only been studied in the past 20 years, after the seminal paper of Tulving.[59] Semantic memory can, however, be assessed through tests devised for other domains (mainly tests also used for the assessment of language disorders). To evaluate the difficulties in word definition some verbal subtests of the Wechsler scales, such as vocabulary and information, can be used. Naming tests can be used as indirect evidence of semantic memory impairment (see language section later). The pyramids and palm tree test[71] was developed specifically to evaluate impairments in the understanding of concepts. There is a verbal and a pictorial version of this task devised for assessing conceptual relations. Limited normative data are available. A further test, the British picture vocabulary test,[72] which uses a word picture matching technique, was first developed for the assessment of language developments between the ages 2 and 18. More recently it has been standardised in a normal healthy elderly population (Clegg and Warrington, unpublished data).

Assessment of language

Language is not a unitary function. The most useful dichotomy is to consider spoken and written language separately.

Spoken language can be characterised as a collection of independent components, each of which is associated with different brain structures. The three main central linguistic components are phonology, syntax, and semantics.[73] Phonological processing analyses the constituent sounds of words. Syntactic processing analyses the grammatical aspects of language—for example, the ordering of the individual words in the sentence. Semantic processing analyses the referential meaning of words. In addition to these three components there are more specialised peripheral systems subserving articulation and prosody. Furthermore, at least for phonology and syntax, receptive and expressive deficits can occur as selective impairments.[74-76] Disruptions in phonological or semantic processing are found at the level of single words whereas disruptions in syntactic processing are found at the level of sentences.

Assessment of spoken language

There are several traditional clinical taxonomies of the acquired aphasias principally inherited from the earliest scientific papers on language disorder.[1-3 19] These taxonomies, based on mixed functional, anatomical, and pathological terms, have inspired the development of classic aphasia batteries. The most widely used are the Boston diagnostic aphasia examination,[76] the western aphasia battery,[77] the Porch index of communicative ability,[78] and the Aachen aphasia test.[79] The traditional taxonomies that form their basis have been questioned in so far as they failed to capture the multidimensional pattern of language breakdown, they are not useful for guiding therapy or for the detailed analysis and under-

189

standing of language disorders.[80] In this section we provide a brief account of the core tests that could provide a framework for the more detailed assessment of a patient's language impairment. We discuss only two areas of language dysfunction: word and sentence comprehension and word and sentence retrieval.

Word and sentence comprehension—Word comprehension deficits can occur as a result of an impairment in auditory perception or as a result of an impairment in word meaning. An auditory word perception deficit can be identified in patients that have a deficit in word repetition that cannot be attributed to a more general articulatory deficit.[81] It can be assessed through phonological discrimination tasks that are usually included in most of the traditional aphasia batteries. Impairment of word meaning is one component of the semantic memory disorders (see earlier) and, as the word retrieval deficit (see later), can be category specific. For example, selective deficits for abstract and concrete concepts and within the concrete domain animate or inanimate reference and even specific word class effects have all been reported.[82] One of the most direct tests of word meaning are synonyms tests (for example, "*timid*" means "*afraid*" or "*quiet*"). Coughlan and Warrington[83] have offered a modest standardisation of one such test. Word meaning comprehension can also be tested by using word-picture matching tests such as the pyramids and palm tree test[71] and the British picture vocabulary test,[72] described in the semantic memory section. In addition, the recent psycholinguistic assessment of language processing in aphasia[84] is a useful research tool for assessing comprehension in the domains of verbal and visual knowledge.

One of the earliest and most commonly used test of sentence comprehension is the token test devised by De Renzi and Vignolo.[85] This test uses tokens of different shapes, sizes, and colours and the patient is given an oral instruction in progressively more complex non-redundant sentences (for example, "put the red circle between the yellow square and the green square"). There have been various modifications of the test including a shortened version by De Renzi and Faglioni and a very abbreviated version by Coughlan and Warrington.[83] Educationally standardised normative data are available. Parisi and Pizzamiglio[86] devised a test specifically for testing syntactic comprehension (for an English version see Lesser[87]). Another test for grammatical comprehension is the test for reception of grammar.[88] This test was developed for the assessment of language developments and has been used also in the context of acquired aphasia investigations. It should be acknowledged that some normative data are available for the sentence comprehension test reviewed here and are undoubtedly very useful for in depth assessment of a patient's aphasic deficit.

Word and sentence retrieval—Word retrieval difficulties are exemplified by the syndrome of amnestic or nominal dysphasia and are often present in other aphasic syndromes and in cortical degenerative conditions. They can be specific for particular categories such as letters, colours, body parts, proper names, and fruits and vegetables.[31] To evaluate word retrieval difficulties naming from verbal description (for example, "what is the name of the large grey animal with a trunk") and picture naming tests can be used. The graded naming test[89] was developed to identify very mild degrees of anomia. It comprises items of low frequency and it has been standardised in a normal population and validated in patients with unilateral lesions. The Boston naming test[90] comprises line drawings of objects and has been widely used in aphasia studies. Only a limited standardisation is available.

Spontaneous language is often elicited by complex picture description. The cookie jar theft picture from the Boston diagnostic aphasia examination is widely used for this purpose. De Renzi and Ferrari[91] devised the reporter test requiring the patient to act as a reporter of the performance carried out by the examiner who acts in accordance with the commands of the token test described earlier. This test is particularly useful for the identification of impairments in grammatical sentence construction, although there are only limited normative data at present.

Written language

In the past 30 years cognitive neuropsychologists have investigated reading and writing disorders in detail and depth. This has resulted in the identification of new syndromes that take the description of reading and writing difficulties well beyond the classic syndrome described by Dejerine[3]: dyslexia with dysgraphia and dyslexia without dysgraphia. Each of these different dyslexic and dysgraphic syndromes corresponds to an identifiable impairment in a subcomponent or subcomponents of the reading and writing process. Shallice and Warrington[92] have proposed a distinction between peripheral and central dyslexic syndromes and this dichotomy applies equally well to the dysgraphia syndromes. Peripheral dyslexias and dysgraphias result from damage to processes responsible for the categorisation of a string of letters or phonemes as orthographic or phonological entities. Central dyslexias and dysgraphias are due to impairment in the comprehension and production of a target stimulus. The study of central dyslexias and dysgraphias has provided evidence that there are at least two parallel forms of processing for reading and writing: one phonologically based and one semantic based. Phonological processing utilises a set of rules for translating print to sound or sound to print. It is used for reading or writing unfamiliar words or non-words. Semantic processing accesses meaningful representations of the words that are in the subject's vocabulary. These two types of processing can break down independently to produce different types of reading and writing impairments.

Assessment of written language

Following the seminal work of Marshall and Newcombe[93] a psycholinguistic method of assessment of written language disorders has gained wide popularity. This method involves the presentation of lists of words that sample contrasting psycholinguistic properties. It is thought that the data on the effect of the psycholinguistic and visual (length, script, and displays) variables coupled with an errors analysis allow conclusions to be drawn about the likely origin of dysfunction within the reading system. In this section we provide a description of some of the standardised and validated formal tests for the assessment of reading and spelling disorders.

Reading—Any assessment of reading skills should include an evaluation of a patient's ability to read both single words and text. In some peripheral dyslexias the ability to read text can be impaired whereas the ability to read single words can be spared. (for example, attentional dyslexia[94]) The Neale test[95] for assessment of prose reading in children is useful in this context. In addition, most of the standard aphasia batteries include a subtest for text reading (for example, Boston diagnostic aphasia examination). For the formal assessment of single words, the two most widely used tests are the NART and the Schonell graded word reading test. Both tests are graded in difficulty and are measures of reading skills; an estimate of premorbid optimal level of functioning can also be obtained (see earlier). When assessing reading skills it is important to evaluate the patient's ability to read aloud non-words. This ability can be selectively impaired despite good word reading as in the case of phonological dyslexia.[96] No formal standardised tests for non-word reading are available; however, several lists have been devised for research purposes.

Oral and written spelling—Written and oral spelling are known to dissociate and therefore are assessed independently. For the assessment of written spelling the Schonell graded spelling test can be used. For the assessment of oral and written spelling, Baxter and Warrington[97] have recently standardised and validated a test that is sensitive to minor degrees of deficit in the general neurological population. This is a graded difficulty test; thus the raw scores can be converted into percentile scores. For patients whose poor eye sight precludes reading, spelling can provide a useful measure of premorbid abilities. The assessment of non-word spelling is also important because patients with phonological dysgraphia might present with some preserved word spelling despite impaired non-word spelling.[98] Several non-word spelling lists have been developed for research purposes.

The use of the standard word reading and spelling tests described combined with assessment of the patient's ability to read and write non-words and an analysis of the errors made by the patient identifies more than the presence of a reading or spelling disorder. It can also provide some preliminary indication of the status of the peripheral and central processing involved in word reading and spelling. This, rather than the description of the presence or absence of a reading or spelling disorder, has a clear clinical and theoretical significance.

Purposes of a neuropsychological assessment

There are at least three main reasons for conducting a neuropsychological assessment: diagnosis, treatment and management, and research.

Diagnosis

A neuropsychological assessment allows the description and evaluation of the major cognitive deficits incurred in neurological patients with possible brain disease. Furthermore, it can indicate possible neuroanatomical correlates of the cognitive impairments. A neuropsychological assessment can, at the very least, provide pointers as to whether there is unilateral, bilateral, or subcortical damage. This information can be useful in diagnosis. Neuropsychological assessment has a key role in differentiating between organic and functional disorders.[14 99–101] There are other neurological conditions—for example, cortical atrophy, frontal and temporal lobe tumours, and undetected temporal lobe seizures—that may manifest themselves with symptoms that can be misinterpreted as functional.[102] For example, patients with visual disorientation disorders due to bilateral occipital disease are often misdiagnosed on the grounds that their visual handicap seems to be disproportionate in the context of normal or near normal acuity.[103]

On the other hand, patients with symptoms of pseudodementia, such as hysteria, malingering, Ganser syndrome, bipolar disorder, and other ill defined psychiatric disorders often present with an abrupt intellectual and memory failure that mimics true cognitive deficits. A neuropsychological assessment can distinguish between organic and functional disorders. It does this by highlighting discrepancies between subjective complaints and objective performance, usually detecting a number of inconsistencies in the patients' performance and a too obvious mismatch between objective performance and daily life activities. Also, the body of neuropsychological knowledge on the organisation and fractionation of cognitive skills is nowadays highly developed. Crucially, the way in which the cognitive functions can fractionate often diverges from the common sense opinion of how a cognitive function can break down. Thus the patient's pattern of performance can be interpreted as neuropsychologically convincing or unconvincing. To consider one example, a neuropsychological assessment is useful in differentiating organic and functional memory loss. Studies of patients with dense organic amnesia have shown that they can still learn new associative information provided that they are tested using implicit learning tasks.[104] For example, they show savings with repeated presentations of fragmented or degraded stimuli (pictures or words) in increasing degrees of completeness.

194

Even quite severely demented patients would show some learning with these tasks. Clearly a patient showing additional impairments on these implicit learning tasks makes no neuropsychological sense. It makes good common sense, however, to also be impaired on these tasks (I have poor memory, I can't remember things). Indeed, a poor performance on these tests may be considered indicative of functional memory loss. On the contrary, a relatively preserved performance on these tasks conforms to an organic pattern.

Another common differential diagnosis where neuropsychological assessment has a key role is between early dementia, anxiety or depressive disorders, or the normal aging process. The diagnosis of probable dementia is usually made by establishing whether there is an acquired deficit of cognition without histopathological evidence obtained from a biopsy or necropsy. Often in the early stages of a dementing illness, the clinical diagnosis cannot be supported by neuroimaging such as CT, MRI, or functional imaging. Patients with depression or anxiety may complain of intellectual or, more often, memory failure similar to the so called "worried well" patients. Usually depressive or anxiety pseudodementia should be suspected when the patient complains of the memory problem more than the carer.[105] In these cases recognition memory tests should be used to determine whether the failure is due to an organic condition or to anxiety or depression. It has been shown that recall tests of memory are vulnerable to the effect of anxiety and depression, whereas recognition memory tests are not.[106]

The aging process itself is associated with cognitive and memory changes. Hence, it is often necessary to differentiate memory failure due to cognitive deterioration rather than benign senescent forgetfulness. In these cases performance in recall memory tests requiring the subjects to engage in elaborative encoding, as opposed to allowing them to devise their own encoding strategy, may discriminate those with brain damage from normal elderly subjects. For example, in word list learning the strategy of performing associations between successive words improves the overall level of recall in normal subjects.

Neuropsychological assessment can also have a central role in diagnosing presymptomatic cognitive impairments in familial neurodegenerative conditions. From the nature of the inheritance and the relatively constant ages of disease onset within a family, asymptomatic at risk subjects below the mean age of onset can be examined. Such studies have shown cognitive abnormalities in apparently asymptomatic subjects with Huntington's and Alzheimer's disease.[33][107]

Treatment and management

The baselines of cognitive functioning provided by the neuropsychological examination allow the monitoring of certain conditions. For example, successive neuropsychological examinations provide reliable indications of whether a pattern of cognitive deficit associated with head injury or stroke is changing and if so, how rapidly and in what way. This information is useful in planning the future medical and social care of the patient. Similarly, repeated neuropsychological testing of patients with degenerative disorders can provide information about their different rates of cognitive decline and thus help them and their family plan for their care. The results of a neuropsychological assessment can also be used in the evaluation of medical and surgical treatments such as those associated with subcortical pathology that is associated with cognitive slowing (for example, Parkinson's disease and hydrocephalus). For instance, obtaining repeated measures of a hydrocephalic patient's performance in a series of psychomotor tests can provide a reliable indication of whether the underlying neurological condition is improving or deteriorating. Psychomotor tests are simple verbal and non-verbal tests that involve verbal and visuomotor responses and the measurement of the patients' speed of responding.[108] Practice effects are minimal in these tests, which are at the same time sensitive to subtle changes in cognitive efficiency. Therefore they can be used at regular and short intervals for monitoring the patient's neurological state. Neuropsychological assessment is also particularly important in monitoring the various treatments for epilepsy.[109][110]

The baselines of cognitive functioning provided by the neuropsychological examination can be important for planning and monitoring rehabilitation programmes. In particular, when planning such programmes, neuropsychological evaluation can provide answers to key questions such as ". . . what are realistic treatment goals and . . . what is the patient's capacity to benefit from available treatment . . .".[12] Moreover, repeated neuropsychological testing can be used to monitor the effects of the rehabilitation programme. Furthermore, the baselines of cognitive functioning provided by neuropsychological examination can be used to explain to patients and their families their relative cognitive problems so that they can both prepare and understand the type of difficulties the patient may face when he leaves the hospital.

Neuropsychological assessment has a central role in the medicolegal context. Neuropsychological data concerning the type and severity of a cognitive deficit, its prognostic value, and the implications for future care are central issues in the litigation over compensation awards.[111] In this context neuropsychological investigation is crucial in assessing the possibility of simulated disability that can sometimes occur before financial settlement.[112]

Research

There are two main neuropsychological research methodologies: the single case study and the group study.[7] For both, neuropsychological assessment procedures are a crucial element. The strength of novel findings and unexpected dissociations can only be evaluated by reference to performance of established tests of cognitive skills. In group studies that explore new hypotheses neuropsychological measures are necessary to obtain baseline data.

Neuropsychological research may consider applied clinical problems or be theoretically driven. In applied research, batteries of neuropsychological tests are commonly given to describe the cognitive profiles associated with particular neurological diseases. For example, specific cognitive profiles have been obtained for diseases such as Parkinson's disease and multiple sclerosis.[113 114] Neuropsychological assessments are also used to identify specific patterns of cognitive deficits associated with Alzheimer's disease and other degenerative dementias.[115-118] In particular, attempts have been made to differentiate various subgroups existing within a category of dementing disorders. The long term aim is to further the understanding of the disease, in particular with regard to early diagnosis and the possibility of pharmacological intervention.[119 120]

Theoretically driven neuropsychological research has proved to be of fundamental importance in the study of the organisation of cerebral functions in the brain and especially in the understanding of normal cognitive functioning. Cognitive neuropsychological single case studies have been used as a legitimate type of evidence to support or criticise information processing models of normal cognition. Furthermore they can provide valuable findings that constrain the development of new theories. Over the years the neuropsychological literature has grown immensely. New cognitive deficits have been identified and important advances have been made in the understanding of the relations between components of complex cognitive skills and the loci of brain lesions. The neuropsychologist's strategy is to harness and incorporate the findings of research investigations to a clinical problem in the form of more specific and more sensitive tests of cognitive function. These improved quantitative techniques for clinical assessment can bring to light new phenomena that in turn promote further theoretical advances.

Summary

Neuropsychological assessment involves the investigation of the cognitive functions of patients with suspected or confirmed cerebral disease. There are three theoretical principles which underlie neuropsychological assessment:

- That the cerebral cortex has a high degree of functional specialisation
- That complex cognitive skills are organised in a broadly modular fashion
- That brain damage can disrupt these cognitive skills selectively.

These theoretical principles underpin the interpretation of the performance on neuropsychological tasks of patients with cerebral damage. A person's neuropsychological investigation should include comprehensive assessments of a wide variety of cognitive functions such as: premorbid ability; general intellectual level; memory; language; calculation; problem solving; alertness and attention, and visual and space perception. Ideally, standardised tests should be used which are: *reliable,* in the same circumstances they produce the same results, *valid,* they measure what they are designed to measure, *of comparable difficulty,* they permit comparison across tasks and, *sensitive to change,* they are graded in difficulty so that changes in cognitive functioning can be monitored and uninformative ceiling and floor effects avoided.

Neuropsychological assessment provides information that is useful for:

Diagnosis—For example, neuropsychological assessment has a key role in differentiating between organic and functional disorders. In addition, neuropsychological assessment can identify the presymptomatic cognitive impairments in familial neurodegenrative conditions.

Treatment and management—Successive neuropsychological examinations are helpful in monitoring the various treatments associated with epilepsy, Parkinson's disease, and hydrocephalus, and the rehabilitation of stroke and head injury patients.

Research—In applied research, "batteries" of neuropsychological tests are given to describe the cognitive profiles associated with Parkinson's disease, multiple sclerosis, Alzheimer's disease, and other degenerative dementias. In theoretical research neuropsychology has proved to be of fundamental importance in the study of the organisation of cerebral functions in the brain and especially in the understanding of normal cognitive functioning.

1 Broca P. Remarques sur le siège de la faculté du langage articulé suivié d'une observation d'aphemie. *Bulletin de la Societé d'Anatomie Paris* 1861;6:330. (Translated in Herrnstein R, Boring EG. *A source book in the history of psychology*. Cambridge, MA: Harvard University Press, 1965.)
2 Wernicke K. Der aphasische Symptomenkomplex. Breslau. (Translated in: *Boston studies in philosophy of science* 1874;4:34–97.)
3 Dejerine J. Contribution a l'étude anatomoclinique et clinique des differentes varietés de cecite verbal. *CR Hebdomadaire des Scances et Memoires de la Societe de Biologie* 1892;4:61–90.
4 Henschen SE. *Klinische und anatomische Betrag zur Pathologie des Gehirns*. Stockholm: Nordiske Bokhandein, 1920.
5 Lissauer H. Ein Fall von Seelenblindheit nebst einem Beitrag zur Theorie derselben. *Archiv fur Psychiatrie* 1890;21:222–270. (Edited and reprinted in translation by M Jackson, Lissauer on agnosia. *Cognitive Neuropsychology* 1988;5:155–92.)
6 Korsakoff SS. Uber eine besondere Form psychischer Storung combiniert mit multipler Neuritis. *Archiv fur Psychiatrie und Nervenkrankheiten* 1889;21:669–704.
7 Shallice T. *From neuropsychology to mental structure*. New York: Cambridge University Press, 1988.
8 Wechsler DA. *Wechsler-Bellevue intelligence scales*. New York: Psychological Corporation, 1939.
9 Wechsler DA. A standardized memory scale for clinical use. *J Psychol* 1945;19:87–95.
10 Raven JC. *Standard progressive matrices*. London: H K Lewis, 1938.
11 Raven JC. *Coloured progressive matrices*. London: H K Lewis, 1956.
12 Lezak MD. *Neuropsychological assessment*. 2nd ed. New York: Oxford University Press, 1983.
13 Crawford JR, Parker DM, McKinlay WW. *A handbook of neuropsychological assessment*. Hove, UK: Erlbaum, 1992.
14 Hodges JR. *Cognitive assessment for clinicians*. Oxford: Oxford University Press, 1994.
15 McKenna P, Warrington EK. The analytical approach to neuropsychological assessment. In: Grant I, Adams KM, eds. *Neuropsychological assessment of neuropsychiatric disorders*. New York: Oxford University Press, 1986:31–47.
16 Gall F, Spurzheim G. Research on the nervous system in general and on that of the brain in particular. 1809. (Reprinted in: Pribram K, ed. *Brain and behaviour: Vol 1. Mood states and mind*. Harmondsworth: Penguin Books, 1969.)

17 Bastian HC. *Aphasia and other speech defects*. London: Lewis, 1898.
18 Jackson JH. Case of large cerebral tumor without optic neuritis and with left hemiplegia and imperception. *Royal Opthalmological Hospital Reports* 1876;**8**:434–44.
19 Lichtheim L. On aphasia. *Brain* 1885;**7**:433–84.
20 Freud S. *Zur Auffassung der Aphasien*. Vienna: Deuticke, 1891.
21 Marie P. Révision de la question de l'aphasie: la troisième convolution frontale gauche ne joue aucun role spéciale dans la fonction du langage. *Semaine Medicale* 1906;**21**:241–7. (Reprinted in Cole MF, Cole M, eds. *Pierre Marie's papers on speech disorders*. New York: Hafner, 1971.)
22 Head H. *Aphasia and kindred disorders of speech*. Cambridge: Cambridge University Press, 1926.
23 Goldstein K. *Language and language disturbances*. New York: Grune and Stratton, 1948.
24 Lashley KS. *Brain mechanisms and intelligence*. Chicago: University of Chicago Press, 1929.
25 Kandel ER, Schwartz JH, Jessell TM. *Principles of neural science*. 3rd ed. New York: Elsevier, 1991.
26 Marr D. *Vision*. San Francisco, CA: Freeman, 1982.
27 Chomsky N. Rules and representations. *Behavioral and Brain Sciences* 1980;**3**:1–61.
28 Morton J. The status of information processing models of language. *Philos Trans Roy Soc Lond Biol* 1981;**295**:387–96.
29 Fodor JA. *The modularity of mind*. Cambridge, MA: MIT Press, 1983.
30 Zeki S, Lamb M. The neurology of kinetic art. *Brain* 1994;**117**:607–36.
31 McCarthy RA, Warrington EK. *Cognitive neuropsychology*. New York: Academic Press, 1990.
32 McCloskey M. Cognitive mechanisms in numerical processing: evidence from acquired dyscalculia. *Cognition* 1992;**44**:107–57.
33 Newman SK, Warrington EK, Kennedy AM, Rossor MN. The earliest cognitive change in a person with familial Alzheimer's disease: presymptomatic neuropsychological features in a pedigree with familial Alzheimer's disease confirmed at necropsy. *J Neurol Neurosurg Psychiatry* 1994;**57**:967–72.
34 Matarazzi JD. *Wechsler's measurement and appraisal of adult intelligence*. 5th ed. Baltimore: Williams and Wilkins, 1972.
35 Crawford JR. Current and premorbid intelligence measures in neuropsychological assessment. In: Crawford JR, Parker DM, McKinley WW, eds. *A handbook of neuropsychological assessment*. Hove, UK: Erlbaum, 1992:21–49.
36 Yates AJ. The use of vocabulary in the measurement of intellectual deterioration. *Journal of Mental Science* 1956;**102**:409–40.
37 Nelson HE, McKenna P. The use of current reading ability in the assessment of dementia. *Br J Soc Clin Psychol* 1975;**14**:259–67.
38 Schonell F. *Backwardness in the basic subjects*. London: Oliver and Boyd, 1942.
39 Nelson HE, O'Connell A. Dementia: the estimation of premorbid intelligence levels using the new adult reading test. *Cortex* 1978;**14**:234–44.
40 Stern W. *Psychologische Methoden der Intelligenz—Prüfung*. Leipzig: Barth, 1912.
41 Nelson HE. *The national adult reading test*. Windsor: NFER-Nelson, 1991.
42 Grober E, Sliwinski M. Development and validation of a model for estimating premorbid verbal intelligence in the elderly. *J Clin Exp Neuropsychol* 1991;**13**:933–49.
43 Patterson K, Graham N, Hodges JR. Reading in Alzheimer's type dementia: a preserved ability? *Neuropsychology* 1994;**8**:395–407.
44 Spearman C. *The abilities of man*. New York: Macmillan, 1927.
45 Thurstone LL. *Primary mental abilities*. Chicago: University of Chicago Press, 1938.
46 Guilford JP. The structure of intellect. *Psychol Bull* 1956;**53**:267–93.
47 Cattell RB. The measurement of adult intelligence. *Psychol Bull* 1943;**40**:153–93.
48 Raven JC. *Advanced progressive matrices, sets I and II*. London: H K Lewis, 1965.
49 Carpenter PA, Just MA, Shell P. What one intelligence test measures: a theoretical account of the processing in the Raven progressive matrices test. *Psychol Rev* 1990;**97**:404–31.
50 Bolin BJ. A comparison of Raven's progressive matrices (1938) with the ACE psychological examination and the Otis gamma mental ability test. *J Consult Psychol* 1955;**19**:400.
51 Wechsler DA. *The Wechsler adult intelligence scale: manual*. New York: Psychological Corporation, 1955.
52 Wechsler DA. *The measurement and appraisal of adult intelligence*. 4th ed. Baltimore:

Williams and Wilkins, 1958.

53 Bornstein RA, Matarazzo JD. Wechsler VIQ versus PIQ differences in cerebral dysfunction: a literature review with emphasis on sex differences. *Journal of Clinical Neuropsychology* 1982;4:319–34.

54 Warrington EK, James M, Maciejewski C. The WAIS as a lateralising and localising diagnostic instrument: a study of 656 patients with unilateral cerebral lesions. *Neuropsychologia* 1986;24:223–39.

55 Ryan JJ, Paolo AM, Brungardt TM. Standardization of the Wechsler adult intelligence scale-revised for persons 75 years and older. *Psychological Assessments: A Journal of Consulting and Clinical Psychology* 1990;2:408–11.

56 Baddeley AD. *Human memory theory and practice*. Hove, UK: Erlbaum, 1990.

57 Schacter DL. Implicit memory: history and current status. *J Exp Psychol Gen* 1987;13: 501–18.

58 Warrington EK, Weiskrantz L. Amnesia: consolidation or retrieval? *Nature* 1970; 228:628–30.

59 Tulving E. Episodic and semantic memory. In: Tulving E, Donaldson W, eds. *Organization of memory*. New York: Academic Press, 1972:382–404.

60 Corsi P. *Interhemispheric differences in the localization of psychological processes in man* [thesis]. University of Montreal, Montreal, 1972.

61 Gathercole SE, McCarthy RA. *Memory tests and techniques*. Hove, UK: Erlbaum, 1994.

62 Coughlan AK, Hollows SE. *The adult memory and information processing battery*. St James's University Hospital, Leeds: A K Coughlan, 1985.

63 Wilson BA, Cockburn J, Baddeley AD. *The Rivermead behavioural memory test*. Bury St Edmunds, UK: Thames Valley Test Company, 1985.

64 Rey A. *L'examen clinique en psychologie*. Paris: Presses Universitaires de France, 1964.

65 Osterreith PA. Le test de copie d'une figure complexe. *Archives de Psychologies* 1944; 30:206–356.

66 Benton AL. *The revised visual retention test*. New York: Psychological Corporation, 1974.

67 Warrington EK. *Recognition memory test*. Windsor, UK: NFER-Nelson, 1984.

68 Clegg F, Warrington EK. Four easy memory tests for older adults. *Memory* 1994; 2:167–82.

69 Kopelman MD, Wilson BA, Baddeley AD. The autobiographical memory interview: a new assessment of autobiographical and personal semantic memory in amnesic patients. *J Clin Exp Neuropsychol* 1989;11:724–44.

70 Warrington EK. The selective impairment of semantic memory. *Q J Exp Psychol* 1975; 27:635–57.

71 Howard D, Patterson KE. *Pyramids and palm trees*. Bury St Edmunds, UK: Thames Valley Test Company, 1992.

72 Dunn LM, Dunn LM, Whetton C, Pintilie D. *The British picture vocabulary scale*. Windsor, UK: NFER-Nelson, 1982.

73 Lesser R. *Linguistic investigations of aphasia*. London: Arnold, 1978.

74 Gainotti G, Caltagirone C, Ibba A. Semantic and phonemic aspects of auditory language comprehension in aphasia. *Linguistics* 1975;154/155:15–29.

75 Miceli G, Gainotti G, Caltagirone C, Masullo C. Some aspects of phonological impairment in aphasia. *Brain Lang* 1980;11:159–69.

76 Goodglass H, Kaplan E. *The assessment of aphasia and related disorders*. Philadelphia, PA: Lea and Febiger, 1972.

77 Kertesz A. *Western aphasia battery*. San Antonio: The Psychological Corporation Inc, 1982.

78 Porch BE. *The Porch index of communicative ability*—theory and development. Palo Alto, USA: Consulting Psychologists Press, 1967 (revised 1971).

79 De Bleser R, Bayer J, Luzzatti C. Die cognitive Neuropsychologie der Schriftsprache. Ein Überblick zwei deutscher Fallbeschreibungen. In: Bayer J, ed. *Grammatik und Cognition. Linguistische Berichte*, Suppl 1. Wiesbaden: Westdeutscher Verlag, 1987:118–62.

80 Caramazza A. The logic of neuropsychological research and the problem of patient classification in aphasia. *Brain Lang* 1984;21:9–20.

81 Auerbach SH, Allard T, Naeser M, Alexander MP, Albert ML. Pure word deafness: an analysis of a case with bilateral lesions and a deficit at the pre-phonemic level. *Brain* 1982;105:271–300.

82 McCarthy RA, Warrington EK. Disorders of semantic memory. *Philos Trans Roy Soc Lond Biol* 1994;346:89–96.

83 Coughlan AK, Warrington EK. Word-comprehension and word-retrieval in patients with localised cerebral lesions. *Brain* 1978;**101**:163–85.
84 Kay J, Lesser R, Coltheart M. *PALPA psycholinguistic assessments of language processing in aphasia.* Hove, UK: Erlbaum, 1992.
85 De Renzi E, Vignolo LA. The token test: a sensitive test to detect receptive disturbances in aphasia. *Brain* 1962;**85**:665–78.
86 Parisi D, Pizzamiglio L. Syntactic comprehension in aphasia. *Cortex* 1970;**6**:204–15.
87 Lesser R. Verbal comprehension in aphasia: an English version of three Italian tests. *Cortex* 1974;**10**:247–63.
88 Bishop D. *Test for reception of grammar.* Oxford: Thomas Leach, 1982.
89 McKenna P, Warrington EK. *The graded naming test.* Windsor, UK: NFER-Nelson, 1980.
90 Kaplan E, Goodglass H, Weintraub S. *Boston naming test* Philadelphia: Lea and Febinger, 1983.
91 De Renzi E, Ferrari C. The reporter's test: a sensitive test to detect expressive disturbances in aphasics. *Cortex* 1978;**14**:279–93.
92 Shallice T, Warrington EK. Single and multiple component central dyslexic syndromes. In: Coltheart M, Patterson KE, Marshall JC, eds. *Deep dyslexia.* London: Routledge and Kegan Paul, 1980:119–45.
93 Marshall JC, Newcombe F. Patterns of paralexia: a psycholinguistic approach. *J Psycholinguist Res* 1973;**2**:175–99.
94 Warrington EK, Cipolotti L, McNeil J. Attentional dyslexia: a single case study. *Neuropsychologia* 1993;**31**:871–85.
95 Neale MD. *The Neale analysis of reading ability.* 2nd ed. London: Macmillan, 1966.
96 Beauvois M-F, Derouesne J. Phonological alexia: three dissociations. *J Neurol Neurosurg Psychiatry* 1979;**42**:1115–24.
97 Baxter DM, Warrington EK. Measuring dysgraphia: a graded-difficulty spelling test (GDST). *Behavioural Neurology* 1994;**71**:107–16.
98 Shallice T. Phonological agraphia and the lexical route in writing. *Brain* 1981;**104**:413–29.
99 Miller E. Cognitive assessment of the older adult. In: Birren JE, Sloane RB, eds. *Handbook of mental health and ageing.* Engelwood Cliffs, NJ: Prentice-Hall, 1980.
100 Kendrick DC. *Kendrick cognitive tests for the elderly.* Windsor, UK: NFER- Nelson, 1985.
101 Caine ED. Pseudodementia: current concepts and future directions. *Arch Gen Psychiatry* 1981;**38**:1359–64.
102 Strub RL, Black FW. *Mental status examination in neurology.* 2nd ed. Philadelphia, PA: Davis, 1985.
103 Godwin-Austin RB. A case of visual disorientation. *J Neurol Neurosurg Psychiatry* 1965;**28**:453–8.
104 Warrington EK, Weiskrantz L. New method of testing long-term retention with special reference to amnesic patients. *Nature* 1968;**277**:972–4.
105 Rossor MN. Management of neurological disorders: dementia. *J Neurol Neurosurg Psychiatry* 1994;**57**:1451–6.
106 Coughlan AK, Hollows SE. The use of memory tests in differentiating organic disorder from depression. *Br J Psychol* 1984;**145**:164–7.
107 Bennett T, Curiel M. Early neuropsychological presentation of Huntington's disease. *Int J Clin Neuropsychol* 1989;**11**:90–5.
108 Willison JR, Warrington EK. Cognitive retardation in a patient with preservation of psychomotor speed. *Behavioural Neurology* 1992;**5**:113–6.
109 Goldstein H. Neuropsychological investigation of temporal lobe epilepsy. *J R Soc Med* 1991;**84**:460–5.
110 Jones-Gotman M. Localization of lesions by neuropsychological testing. *Epilepsia* 1991;**32**(suppl 5):S41–52.
111 McKinlay WW. Assessment of the head-injured for compensation. In: Crawford JR, Parker DM, McKinlay WW, eds. *A handbook of neuropsychological assessment.* Hove, UK: Erlbaum, 1992:381–92.
112 Miller H. Mental after effects of head injury. *Proceedings of the Royal Society of Medicine* 1966;**59**:257–61.
113 Lees J, Smith E. Cognitive deficits in the early stages of Parkinson's disease. *Brain* 1983;**106**:257–270.
114 Grant I, McDonald WI, Trimble MR, Smith E, Reed R. Deficient learning and memory

in early and middle phases of multiple sclerosis. *J Neurol Neurosurg Psychiatry* 1984;**47**:250–5.
115 Cummings J, Benson D, Read S. Aphasia in dementia of the Alzheimer type. *Neurology* 1985;**35**:394–7.
116 Spinnler H, Della Sala S. The role of clinical neuropsychology in the neurological diagnosis of Alzheimer's disease. *J Neurol* 1988;**235**:258–71.
117 Haxby J, Grady C, Koss E, *et al.* Longitudinal study of cerebral metabolic asymmetries and associated neuropsychological patterns in early dementia of the Alzheimer-type. *Arch Neurol* 1990;**47**:753–60.
118 Swearer J, O'Donnell B, Drachman D, Woodward B. Neuropsychological features of familial Alzheimer's disease. *Ann Neurol* 1992;**32**:687–94.
119 Martin A. Neuropsychology of Alzheimer's disease: the case for subgroups. In: Schwartz M, ed. *Modular deficits in Alzheimer type dementia.* Cambridge, MA: MIT Press, 1990:143–75.
120 Rossor MN, Kennedy AK, Newman S. Heterogeneity of familial Alzheimer's disease. In: Boller F, Forette F, Khachaturian Z, eds. *Heterogeneity of Alzheimer's disease.* Berlin: Springer-Verlag, 1992:81–7.

7 Vision

J F ACHESON, M D SANDERS

Before the era of scientific medicine the eye was the window to the soul, and after the invention of the ophthalmoscope, the eye became the window to the brain. Now, in the 1990s, the "decade of the brain", it is no exaggeration to say that it is the neurobiology of the visual sensory apparatus as a whole and not just the eye which offers a window to the brain. As visual function is now increasingly understood in terms of the parallel processing of streams of data concerning form, colour, and motion in parvocellular and magnocellular systems, so is modern clinical practice increasingly based on these concepts. This article offers a guide based on current practice to the clinician faced with a patient with an apparently normal eye but who has poor vision and who therefore starts to cross the threshold from ophthalmology into neurology.[1]

Visual acuity testing

Although acuity testing only measures the central 1 to 2° of field at 100% contrast, this measurement of visual health is almost universally understood and changing levels of performance measured in this way sometimes assume great medicolegal significance. The physiological basis and shortcomings in clinical practice may be less widely appreciated. The minimal resolvable or ordinary acuity is most applicable to everyday practice, involving the correct identification of a target characteristic. In health, there is a remarkable concordance between the observed minimal angle of resolution and the expected resolving capacity of the eye's optics. In disease, the observed minimal angle of resolution will drop not only as a result of defects in optical imagery, but also where abnormalities arise in foveal fixation, photoreceptor structure and function, photopic luminance levels, and full integrity of the neural pathways.[23]

The purest visual acuity test uses a square wave grating comprising black and white stripes of equal width. An acuity of 6/6 equates to a grating made up of stripes each subtending 1 minute of arc at the testing distance, so that the separation between two black and two white stripes is 1 minute; pairs of stripes must therefore be repeated 30 times to subtend a visual angle of 1°. This is termed the spatial frequency and is measured in cycles/degree; the narrower the stripes the higher the spatial frequency. The highest frequency grating which elicits a response is the measure of the visual acuity. Table 7.1 shows the correlation between Snellen values, stripe width, and spatial frequency.

Grating acuities have been shown to be superior to visual acuity based on optotypes especially when there is foveal pathology or dense amblyopia. The stripes can be presented on a TV screen and form the basis for the objective measurement of acuity using optokinetic nystagmus (rotating striped drum to elicit eye movements), visually evoked cortical potentials, and preferential looking techniques. Grating acuity techniques are in standard use in visual science and in the clinical assessment of visual function in infants (figure 7.1).

For the remainder of clinical practice, acuity is measured by presenting a selection of ordinary, recognisable targets or optotypes for the subject to choose between so that guessing is eliminated. A variety of optotype patterns can be used for the determination of the minimal resolvable acuity. The most familiar

Table 7.1   Visual acuity and grating acuity equivalents.

Acuity (m)	Acuity (feet)	Spatial frequency	Stripe width (mm)
6/6	20/20	30 cycles/°	1
6/12	20/40	15	2
6/30	20/100	6	5
6/60	20/200	3	10

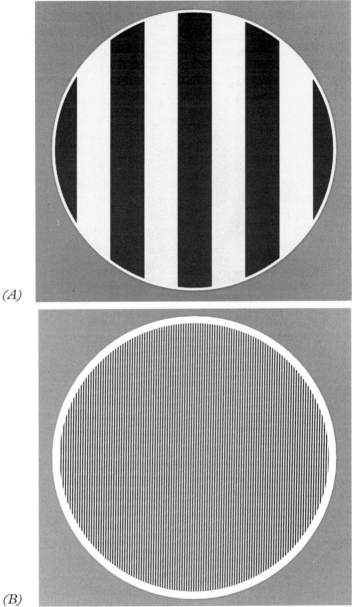

(A)

(B)

Figure 7.1   *Contrast gratings used to obtain grating acuities. (A) 0·29 cycles/° at 38 cm, about equivalent to a Snellen acuity of 6/620. (B) 7·7 cycles/° at 38 cm, about equivalent to a Snellen acuity of 6/24*

is the Snellen chart in which the standard pattern is enlarged so that resolution is achieved (figure 7.2). For a normal observer in best focus the resolution limit is 30 to 60 seconds of arc. The E optotype for 6/6 vision (which uses a sans serif or Gothic typeface) subtends 5 minutes of arc vertically and horizontally, and 1 minute between each stroke when viewed at 6 m (or 20 feet). If the subject can only see at a distance of 6 m an optotype which

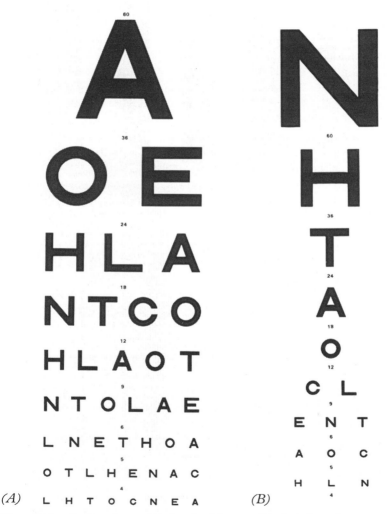

Figure 7.2   *Snellen charts. (A) Standard format. (B) single letter format*

207

would subtend 1 minute of arc at 9 m, then the acuity is said to be 6/9 and so on through to 6/60. Sometimes it is convenient to express acuity in terms of visual efficiency scores (for example, in medicolegal work) or as Snellen ratios (for example, when entering acuity data into automated perimetry equipment) (see table 7.2).

Because some optotypes are easier to see than others, single letter charts have some advantages particularly when assessing patients with cognitive or reading difficulties. In the Landolt C test, the subject must identify the orientation of the C by finding the side of the gap in the curve and in the E test for illiterate patients the direction of the bars must be recognised. If the minimal resolvable optotype size is 1 minute of arc then the acuity is said to be 6/6. These tasks may be easier to perform than that of reading a standard Snellen line alone and are not strictly equivalent. Although the Snellen chart is well understood, the patient's performance may vary simply because of poor illumination and variable optotype complexity. As a general rule the smallest line that the patient can read is used to quantify visual acuity—one or two mistakes per line are often allowed. Changes in visual acuity over time are reported in units of "number of lines lost or gained". This method is subject to a number of limitations: as each line becomes smaller the number of letters becomes greater and therefore harder to read; a two line loss from 6/20 to 6/60 is a tripling of the visual angle but a two line loss from 6/5 to 6/9 is less than double the visual angle and therefore is not comparable. In terms of visual pathophysiology, there may only be a weak correlation between the level of underperformance on a Snellen chart and the level of dysfunction of the visual apparatus and it is not correct to say that an eye with a Snellen fraction of 0·25 (6/24) has a disease process twice as severe as one with a fraction of 0·5 (6/12).

For these reasons the "Logmar" chart is preferable. The working distance is 4 m. Each letter on a line has uniform difficulty, there are the same number of letters on each line, and the size increase from one line to the next is governed by a simple geometrical progression of the log of the minimal angle of resolution (Logmar). In conjunction with standardised illumination systems Logmar charts were first introduced into ophthalmology in 1982 for the Early Treatment of Diabetic Retinopathy Trial and other multicentre prospective trials and are now widely used in clinical practice where accurate follow up data are required (figure 7.3).[4][5]

Table 7.2 Visual acuity equivalents in different notations

Minutes of arc (minimal angle of resolution: MAR)	Logmar	Snellen acuity at 4 m	Snellen acuity at 20 feet	Snellen acuity at 6 m	Visual efficiency (%)	Snellen fraction
0·75	− 0·1	4/3·2	20/15	6/4·5	104	1·33
1·0	0·0	4/4	20/16	6/5	100	1·0
1·25	+ 0·1	4/5	20/20	6/6	96	0·8
1·5			20/25	6/7·5	91	0·67
			20/30	6/9		
			20/32	6/10		
2·0	+ 0·2	4/6·3	20/40	6/12	84	0·5
2·5	+ 0·3	4/8	20/50	6/15	76	0·4
3·0	+ 0·4	4/10	20/60	6/18	70	0·33
			20/63	6/20		
4·0	+ 0·5	4/12·6	20/80	6/24	58	0·25
5·0	+ 0·6	4/16	20/100	6/30	49	0·2
6·0	+ 0·7	4/20	20/120	6/36	41	0·17
			20/125	6/38		
7·5	+ 0·8	4/25	20/160	6/45	31	0·133
				6/48		
10·0	+ 0·9	4/32	20/200	6/60	20	0·10
20·0	+ 1·0	4/40	20/400	6/120 (3/60)	3	0·05

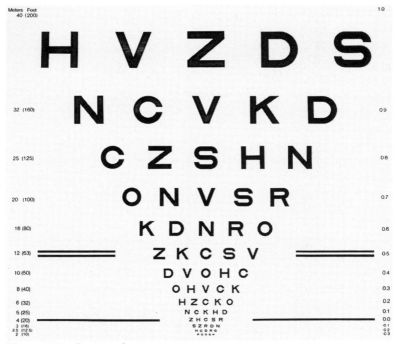

Figure 7.3   *Logmar chart*

Near vision testing

It is often extremely useful to determine acuity for near as well as for distance as some patients experience difficulty in reading out of proportion to their Snellen acuity as a result of parafoveal scotomata (for example, macular degeneration) or to poor foveal fixation in certain eye movement disorders (for example, jerk nystagmus), which prevent the whole word being seen at the same time. The postfixational blindness of a dense bitemporal hemianopia may also be detected by this method, as may cerebral dyslexia. In the United Kingdom, the current standard notation used is the N system where text printed in the Times Roman font is expressed in font sizes as points (multiples of 1/72nd of an inch) and the reading acuity is denoted as the minimum size comfortably seen at a normal reading distance (33 cm) with presbyopic correction when appropriate. This is likely to be replaced by reading versions of the Snellen and Logmar charts in the near future.

210

Factors influencing visual acuity (box 7.1)

To achieve peak performance, referred to as normal visual acuity, all optical, anatomical, and physiological elements must themselves perform normally. For example, acuity is readily degraded by refractive error so that 1 dioptre of defocus will reduce the Snellen fraction to about 0·3. Young hypermetropes (hyperopes) can accommodate to overcome their own refractive error, but myopes and presbyopes cannot. A pinhole is a very helpful method of determining whether acuity is due to refractive error rather than ocular pathology or neurological disease. It is important to remember that a pinhole, however, will only correct to 6/6 up to a maximum of 4 dioptres of spherical and cylindrical error and that an up to date refraction is essential in all cases of unexplained visual loss. Optical quality also depends on pupil size: visual acuity remains roughly constant in the range of 2·5 to 6 mm after which the minimal angle of resolution falls off. In elderly people, as pupil size diminishes and lenticular opacities increase the spatial resolution of the eye may fall even in the absence of specific pathological conditions.

Box 7.1   Testing visual acuity

- A pin-hole only corrects up to a maximum of 4 dioptres of spherical or cylindrical refractive error. Always ensure an accurate recent refraction before proceeding to expensive investigations of unexplained poor vision

- Use grating acuities or Logmar charts in clinical science

- Illiterate E or Lanholt C charts are useful when there are communication difficulties (for example, dysphasia, interpreter, illiteracy)

Pupillary light reflexes (box 7.2)

The assessment of afferent pupil defects is an important part of the neuro-ophthalmic examination and subtle abnormalities may often be clinically significant. A discussion of unequal pupils and efferent pupil defects is beyond the scope of this paper.

Box 7.2 Testing pupillary light reflexes

- Consensual responses and a relative afferent pupil defect can still be elicited when one eye has an abnormal iris (for example, intraocular surgery or penetrating eye injuries)
- The absence of a relative afferent pupil defect makes unilateral optic nerve disease unlikely

---

The pupil of an eye that is blind from retinal or optic nerve disease will fail to react directly to light but will constrict consensually when the other healthy eye is stimulated. The blind eye shows an afferent pupil defect. Much more commonly, however, a disease process will leave one eye with a degree of visual impairment and direct stimulation will still result in pupillary constriction. In these circumstances it is important to perform a swinging light test to look for a relative afferent pupillary defect (Marcus Gunn pupil). Relative afferent pupillary defects are best seen by moving a hand-held light from one eye to the other holding the light to each eye for about one second in a regular symmetric way. As the light shifts from the eye with normal vision to the eye with reduced vision, the direct light stimulus is no longer sufficient to keep both pupils small; thus they both dilate. The test is very quick and easy to perform and is sufficiently sensitive to detect residual optic nerve dysfunction after an episode of retrobular neuritis and recovery of acuity to 6/6. Only one working iris sphincter is necessary to perform this test. For example, a third nerve palsy or anterior ocular segment disruption as a result of trauma, inflammation, or surgery will not stop the examiner from observing the direct and consensual responses of the intact pupil as each is alternately stimulated. A dim side light is invaluable, especially in patients with dark irides, to observe the pupillary movements. The afferent pupil defect may also be quantified by using a series of neutral density filters over the good eye to reduce the stimulus to the point at which a balance is reached.

Afferent pupil defects are absent in functional visual loss and in lesions of the retinal macula, and are either absent or subtle when central visual loss is due to amblyopia. Optic nerve lesions, however, typically produce significant afferent defects and hence the test is of great value in cases of unexplained visual loss. When optic neuritis has been diagnosed and there is no relative afferent pupillary defect, the diagnosis is either wrong or else there is bilateral disease. The acronym PERLA standing for "pupils equal and reacting to light (and accommodation)" is often used in clinical notes but does not indicate whether the consensual reflex has been tested, or whether a relative afferent defect is present.

Colour vision (see boxes 7.3 and 7.4)

It is a characteristic of certain disorders of the anterior visual pathways that sensitivity to hue discrimination (colour vision) may be impaired whereas luminance and contrast based functions (acuity) are preserved.[67] At the level of retinal photoreceptors, colour vision is a function of three classes of cones of overlapping spectral sensitivities for red, green, and blue so that colours are represented by differential matching of the output of each group. At a neural level, colour vision is processed according to a colour-opponent code whereby certain colour pairs appear as mutually exclusive opposites such as red-green and blue-yellow. The physiological substrate for colour opponent encoding lies within the neural elements of the retina. In clinical terms, these concepts are reflected in the classification of congenital defects of colour vision according to whether one or more classes of photoreceptor are missing (dichromats and monochromats) or have anomolous sensitivity to specific wavelengths of light (anomalous trichromats). The inherited dyschromatopsias are binocular, symmetric, and do not change over time. Monochromats have major cone defects and also have poor acuity. Dichromats and anomalous trichromats have normal acuity.

Acquired dyschromatopsias are different from congenital defects in several respects. Firstly, they are noticeable to the observer. Secondly they may be monocular or even restricted to one part of the visual field. Thirdly, although colour defects may be much more pronounced than acuity defects, acuity is generally reduced to some degree. It is helpful to classify acquired defects of colour vision as follows:

According to Kollner's rule patients with neural disorders have a preponderance of damage to red-green discrimination with preservation of blue-yellow discrimination (type I and II defects), whereas those with retinal and choroidal disease may show selective loss of blue-yellow discrimination (type III defects). However, some optic neuropathies—especially those associated with pre-

213

served acuity—may show type III defects. Cones sensitive to blue are not found in the central 0·5° of the field, so that disease processes that selectively damage the extrafoveal visual field will leave the patient with normal acuity and normal red-green discrimination. Examples of this include glaucoma, dominant optic atrophy, chronic papilloedema, and early chloroquine retinal toxicity. More typically, optic neuropathies that involve the fibres of the papillomacular bundle such as retrobulbar neuritis, Leber's disease, and extrinsic compression will damage neural elements serving foveal function and green-red discrimination will be damaged, often out of proportion to acuity loss. Box 7.3 summarises the classifications of colour deficiency.

Box 7.3 Classification of colour deficiencies

Congenital colour deficiency	Red deficient	Green deficient	Blue deficient
Anomalous trichomats	Protanomal	Deuteranomal	Tritanomal
Dichromats	Protanope	Deuteranope	Tritanope
Monochromats	Blue-cone monchromats/rod monochromats		

Acquired colour deficiency	Alternative name	Hue discrimination defect	Visual acuity loss
Type I	Red/green "protan-like"	Red/green discrimination loss: preserved blue/yellow discrimination	Moderate to severe
Type II	Red/green "deutan-like"	Red/green discrimination loss plus mild blue/yellow impairment	Moderate to severe
Type III	Blue/yellow "tritan-like"	Blue-yellow confusion	Mild to moderate

---

Formal colour vision testing with spectral light sources graded for luminance changes is very demanding and time consuming, and not very practical in the clinical setting. Pseudoisochromatic plates are very widely used because of their portable nature, low cost, and ease of use. The plates consist of a series of dots of various colours and sizes that are clustered together into carefully arranged patterns of various hues. These hues can readily be distinguished by normal trichromats but not by those with defective colour vision. The patterns form highly legible figures that are visible even to those with poor acuity. An initial test plate excludes subjects whose acuity or reading skills do not allow them to perform the test. Commercially available pseudoisochromatic plates (Ishihara and Hardy, Ritter, Read (HRR) plates) are designed to detect those with congenital dyschromatopsias, but do not allow protan-deutran distinctions or the separation of anomalous trichromats from dichromats. They may be used in the qualitative assessment of acquired colour defects. A greater quantitative element is supplied by the Farnsworth-Munsell 100 hue test in which the subject is required to arrange a series of coloured discs in sequence between pairs of reference discs.[6] The order of discs is then plotted in a circular diagram so that the degree of error is represented by points far away from the centre of the diagram. Characteristic patterns for errors along the red-green and blue-yellow axis will emerge allowing full characterisation of the dyschromatopsia. Even with automated, computer assisted versions, this test remains inconvenient and time consuming and is not greatly used. The Farnsworth D-15 (dichotomous) panel test simplifies matters by recording confusions in the allocation of non-adjacent hues into their correct colour grouping.

Other techniques include the Pickford-Nicholson anomaloscope in which the subject views a translucent panel through a monocular objective and has to match pairs of coloured lights. A more modern alternative is provided by computer assisted colour contrast sensitivity systems in which standard optotypes are presented in colour against a coloured background and the contrast thresholds measured in each of the colour confusion axes. It is likely that in many clinics a psychophysical central vision assessment package can be used where thresholds for acuity tasks, contrast sensitivity, and colour contrast sensitivity can all be presented in a sequence of quick user friendly formats with a microprocessor and standard computer monitor.[7]

Box 7.4   Testing colour vision

- Colour vision defects appear early in the course of optic nerve disease (even when Snellen acuity is normal)

- The subjective appreciation of colour desaturation between one eye and the other (or between different parts of the visual field: see below) is a very sensitive qualitative test of colour vision

- Ishihara plates are a useful semiquantitative guide to the integrity of colour vision but are less sensitive than testing subjective colour desaturation

---

Visual field testing

The analysis of the visual fields retains central importance in the localisation of defects in the visual system, and for monitoring the natural history of a condition and responses to treatment.[8] Simple confrontation testing (qualitative) remains useful in clinic based and bedside topical diagnosis, but semiquantitative and quantitative methods are essential for accurate documentation, detection of more subtle defects, and for assessing progress. The diagnostic value of field testing rests on the principle of the retinotopic organisation of the afferent visual system whereby nerve fibres from retinal ganglion cells serving defined parts of the visual field project in an anatomically consistent arrangement. Fibres from the inferior retina pass inferiorly in the optic nerve and chiasm. Fibres serving central vision (the papillomacular bundle) tend to move from the temporal or lateral side of the optic nerve anteriorly to occupy the central core posteriorly. As these fibres make up most fibres in the optic nerve, the hallmark of optic nerve lesions is a central scotoma, together with acuity loss and defects in colour vision. At the chiasm, fibres deriving from retinal elements serving the nasal hemiretina move centrally to decussate with those serving the upper temporal field looping anteriorly into the distal contralateral optic nerve (von Willbrand's knee) before passing into the contralateral optic tract. Crossing fibres at the chiasm seem to be more sensitive to pathological processes than non-crossing fibres and the hallmark of chiasmal disease is the bitemporal hemianopia or one of its variants. It is at the chiasm that the visual system becomes functionally divided about the vertical through the fixation point (represented in the fundus by the fovea, not the optic nerve head). At the chiasm and posteriorly in projections throughout the optic radiations to the cortex, the lateral separation of blended hemifields from each side is inviolate. In any technique of assessing the visual field for suspected abnormalities of the visual pathways it is therefore essential to pay close attention to the vertical meridian. As a rule monocular field defects which are monocular with a central, peripheral, horizontal, or arcuate pattern are due to lesions anterior to the chiasm, whereas defects which are homonymous and respect the vertical meridian relate to lesions of the chiasm or posterior visual pathways.

In testing the visual field it is helpful to employ Traquair's analogy of the hill of vision. The field is represented as a three dimensional hill with the base plane representing the horizontal and vertical dimensions of visual space and the hill representing the sensitivity of the retina to stimulation by a focal light at different places. At the pinnacle of the hill is the fovea where even the dimmest and smallest target can be detected. This concept allows for the representation of relative field loss as alteration in the slope of the hill, as well as constriction ("coast erosion") and absolute loss (the blind spot, for example). Lines joining points of equal sensitivity are isopters, and using the standard manual perimeter (Goldmann), the isopters are determined either by moving a spot of light from periphery to centre until it hits the hill and is perceived (kinetic testing), or by increasing the intensity of stimulus at one spot until threshold is reached (static testing). The concept of the hill of vision is also useful in confrontation testing, in which relative defects can be detected by eliciting differential brightness of say a hand, or a red bottle top in opposite hemifields. In obtunded patients an involuntary saccadic eye movement to fixate on a peripherally placed stimulus may serve as a sensitive test.

In quantitative perimetry the task is always hampered by the need for highly trained and experienced perimetrists who can reliably distinguish between pathology and artefact. Enormous efforts have been devoted to the task of replacing perimetrists with computers and now automated perimetry machines are widely available (figure 7.4).[9-11] These can now generate numerical indices of point by point deviations in retinal thresholds supported by reliability scores and by statistical analysis packages to help to determine the significance of any departure from age matched controls.

Box 7.5   Techniques for assessing the visual field

Method	Variants	Comments
Qualitative methods	Confrontation with fingers or neurological pin heads	
	Visually elicited eye movements	Infants and obtunded adults
	Finger mimicking	Preverbal children and dysphasic adults
	Hand and colour comparison	Children and adults
	Blinking to menace and flashing lights	Children and obtunded adults
Semiquantitative methods	Tangent screen perimetry (Bjerrum)	Very rapid: suitable for all patients with steady fixation. Good for topical diagnosis of neuro-ophthalamic disease
Quantitative methods	Goldmann kinetic and static perimetry	Standard reference method: very operator dependent
	Automated perimetry	Excellent for detecting early bitemporal defects. Unsuitable for ill patients, or those with poor· concentration, poor acuity, or functional visual loss

Ease of data storage and standardisation of presentation are advantages. With increasing sensitivity, however, specificity is lost. Although it is now possible to explore the visual field at the limits of complex physiological measurement—even to the extent of measuring differential function in ganglion cell subpopulations according to their motion detection and luminance functions—it is important to deploy strategies that support practical management decisions. Automated systems measuring static or motion

218

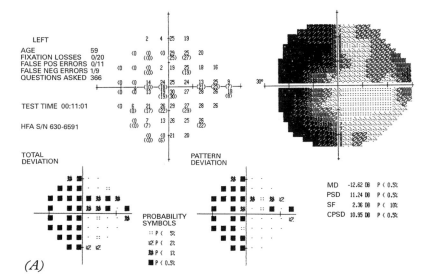

(A)

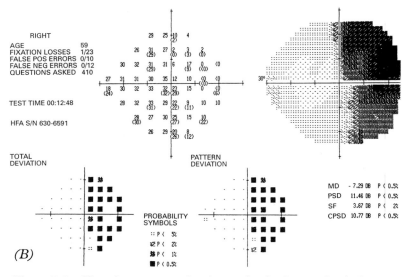

(B)

Figure 7.4   *Humphrey automated perimetry showing increased retinal thresholds to static testing in the central (24°) temporal hemifields of each eye representing a bitemporal hemianopia*

detection thresholds are primarily designed for the detection of subclinical disease states not detectable by confrontation, in particular early glaucomatous optic neuropathy and are not necessarily suitable for characterising patterns of field defect, which are so important in neuro-ophthalmic diagnosis.[12] Other problems include patient learning effects, physiological variation in field performance over time,[13-16] and fatigue.[17] Also, test strategies emphasise threshold changes across the horizontal meridian, but in neuro-ophthalmic assessment, the vertical meridian is of crucial diagnostic importance, and fixation testing strategies rely on repeated blind spot checking; this is of course lost in bitemporal defects with chiasmal disease.[18 19] Box 7.5 summarises these techniques for assessing the visual field.

Colour perimetry (box 7.6)

As described in the section on colour vision testing, acquired lesions of the optic nerve characteristically show chromatic defects that may precede luminance defects. It follows that in some circumstances colour visual field testing is more sensitive than using white test targets of differing sizes and light intensities. From Kollner's rule, optic neuropathies often manifest red-green discrimination defects which are readily picked up with a red target and confrontation methods ("in which hemifield is the colour brighter?"), especially with the tangent screen.

Box 7.6   Testing visual fields

- Tangent screen testing with a red target and testing subjective appreciation of hue differences across the vertical meridian are very sensitive semiquantitative tests

- Formal perimetry is essential for quantitative assessment and follow up. Automated perimetry is useful but fallible (in particular susceptible to patient learning effects, and poor concentration)

- Bitemporal hemianopias which respect the vertical meridian can only be produced by chiasmal lesions: bitemporal field defects which do not obey the vertical meridian can be produced by very large blind spots, caecocentral scotomas, retinal lesions, uncorrected refractive error, and overhanging eyelids

---

Fundoscopy: direct and indirect ophthalmoscopy, special techniques (see box 7.7)

The direct ophthalmoscope incorporates a light source focused directly on to the retina through a small angled mirror that fills either half or the whole of the aperture. The mirror centre is unsilvered so that the illuminated fundus can be seen through it. Between the returning light rays and the examiner's eye there is a revolving magazine of lenses that usually range from -30 to $+30$ dioptres to correct any inherent refractive error in either the patient or the examiner. In practice, it may be easier to view the fundus of a patient with a larger refractive error by leaving the glasses on and turning the ophthalmoscope lens to zero. Changing the ophthalmoscope lens power will also change the depth of focus within the eye and allow examination of media opacities, especially in the lens. The field of view with the direct ophthalmoscope is small, about 6° with a magnification of × 15; the image is erect and real. A green or "red free" filter is useful for examining nerve fibre detail, retinal vessels, haemorrhages, and microaneurysms. The examiner views the patient's right eye with his right eye and changes eyes to view the left. Pupillary dilatation with 1% tropicamide drops is essential for the best retinal view. The risk of precipitating an attack of acute angle closure glaucoma by using dilating drops is very low and is usually outweighed by the benefits of achieving an adequate view. Red-free (green) illumination is helpful to observe the retinal nerve fibre layer and note vascular

---

Box 7.7 Examining the fundus

- The use of tropicamide 1% to dilate the pupils can be essential to obtain an adequate view of the optic disc, and posterior and mid-peripheral retina

- This is only contraindicated in acute neurological illness where surgical intervention is a possibility (head injury for example). The risk of precipitating acute angle closure glaucoma is low

- Fluorescein angiography is useful in the elucidation of observed pathology but is seldom helpful when adequate fundoscopy is normal

abnormalities including haemorrhages, microneurysms, and vessel attenuation.

The direct ophthalmoscope, by virtue of its small field and high magnification, is very suitable for viewing the optic nerve head. When a wider field and an appreciation of stereoscopic depth detail is required, indirect ophthalmoscopy is used. In this technique a light source is directed into the eye and the reflected light is gathered by a hand held condensing lens to form a virtual inverted image of the retina. The size of the image varies according to the power of the condensing lens: the greater the power the smaller the image. A +13D lens magnifies the retina about four times and a +30D lens by two. Indirect ophthalmoscopy has the advantage of providing high intensity illumination, stereopsis, and a wide field of view as well as allowing dynamic assessment of vitreoretinal pathology. Disadvantages include the inverted image, the requirement for wide pupillary dilatation, and the considerable practice needed to master the technique.

Other methods for viewing the fundus require a slit lamp and are especially helpful in the assessment of stereo detail in macular pathology. These include fundus contact lenses and the non-contact Hruby and Volk lenses.

Fluorescein angiography

Fluorescein angiography provides an important adjunct to the ophthalmoscopy of diseases of the retina and the optic nerve head by showing evidence of disease activity and by providing a permanent record (figure 7.5). After an intravenous injection, a dilute solution of fluorescein in the blood will absorb blue light at a peak of 480 nm and emit it as green-yellow at a peak frequency of 530 nm. With appropriate filters on flash fundus photography the exciting blue light can be separated from the emitted light and the retinal and choroidal circulations studied. Dynamic studies of the passage of dye from the arterial to venous sides of the circulation in the two vascular beds are obtained. In the evaluation of optic disc swelling, true disc oedema can be distinguished from the pseudopapilloedema of buried optic disc drusen or elevated discs in hypermetropic eyes by demonstrating the presence of dilated capillaries on the disc surface during the arterial phase of the angiogram, and hyperfluorescence in the late venous phase. Also, buried disc drusen may fluoresce without any injection of dye—a phenomenon known as autofluorescence. This avoids unnecessary

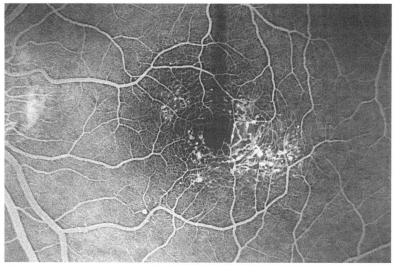

Figure 7.5   *Fundus fluorescein angiogram showing abnormal microvascular perfusion at the macula in a patient with central visual loss due to a branch retinal vein occlusion*

imaging and CSF studies, and even shunting procedures. Box 7.8 gives further examples.

It is important to remember that fluorescein angiography is an invasive study. Patients often experience nausea and occasionally vomit shortly after injection. They should be warned that the skin (but not the sclera) appears icteric for a few hours and that urine passed during this time will fluoresce. Rarely, hypersensitivity reactions occur—probably due to the presence of macromolecular impurities because fluorescein itself has a low molecular weight and does not provoke an antigen-antibody reaction. This usually takes the form of urticaria and transient bronchospasm but may occasionally give rise to anaphylactic shock. Full resuscitation equipment is mandatory and the investigation is contraindicated in patients with a history of asthma or adverse reactions to radiological contrast media.

Contrast sensitivity

In visual science contrast sensitivity forms the basis of one of the most important psychophysical methods for measuring visual

223

Box 7.8   Common indications for fluorescein angiography in neuro-ophthalmology

Clinical problem	Comment
Optic disc swelling	Distinction between true acquired pathological disc swelling of raised intracranial pressure or local disease and pseudopapilloedema of hypermetropic eyes, buried disc drusen, and other anomalies
Multifocal white matter lesions or unexplained optic neuropathy	Subtle or subclinical retinal vasculitis indicates an inflammatory cause (multiple sclerosis, sarcoidosis, or Behçet's)
Unexplained visual acuity loss with a central scotoma	Subtle macular pathology (age related macular degeneration, branch retinal vein occlusion, retinal dystrophies) well demonstrated
Unexplained neuro-muscular disease	Mild or severe forms of retinal pigment epithelial degeneration well shown in the mitochondrial myopathies (Kearns-Sayre syndrome)
Unexplained (aseptic) meningitis	Demonstration of choroidal abnormalities in the uveomeningeal syndromes (Vogt-Koyanagi-Harada disease), Behçet's sarcoidosis, non-Hodgkin's lymphoma, metastatic carcinoma)

function—for example, allowing the demonstration that neurons of the visual system are sensitive to limited ranges of spatial frequency and orientation. In clinical practice these methods allow the detection of otherwise subclinical pathology and offer a sensitive way of following up patients with chronic disease such as optic nerve function after an episode of optic neuritis (figure 7.6).

The patient who complains of "faded" vision but who has a normal (high contrast) Snellen acuity may have defects in contrast sensitivity.[20] The level of contrast at which a light and dark pattern is first discriminated is the contrast threshold. No consistent discrimination occurs for contrast below the subject's threshold for a particular spatial frequency. High and very low spatial frequencies require higher contrast for resolution. Contrast sensitivity is the reciprocal of the contrast threshold and is measured with sine wave (sinusoidal) gratings that show gradual change from light to dark. Measurement aims to record the patient's contrast threshold over a range of spatial frequencies with gratings of different contrast levels. Because two variables are involved (spatial frequency and contrast threshold) a graph is constructed that sets out the contrast threshold for each spatial frequency, and results in a contrast sensitivity curve. Pathological reduction in contrast sensitivity occurs in developmental and acquired visual defects when the contrast threshold can be raised for low, high, or all spatial frequencies depending on the underlying cause.

In formal systems, spatial vision is represented by sinusoidal or square wave gratings presented on a TV monitor with frequencies ranging between 0·1 and 25 cycles/°, with standardised visual angles of 5° height and 32° width and with additional counterphasing at a frequency of 0·6/s to prevent after images. User friendly book mounted and wall mounted charts are available—for example, the Vis Tech and Pelli-Robson systems.[21-24] In a Vis Tech chart photographs of sinusoidal gratings are presented and thresholds for different spatial frequencies are determined by the subject recognising the correct orientation of the stripes whereas in the simpler Pelli-Robson chart (figure 7.6) standard sized optotypes of uniform spatial frequency are presented with decreasing contrast as the patient reads along a line allowing threshold detection. Computer generated presentations have the advantage of a capability to assess temporal effects (loss of contrast sensitivity with time), and colour contrast sensitivity.[25-29]

Macular pathology and amblyopia

In all instances of deficient vision the clinician must ask whether the observed pathology matches the degree of visual loss. Normally this question lies within the province of the general ophthalmologist, but it is not unusual for a patient to have an apparently normal eye and yet still have poor vision raising the question of a retrobulbar optic neuropathy. Localisation to the optic nerve is supported by the presence of dyschromatopsia, a central scotoma or altitudinal field loss, and a relative afferent pupil defect.

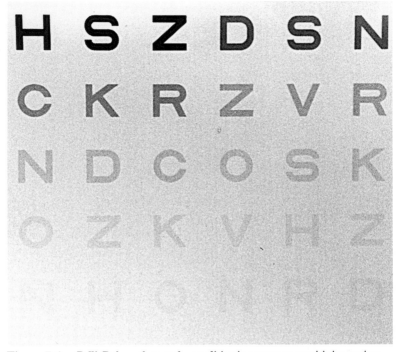

Figure 7.6   *Pelli-Robson format for qualititative contrast sensitivity testing*

A central scotoma (but **not** a relative afferent pupil defect) may also be due to retinal pathology at the macula and subtle pathology may be overlooked. Sometimes the scotoma is too small to be detected by confrontation or perimetry. The Amsler grid is a coarse high contrast grid against which the small paracentral scotomas and central distortions (metamorphopsia, micropsia, macropsia) of macular disease can readily be seen. In the photostress test the subject fixates on a bright light for a defined period of time (about 30 seconds) and the time to recovery of acuity to the pretest level after eventual disappearance of the induced positive scotoma is measured. In lesions of the choroid, pigment epithelium, or photoreceptors, recovery from this bleaching is greatly prolonged, whereas in optic nerve disease recovery is normal as function is not dependent on the rapid functioning of the visual cycle.

226

Amblyopia (box 7.9)

An additional common difficulty arises in the discrimination between poor uniocular vision due to amblyopia ("lazy eye"), which the adult patient may suddenly become aware of, and an acquired cause of visual loss without evident intraocular pathology. Amblyopia arises from a failure to establish normal cortical representation of the visual input from one eye during the critical period for visual maturation in childhood (six months to nine years) as a result of strabismus, stimulus deprivation, or uncorrected refractive error. Amblyopic eyes may have a small relative afferent pupil defect. When illumination is reduced (for example, by using a standard neutral density filter), acuity is preserved in eyes with amblyopia, but is profoundly degraded in an acquired optic neuropathy. Another characteristic of the amblyopic eye is that acuity improves on testing with a single letter per line format on the Snellen chart compared with a chart with four to five letters per line: this phenomenon is known as crowding. Because amblyopia is often associated with some degree of concomitant squint, the demonstration of reduced motor and sensory fusion by an orthoptist can be invaluable. A squint can be shown by the cover-uncover test where an occluder is placed over one eye and the patient fixates with the other eye. Then the occluder is placed in front of the eye initially fixating—in a patient with manifest squint the uncovered eye will move to take up fixation.

Box 7.9   Macular pathology and amblyopia

- Visual loss due to optic nerve disease is commonly mistaken for macular pathology and vice versa. Macular lesions are not associated with a relative afferent pupil defect and may cause scotomas which are two small to be detected without an Amsler grid

- Mascular lesions do not usually degrade colour vision until late in a disease process

- A patient may become aware of amblyopia for the first time in adulthood

Electrophysiological assessment of visual function (box 7.10)

Psychophysical methods of acuity measurement, contrast function, motion detection, perimetry, and colour vision all depend on a stimulus-response paradigm that is mediated by the subject's conscious understanding of the test, and certain assumptions must be made about the correlation of these stimulus-response properties to physiological events. The clinical electrophysiology of vision bypasses this area of theoretical and practical complexity and allows closer correlation with physiological functions. There is the added advantage of being suitable for the assessment of vision in preverbal children, and in cognitively impaired patients.

Visual evoked potentials

After repetitive visual stimulation using flashes of light or sudden changes in a grid pattern, a cortical potential is detectable that may be summated and averaged using microprocessors after repeated testing to yield the visually evoked cortical potential or visual evoked response (VER).[30 31] The VER reflects the integrity of the central visual field throughout the entire afferent visual system but is non-specific in localising a lesion to the retina, optic nerve or cortex. A flash generated VER is stimulated by luminance change whereas a pattern VER is stimulated by contrast change. The complex wave form is described in terms of amplitude and latency according to characteristics of the P_1 wave, which is a large positive deflection occurring at around 100 ms. Amplitude varies

---

Box 7.10   Electrophysiological testing

- When assesssing unexplained visual loss, an assessment of refraction, pupils, fields, and colour vision should be obtained before electrophysiological data becomes useful. Pattern and flash VEPs can be abnormal with refractive, optical, and retinal abnormalities
- Pattern and flash VEP data can only be fully interpreted when ERG data are also available. The pattern ERG can be very useful in selected cases of unexplained central field or acuity loss

---

widely among normal subjects but latency is constant. Pathological conditions of the anterior visual pathways yield relatively non-specific abnormalities of the VER, but the test is none the less useful, especially when carried out in conjunction with flash and pattern generated electroretinograms (see later). Latency delay with relative amplitude preservation is found in demyelination, even long after the acute episode and after visual recovery, and also in optic nerve compression. Amplitude reduction is a feature of ischaemic optic neuropathy and other conditions where axonal loss is prominent compared with conduction block. By careful choice of stimulus variables (check size and reversal speed in the pattern generated VER), the effects of optical blurring can be minimised and the test made sufficiently sensitive to be useful in moderate or minimal acuity loss. For example, the persistent latency changes of optic neuritis are best demonstrated and the effects of optical defocus minimised by using high contrast squares. Additional specificity can be achieved by half field testing whereby differences in amplitude and latency recorded from each hemisphere after uniocular stimulation can be used to assess abnormalities of the optic chiasm. Further refinements in VER techniques, which are currently undergoing clinical evaluation, include differential testing of the parvo and magnocellular systems by the use of test targets that selectively stimulate chromatic, temporal, and spatial functions, and also the discrimination between striate, extrastriate, and subcortical responses. These are likely to be of value in the early detection of subclinical abnormalities such as glaucomatous optic neuropathy and in the assessment of residual vision in those with cortical visual impairment, especially children.[32]

Electroretinography

Stimulation of the eye with either a flash or a pattern reversal system results in a recordable potential from the retina which has two principal components[33][34]: the "a" wave, which depends on the activity of the photoreceptors, and the "b" wave, which arises from the inner nuclear layer and the Müller cells. Disorders predominantly involving cones can be distinguished from those involving rods by performing the test in light (photopic) and dark (scotopic) conditions. In primary retinal diseases, such as diabetic retinopathy, pigmentary retinopathies, and dystrophies, and in toxic

229

degenerations, both the a wave and the b wave are abnormal. Exceptions to this are seen in central retinal artery occlusion where in the acute phase the photoceptors which derive their blood supply from the choroidal circulation are preserved and therefore the a wave persists while the b wave is extinguished. Superimposed on the b wave in a normal retina are a series of rhythmic oscillations referred to as oscillatory potentials. These may be of diagnostic importance when lost in the early stages of both diabetic retinopathy and in pigmentary retinopathies. When visual loss results from diseases which involve the ganglion cells or optic nerve, such as Tay-Sachs disease, glaucoma, or optic neuritis, the electroetinogram (ERG) in response to flashes of light is normal. In clinical practice the distinction between loss of visual acuity as a result of an optic neuropathy and visual loss of retinal origin may be difficult as each may be associated with loss of retinal ganglion cells and optic disc pallor. In advanced disease, the flash ERG will be abnormal whereas in a primary optic neuropathy it will be unaffected unless secondary trans-synaptic degeneration of outer retinal cells has taken place. The flash ERG, however, is a mass retinal response to luminance change, and just as the use of pattern reversal stimuli offers greater sensitivity in the VER, so it does in the ERG. Although origins of the pattern ERG are not entirely clear, it is accepted that the response does arise from retinal structures proximal to the photoreceptors, and it is this anatomical localisation which, together with the fact that pattern reversal stimuli test the central retina only, gives the test its potential power. Unlike the flash ERG, the late components of the pattern ERG are abnormal in disorders of the optic nerve and retinal ganglion cell layer. Therefore, the pattern ERG may be of value in discriminating subtle cases of central visual loss of central retinal origin, when early and late components will be abnormal, from visual loss of optic nerve origin when the late component alone is abnormal. With the increasing recognition that subclinical abnormalities of retinal function may be of diagnostic importance in, for example, the tapetoretinal degenerations and in the mitochondrial cytopathies, the use of electroretinography is likely to gain in importance in clinical neuro-ophthalmology.[35-40]

We are grateful to Dr Malcolm Steiger for helpful comments on an earlier version of the manuscript.

Standard texts for further reading

Spalton DJ, Hitchings RA, Hunter P. *A colour atlas of clinical ophthalmology.* London: Gower, 1985.
Vaughan DG, Astbury T, Riordan-Eva P. *General ophthalmology.* 13th ed. Norwalk: Appleton and Lange 1992.
Hart WM. *Adler's physiology of the eye.* 9th ed. St Louis: Mosby Year Book, 1992.
Glaser JS. *Clinical neuro-ophthalmology.* 2nd ed. Philadelphia: JB Lippincott, 1991.
Frisén L. *Clinical tests of vision.* New York: Raven Press, 1990.

1 van Essen DC, Anderson CH, Felleman DJ. Information processing in the primate visual system: an integrated systems perspective. *Science* 1992;**255**:419–23.
2 Frisén L, Frisén M. How good is normal visual acuity? *Graefes Arch Exp Ophthalmology* 1981;**215**:149.
3 Wetherill JR. Visual acuity assessment. *Eye* 1993;7:26–9.
4 Ferris FL III, Kassof KA, Brenick GH, Bailey I. New visual acuity charts for clinical research. *Am J Ophthalmol* 1982;**94**:91–6.
5 Ferris FL III, Sperduto RD. Standardised illumination for visual acuity testing in clinical research. *Am J Ophthalmol* 1982;**94**:97–8.
6 Hart WM. Acquired dyschromatopsias. *Surv Ophthalmol* 1987;**32**:10–31.
7 Lanthony PH. Clinical examination of the chromatic saturation. *Neuro-ophthalmology* 1990;**10**:119-28.
8 Wellings PC. Detection and recognition of visual field defects resulting from lesions involving the visual pathways. *Aust NZ J Ophthalmol* 1989;**17**:331–5.
9 Beck RW. Automated perimetry: principles and practice. *Int Ophthalmol Clin* 1986;**26**: 163–73.
10 Beck RW, Bergstrom TJ, Lichter PR. A clinical comparison of visual field testing with a new automated perimeter, the Humphrey field analyser, and the Goldmann perimeter. *Ophthalmology* 1985;**92**:77–82.
11 Mills R. Automated perimetry in neuro-ophthalmology. *Int Ophthalmol Clin* 1991;**31**: 51–70.
12 Hitchings RA, Migdal CS, Wormald R, Pooinooswamy D, Fitzke F. The (Glaucoma) Primary Treatment Trial: changes in visual field analysis by computer assisted perimetry. *Eye* 1994;**8**:117–20.
13 Lachemeyer BJ, Drance SM, Douglas GR, Mikelberg FS. Light sense, flicker and resolution perimetry in glaucoma. A comparative study. *Graefes Arch Clin Ophthalmol* 1991; **29**:1246–51.
14 Searle AET, Wild JM, Shaw DE, O'Neill EC. Time-related variation in normal automated static perimetry. *Ophthalmology* 1991;**98**:701–7.
15 Glovinsky Y, Quigley HA, Bissett RA, Miller NR. Artificially produced quadrantanopsia in computed vision testing. *Am J Ophthalmol* 1990;**110**:90–1.
16 Safran AB, Glaser JS. Statokinetic dissociation in lesions of the anterior visual pathways. *Arch Ophthalmol* 1980;**98**:291–5.
17 Wilderberger H, Robert Y. Visual fatigue during prolonged visual field testing in optic neuropathies. *Neuro-ophthalmology* 1993;**8**:167–74.
18 Keltner JL, Johnson CA. Current status of automated perimetry. Is the ideal automated perimeter available? *Arch Ophthalmol* 1986;**104**:347–9.
19 Sanabria O, Feuer WJ, Anderson DR. Pseudo-loss of fixation in automated perimetry. *Ophthalmology* 1991;**98**:76–8.
20 Arden GB. Testing contrast sensitivity in clinical practice. *Clinical Vision Science* 1988;**2**:213–24.
21 Pelli DG, Robson JG, Wilkins AJ. The design of a new letter chart for measuring contrast sensitivity. *Clinical Vision Science* 1988;2:187.
22 Regan D, Neiman D. Low-contrast letter charts as a test of visual function. *Ophthalmology* 1983;**90**:1192–200.
23 Pardhan S. Binocular performance in patients with unilateral cataract using the Regan test. *Eye* 1990;**4**:702–17.
24 Arden GB, Jacobsen JJ. A simple grating test for contrast sensitivity: preliminary results indicate value in screening for glaucoma. *Invest Ophthalmol Vis Sci* 1978;**17**:23–32.

25 Arden GB, Grundez K, Perry S. Colour vision testing with a computer graphics system. *Clinical Vision Science* 1988;2:303–20.
26 Hess RF, Zihl J, Pointer JS, Schmid C. The contrast sensitivity in patients with cerebral lesions. *Clinical Vision Science* 1990;5:203–15.
27 Potts M, Fells P, Falcano-Reis F, Arden GB. Colour contrast sensitivity, pattern electroretinography and cortical VEP's in dysthyroid optic neuropathy. *Invest Ophthalmol Vis Sci* 1990;31(suppl):189.
28 Travis D, Thompson P. Spatiotemporal contrast sensitivity and colour vision in multiple sclerosis. *Brain* 1989;112:283–303.
29 Verplank M, Kaufman DJ, Parono T, Yedavally S, Kokinakis D. Electrophysiology versus contrast sensitivity in the detection of visual loss in pseudotumour cerebri. *Neurology* 1978;38:1789–92.
30 Halliday AM, Halliday E, Kriss A, et al. The pattern evoked potential in compression of the anterior visual pathways. *Brain* 1976;99:357–74.
31 Frederiksen JL, Larsson HB, Ottovay E, Stigsby B, Olesen J. Acute optic neuritis with normal visual acuity: comparison of symptoms and signs with psychophysical, electrophysiological and magnetic resonance imaging data. *Acta Ophthalmol* 1991;69:357–66.
32 Sanders EACM, Volkers ACW, van der Poel JC, Lith GHM. Visual function and pattern visual evoked potentials in optic neuritis. *Br J Ophthalmol* 1987;71:602–8.
33 Berninger TA, Arden GB, Hogg CR, Franto T. Separable evoked retinal and cortical potentials from each major visual pathway: preliminary results. *Br J Ophthalmol* 1989;73:502–11.
34 International standardisation committee of the international society for the clinical electrophysiology of vision. Standard for clinical electroretinography. *Arch Ophthalmol* 1989;107:816–9.
35 Plant G, Hess R, Thomas S. The pattern evoked electroretinogram in optic neuritis. A combined psychophysical and electrophysiological study. *Brain* 1986;109:469–90.
36 Holder GE. Significance of abnormal pattern electroretinography in anterior visual pathway dysfunction. *Br J Ophthalmol* 1987;71:166–71.
37 Lorenz R, Dodt E, Heider W. Pattern electroretinogram peak times as a clinical means of discriminating retinal from optic nerve disease. *Doc Ophthalmol* 1989;71:307–20.
38 Holder GE, Acheson JF, Griffiths MFP, Green W, Shilling WE. Pattern electroretinography in patients with branch retinal vein occlusion. *J Physiol* 1991;438:295.
39 Berninger TA, Arden GB. The pattern electroretinogram. *Eye* 1988;2:257–83.
40 Ryan S, Arden GB. Electrophysiological discrimination between retinal and optic nerve disorders. *Doc Ophthalmol* 1988;68:247–55.

8 Investigation of visual loss: neuro-ophthalmology from a neurologist's perspective

CHRISTIAN J LUECK

A large proportion of the human nervous system is devoted to receiving and processing visual information.[1] This means that the potential for CNS disease to produce visual disturbance of one sort or another is therefore enormous. The great advantage to the clinician dealing with a visual disturbance is that the visual pathways are organised very precisely, with preservation of topographic relation from retina through optic nerves, chiasm, tracts, geniculate nuclei, radiations, and on into the visual cortex.[2] Hence, careful attention to visual field disturbance is likely to give a fairly precise clue as to what part of the visual system is being affected.

Because certain diseases are more likely to affect some parts of the visual system than others, it is often possible to narrow down a differential diagnosis simply on the basis of site of lesion. This process of restricting the differential is further enhanced by knowing the time course over which visual disturbance has developed. These two considerations make the investigation of such disturbances much more straightforward.

Differential diagnosis of visual loss

Visual loss has a wide differential diagnosis (box 8.1). Visual loss secondary to trauma, or longstanding, non-progressive visual loss (for example, amblyopia) will not be considered further; the interested reader is referred to textbooks of neuro-ophthalmology.[2 3] It is assumed that visual loss secondary to diseases of the eye itself or to visible disturbance of the retina will be detected

233

Box 8.1 Differential diagnosis of visual loss based on site and timing of lesion

Continued opposite

| *Site of lesion* | *Time course* | | | |
	Transient	*Seconds to minutes*	*Hours to days*	*Days to months +*
●Retinal	Amaurosis fugax:	CRAO/BRAO	"Phlebitis"	Macular degenerations
	●Thromboembolic	CRVO/BRVO	ischaemia	Hereditary retinal disease:
	●Benign (young)			●Retinitis pigmentosa
	Retinal migraine			●Cone/rod dystrophies
	Photostress (ischaemia)			Storage disorders
	Hemeralopia (cone dystrophies)			Neurodegenerative conditions
	Angle closure glaucoma			Uveomeningeal syndromes
				Carcinoma associated retinopathy
●Optic nerve/ optic disc	AION (vasculitic)	Abnormal fundus:	Typical ON	Compressive:
	Obscurations	●AION:	Atypical ON:	●Neoplasm
	(papilloedema)	●Vasculitic	●Immune	●Thyroid eye disease
		●Non-vasculitic	●Infective	●Aneurysm
		●Leber's HON	●Leber's HON	●Granuloma
		●Disc haemorrhage	Neuroretinitis	●Paget's disease
		●Diabetic papillopathy	Paraneoplastic	Infective/inflammatory:
		●Big blind spot syndrome	Toxic	●Syphilis
		●Neuroretinitis		●HTLV 1 (TSP)
		●Optic nerve head drusen		●Tuberculosis
		Normal fundus:		●Orbital/paranasal sinus infection
		●PION		●Sarcoidosis
		(compressive lesion)		Leber's HON
				Infiltrative
				Toxic/nutritional (B12)
				Hereditary neuropathy
				Chronic papilloedema
				Postirradiation
				AV malformation
				Optic disc dysplasia

Box 8.1 Differential diagnosis of visual loss based on site and timing of lesion—continued

Site of lesion	Transient	Time course Seconds to minutes	Hours to days	Days to months +
Optic chiasm	Cystic tumours •Craniopharyngioma •Mucocele	Pituitary apoplexy Ruptured AVM	Pituitary tumour (pregnancy) Pituitary abscess Sphenoidal abscess Demyelination Adenohypophysitis	Compressive: •Neoplasm •Sphenoidal mucocele •Dilated IIIrd ventricle •Granuloma (sarcoid, TB) •Aneurysm •Primary hypothyroidism •Thalassaemia Postradiation damage Subacute/chronic meningitis Septo-optic dysplasia Empty sella syndrome
Retrochiasmal pathways	TIA Migraine Epilepsy Trauma (children)	CVA: •Thromboembolic •Haemorrhage (tumour) •Spasm (angiography) Migraine Impaired cerebral Perfusion	Demyelination Cerebral abscess Tumour Poisoning Meningitis Encephalitis	Tumour: •Intrinsic •Extrinsic AV malformation Creutzfeldt-Jakob Pelizaeus-Merzbacher Metachromatic leukodystrophy Progressive multifocal leukoencephalopathy Subacute sclerosing panencephalitis Schilder's disease

AION = anterior ischaemic optic neuropathy; AVM = arteriovenous malformation; BRAO = branch retinal artery occlusion; BRVO = branch retinal vein occlusion; CRAO = central retinal artery occlusion; CRVO = central retinal vein occlusion; CVA = cerebrovascular accident; HON = hereditary optic neuropathy; HTLV 1 = human T lymphocytic virus, type I; ON = optic neuritis; PION = posterior ischaemic optic neuropathy; TB = tuberculosis; TIA = transient ischaemic attack; TSP = tropical spastic paraparesis.

and referred appropriately to an ophthalmologist. Visual loss as a result of psychogenic causes is considered at the end of this chapter.[23]

Visual field loss

Visual loss without visual field loss is most often due to an ophthalmological cause, typically a disturbance of the ocular media. In neurological practice, the vast majority of visual loss is associated with disturbance of the visual field. Box 8.2 gives the differential diagnosis of visual loss without field loss.

The methods for assessing visual fields have been dealt with in chapter 7.[4] For the purposes of this discussion, it is assumed that the clinician has access to accurate visual fields.

In constructing box 8.1, four broad divisions of lesion site are considered. Corresponding diagrammatic representations of possible visual field loss referable to each division are shown in figure 8.1.

Retina/optic disc

Ophthalmoscopically visible lesions of the retina or choroid are likely to produce focal scotomatous field loss, and these will not be discussed further here. Patterns of visual field loss likely to be encountered by a neurologist and referable to disorders of the retina or optic disc include central visual field loss (macular

---

Box 8.2   Causes of visual loss without visual field disturbance

- Transient visual loss
- Refractive error/accommodation failure
- Disturbance of ocular media
- Amblyopia
- Disturbance of higher visual function (cognitive)
- Subtle oculomotor disturbance (including nystagmus)
- Failure to detect visual field loss:
  - Subclinical optic neuropathy or maculopathy
  - Technical difficulty
- Functional visual loss

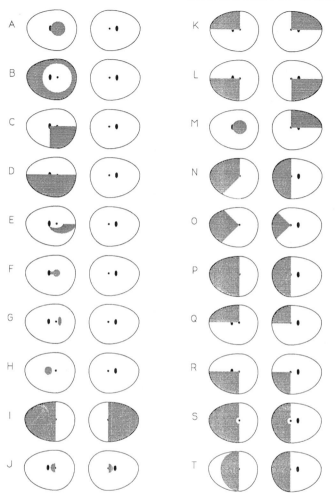

Figure 8.1   *Schematic representation of visual field disturbance of various possible types, referred to in the text. Against each letter are represented the visual fields of the two eyes along with fixation points and the blind spots. (A) central scotoma; (B) concentric visual field reduction; (C) sectoral field loss; (D) altitudinal field loss; (E) arcuate scotoma; (F) centrocaecal scotoma; (G) paracentral scotoma; (H) enlarged blind spot; (I) full field bitemporal hemianopia; (J) central field bitemporal hemianopia; (K) bitemporal upper quadrantanopia; (L) bitemporal lower quadrantanopia; (M) junctional scotoma; (N) incongruous homonymous hemianopia; (O) wedge hemianopia; (P) congruous homonymous hemianopia; (Q) homonymous upper quadrantanopia; (R) homonymous lower quadrantanopia; (S) macular sparing homonymous hemianopia; (T) homonymous hemianopia with sparing of temporal crescent*

237

lesion), concentric visual field loss, sectoral visual field loss, altitudinal field loss, and arcuate scotomata. Bilateral macular sparing homonymous hemianopias may masquerade as bilateral concentric field reduction. There is usually a small step at the vertical meridian if visual fields are performed carefully.

Optic nerve/disc

The classic visual field loss is a central scotoma. In certain situations (especially toxic/nutritional ambylopias) the papillomacular bundle, if such an anatomically distinct structure exists,[4] seems to be particularly affected, giving rise to a centrocaecal scotoma. It should be noted that optic nerve disease can give rise to various field defects including arcuate scotoma, paracentral scotoma, and altitudinal field defects, and the pattern of monocular visual field loss is of limited utility in distinguishing one disease from another.[5] Swelling of the optic nerve head may give rise to an enlarged blind spot. Involvement of the optic nerves may, of course, be bilateral.

Optic chiasm

The crossing of nasal nerve fibres in the chiasm means that compression of the central chiasm typically gives rise to a bitemporal hemianopia. There are, however, considerable variations on this, including bitemporal partial field defects (which may be considerably asymmetric), and junctional scotomata. For this reason it is most important to examine the temporal visual field of the "good eye" in a patient presenting with apparent unilateral visual loss. A binasal visual field defect has been reported to occur with sideways compression of the chiasm (in theory picking out the uncrossed fibres of each side), but this is rare,[6] and strongly raises the suspicion of glaucoma or functional visual loss. Damage to the whole optic chiasm will, of course, give rise to total bilateral visual field loss.

Retrochiasmal lesions

The hallmark of such lesions is that the field defects are homonymous. Congruity of homonymous defects tends to increase as the lesion becomes more posterior, but this is by no means an absolute rule. Typically, optic tract lesions are relatively incongruous. Lateral geniculate lesions tend to give rise to "wedge hemianopias"; it is suggested that congruity in a geniculate hemi-

238

anopia implies infarction, but this is not always the case.[3] Lesions in the optic radiation can give rise to homonymous quadrantanopias, either in the upper visual field (temporal lobe lesions), or lower visual field (parietal lobe lesions). Occipital lobe lesions typically produce congruous hemianopias which may or may not be macular sparing. If the lesion in the occipital lobe is very posterior, it may spare the cortical representation of the far lateral visual field, thereby producing sparing of the temporal crescent of the contralateral eye.

Time course

For current purposes, the temporal evolution of visual loss will be divided up into four groups: transient (reversible); irreversible onset over seconds to minutes; progressive onset over hours to days; progressive onset over days to months or longer.

It may be difficult to be confident in allocating the patient's symptoms to one specific group, and more than one differential diagnostic category may therefore have to be considered. A typical example of this would be when a patient awoke with visual loss in one eye—this could have arisen suddenly over seconds/minutes during the night, or, alternatively, have developed over several hours. All possible diagnoses in both groups would then have to be considered.

Investigation of visual loss

Transient visual loss in one eye

By definition, the visual fields will be normal in relation to a transient attack. It is therefore crucial to try to determine the nature of the visual field disturbance on the basis of the history. Patients are notoriously unable to tell the difference between visual disturbance in *one visual hemifield* versus that in *one eye* (amaurosis fugax), and it can be very difficult to sort this out. Apart from asking the patient whether alternate eye closure was attempted, it is often helpful to ask them what their vision was like during the attack: I usually ask them if, were they to look directly at my face during an attack, would the whole face be normal or would one half of it be affected?

Whether or not the transient visual field loss was referable to the eye or to the occipital cortex, preliminary investigations are simi-

239

lar, looking for causes of transient ischaemic attack.[7 8] The indications and value of these investigations have been dealt with elsewhere[7 8] and box 8.3 gives a summary.

Carotid ultrasound (Doppler or duplex) examination is appropriate if the visual loss affected one eye, assuming that the patient would entertain the idea of an endarterectomy. If the examination indicates that a carotid stenosis is present, it is likely that endarterectomy will improve the patient's risk of stroke if the stenosis is greater than 70%,[9 10] but even then other factors may have to be taken into account,[11] not least of which is the fact that the risk of stroke is considerably less after amaurosis fugax than after other types of transient ischaemic attack.[12 13] The finding of an ulcerated plaque probably increases the risk of stroke[15] without increasing surgical mortality[14] and there may be an effect of the type of plaque as determined by its echogenicity.[8] The degree of stenosis must be more firmly established with further imaging, such as selective carotid angiography, but some centres are increasingly using MR angiography.[8] Which technique is considered acceptable by way of preoperative anatomical definition currently varies somewhat from centre to centre.

Amaurosis fugax may occasionally be the harbinger of irreversible visual loss in patients with giant cell arteritis. If there is any suggestion of headache, jaw claudication, or general malaise, an erythrocyte sedimentation rate should be performed as an emergency. If it is not raised, but the story is suggestive, strong consideration should be given to temporal artery biopsy because up to 17% of cases are not associated with raised erythrocyte sedimentation rate.[16]

In young people, recurrent monocular visual loss is often a benign condition, unassociated with an increased risk of stroke.[17] It is probably due to vascular spasm, and may be pathogenetically related to migraine.[17] It is usually regarded as a diagnosis of exclusion, and only applicable after the above investigations and imaging of the optic nerve or visual pathways have come back negative.[17 18]

Obscurations are transient disturbances of vision which occur in association with papilloedema secondary to raised intracranial pressure of whatever cause. This usually results in bilateral visual symptoms, but if the papilloedema is unilateral, monocular symptoms can result. Typically patients do not lose vision entirely (vision does not go "black"), but complain of greying of vision,

Box 8.3 Investigation of transient ischaemic attacks[78]

Group I	Group II	Group III
Appropriate for all patients with suspected TIAs	*Appropriate in selected patients only*	*Appropriate only if clinical evaluation, and tests in groups I and II have not yielded answer, or clinical features suggest specific test*
FBC, ESR	Urea and electrolytes	Thrombophilia screen (proteins S, C, antithrombin III, etc)
Serum glucose	Thyroid function	Blood cultures
Serum cholesterol	Antiphospholipid antibodies	HIV serology
Syphilis serology	Antinuclear antibodies	Lipoprotein fractionation
Urinalysis	Protein electrophoresis	Serum homocysteine
Electrocardiogram	Plasma viscosity	WBC galactosidase
	Sickle test/haemoglobin EPS	CSF
	Chest radiograph	Urinary VMA
	Echocardiogram (transthoracic or oesophageal)	24 hour electrocardiogram
	Carotid ultrasound	Temporal artery biopsy
	Carotid angiography	
	Cranial CT	
	Electroencephalogram	

FBC = full blood count; ESR = erythrocyte sedimentation rate; EPS = electrophoresis; VMA = vanillylmandelic acid.

often in association with change in posture. In this situation, it is obviously mandatory to image the head (MRI or CT[19]) to look for a cause of raised pressure. If imaging shows no space occupying lesion, lumbar puncture is indicated. There are many causes of a raised CSF pressure in the absence of a space occupying lesion (pseudotumour cerebri),[3] but one important condition is sagittal sinus thrombosis. Nowadays, this can often be detected by MR angiography, but formal angiography may still be required, depending on local facilities. This condition and its management have been considered recently.[20]

There are a few unusual causes. Ocular ischaemia can present with transient visual loss provoked by exposure to bright light (photostress). There are usually ophthalmoscopic changes to suggest the diagnosis, including peripheral exudates and haemorrhages, microaneurysms, and new vessels. A photostress test[3] is useful in this circumstance, and further investigation will include carotid ultrasound, with tests as in box 8.3 as appropriate. Transient visual disturbance provoked by changes in ambient lighting can also be produced by retinal diseases such as cone dystrophies, and diagnosis can be aided by the use of electroretinography (see chapter 7 and Armington[21]). Finally, if the diagnosis remains obscure, an attempt should be made to measure intraocular pressure during an attack as acute closed angle glaucoma can rarely present with transient visual loss.[22]

Sudden, irreversible visual loss in one eye

As mentioned above, conditions referable to primary ocular structures such as acute angle-closure glaucoma or vitreous haemorrhage will not be discussed here. Nevertheless, it is likely that there will be abnormalities on ophthalmoscopy to aid diagnosis, especially if the patient is seen within a day or so of the acute event. If possible, pupil dilatation should be performed as failure to perform this often results in missing ophthalmoscopic clues to diagnosis. If ophthalmoscopy is completely normal, then the possibility of posterior ischaemic optic neuropathy should be considered, although this condition is rare.[2] Other rare conditions which might produce this picture include haemorrhage of an orbital arteriovenous malformation, or into a tumour next to the optic nerve, either in the orbit or in its prechiasmal intracranial portion.

Usually, however, ophthalmoscopy shows changes which suggest a diagnosis, provided the patient is seen within 24 hours of visual loss. Such diagnoses include retinal arterial infarction, venous occlusion, optic nerve head infarction (anterior ischaemic optic neuropathy), haemorrhage, or acute disc swelling. The last may be associated with sudden visual loss in acute papilloedema, or Leber's hereditary optic neuropathy. Visual disturbance with field loss usually confined to an enlarged blind spot can also be seen in diabetic papillopathy,[23 24] or the big blind spot syndrome,[2 25] although these conditions more commonly present with minimal visual symptoms. Box 8.4 lists the various ophthalmoscopic findings seen in each of the above diagnoses.

Box 8.4 also lists appropriate investigations. Certain points are amplified here.

(1) If there are no abnormalities in the retina, posterior ischaemic optic neuropathy is a possibility, but imaging the orbit would be required to exclude a compressive lesion. Other investigations would be similar to those for anterior ischaemic optic neuropathy (AION).[2]

(2) The investigation of central retinal artery occlusion is similar to that for amaurosis fugax (see above), although local retinal causes such as radiation retinopathy[34] may contribute to its aetiology.

(3) In central retinal vein occlusion, search for anticardiolipin antibodies is probably not worthwhile unless the patient has other features of systemic lupus erythematosus.[35 36]

(4) Anterior ischaemic optic neuropathy (AION) may be arteritic or non-arteritic. An erythrocyte sedimentation rate is required as an emergency, and, if any other feature suggests temporal arteritis, a temporal artery biopsy should be performed, even if the sedimentation rate is normal (see above). The role of ophthalmic colour Doppler is as yet undetermined, but it may be of use in differentiating arteritic from non-arteritic AION.[37 38] In the absence of clinical features of temporal arteritis or a raised erythrocyte sedimentation rate, biopsy is unlikely to be positive, and is therefore unnecessarily invasive. The exception to this is in bilateral simultaneous AION in which a large proportion of patients have evidence of systemic connective tissue disease.[2] In younger patients or those with bilateral disease, investigation for coagulation abnormalities is appropriate.[30] The history may point to one of the rarely encountered associations between AION and other diseases,[2] but routine investigation beyond that indicated in box 8.4 is probably not worthwhile unless it does.

Box 8.4 Ophthalmoscopic findings and investigations in acute monocular visual loss

Condition	Ophthalmoscopic findings	Appropriate investigations
Central retinal artery occlusion	Opacification of nerve fibre layer Cherry red spot (cholesterol) embolus/microemboli Attenuation of arterial tree	ESR Fluorescein angiography See box 8.3 Carotid ultrasound/angiography
Central retinal vein occlusion[26,27]	Retinal venous dilatation Scattered retinal haemorrhages (several disc diameters from optic disc)	FBC, ESR, fibrinogen, glucose Lipid profile (fluorescein angiography) (BP, intraocular pressure)
Anterior ischaemic optic neuropathy (AION)	Sectoral/complete optic disc swelling Disc haemorrhages Exudates/macular star (small optic discs)[28] (buried drusen)[29]	ESR, ? temporal artery biopsy Fluorescein angiography FBC, fibrinogen, glucose Protein electrophoresis Lipid profile (coagulopathy screen)[30]
Neuroretinitis[31,32]	Disc swelling, peripapillary exudates Macular star formation Possibly vitreous cells[31]	(As for AION) VDRL, ANA, serum ACE Viral titres, Lyme serology
Leber's hereditary optic neuropathy	Circumpapillary telangiectatic microangiopathy (non-oedematous) elevation of optic disc	Fluorescein angiography Mitochondrial DNA
Infiltrative optic neuropathy	Optic disc swelling Haemorrhages/exudates	B mode ultrasonography MRI/CT, LP, chest radiograph Bence Jones protein, serum ACE Bone marrow, abdominal CT
Diabetic papillopathy[23,24]	Disc swelling, usually bilateral Haemorrhages/exudates	Glucose, haemoglobin A1c Fluorescein angiography
Big blind spot syndrome[2,25]	Swollen optic disc (?absent) Venous overfilling, occasional haemorrhage Multiple evanescent white dots[33]	MRI/CT, lumbar puncture Fluorescein angiography

ANA = antinuclear antibody; ESR = erythrocyte sedimentation rate; BP = blood pressure; FBC = full blood count; VDRL = venereal disease research laboratory test.

(5) Neuroretinitis is generally thought of as a relatively benign condition in which central visual loss occurs over hours and is associated with a central scotoma and a macular star on ophthalmoscopy.[31][39] However, it may present acutely, and have a poor prognosis.[32] In this situation, investigation should include tests for vasculitic and infective diseases (particularly cat scratch fever) as well as those tests listed for AION, but in most cases investigation is negative.[32]

(6) In Leber's hereditary optic neuropathy, fluorescein angiography shows peripapillary telangiectasia and an apparently swollen disc which paradoxically does not leak,[40] although these findings are not always present.[41] This finding should be followed by mitochondrial DNA analysis.[41] Interestingly, there may be surprisingly little by way of relative afferent pupillary defect.[42]

(7) Occasionally optic nerve head drusen can present as acute visual loss, often with inferior nasal field defect.[29] This diagnosis is generally taken to be a diagnosis of exclusion after full investigation in the form of CT/MRI, lumbar puncture, and investigations as for AION. The drusen themselves may be more specifically detected by CT, MRI, fluorescein angiography, or ocular ultrasound.[19][43]

Optic nerve pathology developing over hours to days

The natural history of typical optic neuritis is as follows: a previously fit patient, aged between 20 and 50, experiences pain in the eye or orbit, often exacerbated by eye movement, for hours or a few days before visual loss occurs. The visual loss then develops gradually (usually several hours) with loss of colour saturation, central visual acuity, and then the development of a scotoma which may expand to fill the entire visual field. The exact nature of the scotoma is extremely variable.[5] Visual loss usually remains static for a few days, and then starts to improve, although it may not improve back to the premorbid level. The typical signs include loss of visual acuity, impaired colour perception, central visual field loss, possible disc swelling (papillitis), and a relative afferent pupillary defect.[2][3][18]

If a patient presents with the typical history and signs of optic neuritis, standard wisdom has been that there is no need to image the patient, provided there are no clinical features to suggest a diagnosis of multiple sclerosis.[3] Recently, however, this view has been changed somewhat by two developments. Firstly, the recent optic neuritis trial suggested that patients with typical optic neuritis should be treated with intravenous methyl prednisolone (whatever the severity) as this significantly reduced the likelihood of progressing to diagnosable multiple sclerosis at two years[44] (although the most recent report from the optic neuritis study group suggests that the two year benefit is not maintained at three years)[45]. Secondly, recent studies have suggested that the prognosis for going on to develop multiple sclerosis is much less if MRI does not show multiple lesions.[46] For these reasons, it has been advocated that all cases of typical optic neuritis should have MRI.[47] However, this remains controversial, and depends critically on the ability of scanning facilities to cope with local demand. There is no role for visual evoked potentials, CT, or lumbar puncture in the clinical management of *typical* isolated optic neuritis.

If any of the features of typical optic neuritis are missing, both optic nerves are affected, there is no evidence of recovery after four weeks, or there are additional features, then further investigation is warranted. In the first instance, it is appropriate to image the orbits, paranasal sinuses, sphenoid, and pituitary fossa to detect compressive lesions (which may have acutely decompensated) or infective processes such as paranasal sinus disease. As a first line investigation, contrast enhanced orbital CT is probably still the investigation of choice,[19 48] but intrinsic and inflammatory optic nerve lesions are better shown on MRI,[49] and both may be required. Skull radiography is not a useful tool in the investigation of visual loss.[50] Lumbar puncture is indicated if imaging does not yield a diagnosis.

Previous or concurrent symptoms of infective illness raise the possibility of viral, paraviral, or postviral syndromes, or active bacterial or fungal infection. It is thus worth considering screening blood and CSF for viruses (measles, rubella, mumps, chicken pox, influenza, herpes simplex, herpes zoster, cytomegalovirus, E-B virus, hepatitis (A or B), HIV), bacterial infections (syphilis, borrelia, tuberculosis), and fungal infections (aspergillus, cryptococcus, coccidioidomycosis) as appropriate to the clinical picture. Presumed "viral" illnesses or cat scratch fever are often reported in patients with neuroretinitis in whom there is typically a macular star on ophthalmoscopy (see above); investigations usually, however, prove negative.[31]

Optic neuritis has been reported in systemic lupus erythematosus, and other immune mediated conditions such as Sjögren's syndrome and ulcerative colitis.[18] If the optic neuritis is atypical in any way, antinuclear antigen and anti-dsDNA antibodies, along with extractable nuclear antigen, should be checked.

Perhaps the most common "look alike" of optic neuritis is sarcoidosis affecting the optic nerve. Suspicion should be raised by failure of the visual loss to improve, or any evidence of past or present iritis or uveitis. Initial investigation in the form of a chest radiograph, serum angiotensin converting enzyme, and lumbar puncture is appropriate. Unfortunately, Kveim testing is no longer available as a diagnostic test. In the absence of any other clinical features, my experience has been that further tests such as pulmonary function tests or gallium scans are unlikely to be rewarding, but could be considered.

About 20% of simultaneous bilateral optic neuritis in adults turns out to be due to Leber's hereditary optic neuropathy, even in the absence of affected relatives,[51] and in this circumstance, mitochondrial DNA analysis should be performed. A further 20% turns out to be due to multiple sclerosis.[51] Other possibilities include toxic neuropathy. This could be due to the medication the patient is taking, or possibly to an external agent such as lead. Serum lead, B12, and a toxicology screen should be added to the above tests, along with careful questioning of the patient regarding drugs (prescribed and "recreational"), diet, and work exposure.

Optic nerve pathology developing over days or months

In this situation, imaging is mandatory, and should include good views of the optic nerves (intraorbital, intracanalicular, and intracranial) including the pituitary fossa region. As mentioned above, there is some debate as to whether high quality enhanced orbital CT, or gadolinium enhanced MRI is superior as a first line investigation,[19 48 49] but it is not uncommon for both to be required eventually. Practically, it depends on local facilities. Most lesions large enough to cause visual loss by optic nerve compression will be visible, but it is not uncommon for optic nerve sheath meningiomas to be missed: repeated scans may be necessary, and are especially indicated if there is evidence of optic disc swelling or optociliary shunt vessels on fundoscopy.[52]

Further investigation of any lesion found will, of course, depend on the nature of the lesion. Imaging in the form of angiography may be necessary, or it might be appropriate to proceed to biopsy.

247

Likewise, thyroid function tests may be appropriate, but these are often normal in thyroid eye disease; the use of a thyrotrophin releasing hormone test considerably improves the diagnostic yield.[53]

If imaging of the optic nerve fails to show a reason for the visual loss, infective and inflammatory causes should be screened for with VDRL, HTLV I titres, serum angiotensin converting enzyme, and autoantibody screen, and consideration should be given to an HIV test. Nutritional optic neuropathy can be screened for by checking folate and B12, in combination with a careful dietary history. Sudden weight loss or protracted vomiting of any cause may be associated with nutritional amblyopia. Smoking, alcohol, drugs (prescribed, "recreational", or otherwise—for example, methanol) are causes of toxic amblyopia and must be looked for, possibly with the help of a toxicology screen. Bilateral centrocaecal scotomata strongly suggest nutritional/toxic amblyopia.

If visual field testing suggests a lesion of the optic nerve and there is disc swelling on fundoscopy, further thought is required. Papilloedema (disc swelling due to raised intracranial pressure) does not typically cause central visual field loss. Therefore, if there is raised intracranial pressure, this must be due to a structural cause which is associated with optic nerve disease/compression, but imaging should already have detected such a cause. If imaging is normal and the discs are swollen, the next test should be a lumbar puncture. In this circumstance, raised pressure should not be regarded as the cause of the visual loss. An alternative cause in the form of inflammatory disease such as sarcoidosis must be considered and investigated as above. Failing this, carcinomatous meningitis or direct optic disc infiltration by haematological malignancy should be considered, and investigated appropriately (box 8.4).

Hereditary optic neuropathies may be diagnosed on the basis of a positive family history, but occasionally Leber's hereditary optic neuropathy can be surprising, and searching for the known mitochondrial DNA mutations is worthwhile at this point.[41]

Two other reasons for progressive anterior pathway visual failure may have to be considered. Dysplasia of the optic disc may be associated with visual field disturbance. This is often longstanding, but occasionally comes to the attention of the patient and requires explanation. Typical examples include tilted optic discs, which are usually associated with superotemporal field loss,[2] or optic nerve head drusen (hyaline bodies).[54] Diagnosis of the drusen is suggested by anomalous optic disc vasculature, and can be quite difficult, particularly if the drusen are buried. Help may be required in the form of fluorescein angiography (looking for autofluorescence), or B mode ultrasonography.[19 43] Occasionally calcification of the optic nerve head can be seen on unenhanced CT.[19 43]

Psychogenic visual loss

Occasionally the clinician is faced with a patient in whom investigation is normal or negative, and there is some doubt as to whether visual loss is as severe as is claimed. A clue to this is often given by the fact that the patient has markedly preserved "navigational abilities" in relation to pronounced visual field loss. Alternatively, certain behaviours such as going slightly out of the way to "bump into" objects which are not quite in the patient's path may suggest elaboration of visual loss. As with all fields of neurology, making a diagnosis of functional/elaborated visual loss must be made with extreme care: patients with dense central scotomata may have well preserved peripheral fields allowing relatively "unimpaired" navigation, and all elaborated visual loss may have an underlying genuine component which must not be missed.

Nevertheless, there are some useful diagnostic pointers in the examination/investigation

- General demeanour and navigational ability have already been discussed. As a patient walks into the room it can be useful to fix their eye, and extend your own hand, as though to shake theirs. If the patient is fixing your eye, but responds with appropriate hand movement, the visual field must be appropriately large

- With the help of trial lenses, patients can sometimes be persuaded to continue reading down the Snellen chart with the "bad" eye if the "good" eye is suddenly covered with a strongly positive lens, or an occluder

- Gross inconsistency of near and far acuities, and colour vision as assessed by Ishihara plates may suggest elaboration, particularly if there is no corresponding visual field loss or pupillary abnormality. Extreme caution must be taken to ensure that this situation is not the result of correctable refractive error.

- Assessment of visual fields by Goldmann perimetry may yield "spiral visual fields"; this strongly suggests elaboration. Similarly, a hemianopia present with both eyes viewing, but absent in the field of the "good" eye also suggests elaboration.
- Feigned complete blindness can sometimes be detected by the use of an optokinetic drum to generate nystagmus, or the use of a mirror placed in front of the patient's eyes and then moved suddenly. As above, eye movements seen in these circumstances must be interpreted with caution as cortical visual loss can be associated with some preservation of visually induced eye movements mediated by brainstem pathways.
- Similar reasoning applies to the use of visual evoked potentials. A normal visual evoked potential in the presence of apparent total visual loss is unlikely, but conceivably could occur if the primary visual cortex were intact in the presence of damage to its onward connections. Visual evoked potentials are significantly degraded by lack of visual fixation on the part of the patient, and my personal experience is that they are not much help in these circumstances.

There are numerous other clues to non-organic visual loss, but space does not permit discussion of them here. The interested reader is referred to a recent review for further details.[55]

Finally, it is not unheard of for a neurologist or neuro-ophthalmologist to be referred a patient who actually has an ophthalmological diagnosis, even if the source of referral is an ophthalmologist. The most common situation in which this arises is that of a maculopathy being misdiagnosed as possible optic nerve disease. It is always worth re-examining the ocular fundus in the case of monocular visual disturbance, particularly if there is no associated relative afferent pupillary defect, so as not to be led into inappropriate investigations.

1 Zeki S. *A vision of the brain*. Oxford: Blackwell, 1993.
2 Miller NR. *Walsh and Hoyt's clinical neuro-ophthalmology*. 4th ed. Vol 1. Baltimore: Williams and Wilkins, 1982.
3 Glaser JS. *Clinical neuro-ophthalmology*. 2nd ed. Philadelphia: JB Lippincott, 1991.
4 Plant GT, Perry VH. The anatomical basis of the caecocentral scotoma. New observations and a review. *Brain* 1990;113:441–57.
5 Keltner JC, Johnson CA, Spurr JO, Beck RW, Optic Neuritis Study Group. Baseline visual field profile of optic neuritis. The experience of the optic neuritis treatment trial. *Arch Ophthalmol* 1993;111:231–4.
6 O'Connell JEA, du Boulay EPGH. Binasal hemianopia. *J Neurol Neurosurg Psychiatry* 1973;36:697–709.

7 Hankey GJ, Warlow CP. Cost-effective investigation of patients with suspected transient ischaemic attacks. *J Neurol Neurosurg Psychiatry* 1992;**55**:171–6.

8 Hankey GJ, Warlow CP. *Major problems in neurology 27: transient ischaemic attacks of the brain and eye.* London: WB Saunders, 1994.

9 North American Symptomatic Carotid Endarterectomy Trial Collaborators. Beneficial effect of carotid endarterectomy in symptomatic patients with high-grade carotid stenosis. *N Engl J Med* 1991;**325**:445–53.

10 European Carotid Surgery Trialists' Collaborative Group. MRC European carotid surgery trial: interim results for symptomatic patients with severe (70–99%) or with mild (0–29%) carotid stenosis. *Lancet* 1991;**337**:1235–43.

11 Trobe JD. Carotid endarterectomy. Who needs it? *Ophthalmology* 1987;**94**:725.

12 Hankey GJ, Slattery JM, Warlow CP. Transient ischaemic attacks: which patients are at high (and low) risk of serious vascular events? *J Neurol Neurosurg Psychiatry* 1992;**55**: 640–52.

13 Streifler JY, Eliasziw M, Benavente OR, Harbison JW, Hachinski VC, Barnett HJM, Simard D for the North American Symptomatic Carotid Endarterctomy trial. The risk of stroke in patients with first-ever retinal vs hemispheric transient ischemic attacks and high-grade carotid stenosis. *Arch Neurol* 1995;**52**:246–9.

14 Eliasziw M, Streifler JY, Fox AJ, Hachinski VC, Ferguson GG, Barnett HJM, for the North American Symptomatic Carotid Endartevectomy Trial. Significance of plaque ulceration in symptomatic patients with high grade carotid stenosis. *Stroke* 1994;**25**:304–8.

15 Goldstein LB, McCrory DC, Landsman PB, Samsa GP, Ancukiewicz M, Oddone EZ, Matchar DB. Multicenter review of preoperative risk factors for carotid endarterectomy in patients with ipsilateral symptoms. *Stroke* 1994;**25**:1116–21.

16 Jacobson DM, Slamovits TL. Erythrocyte sedimentation rate and its relationship to hematocrit in giant cell arteritis. *Arch Ophthalmol* 1987;**105**:965–7.

17 Tippin J, Corbett JJ, Kerber RE, Schroeder E, Thompson HS. Amaurosis fugax and ocular infarction in adolescents and young adults. *Ann Neurol* 1989;**26**:69–77.

18 Burde RM, Savino PJ, Trobe JD. *Clinical decisions in neuro-ophthalmology.* 2nd ed. St Louis: Mosby Year Book, 1992.

19 Moseley IF. Diagnostic imaging in visual loss: a problem-oriented approach. *Imaging* 1992;**4**:151–6.

20 Perkin GD. Cerebral venous thrombosis: developments in imaging and treatment. *J Neurol Neurosurg Psychiatry* 1995;**59**:1–3.

21 Armington JC. Electroretinography. In: Aminoff MJ, ed. *Electrodiagnosis in clinical neurology.* New York: Churchill Livingstone, 1992:433–66.

22 O'Sullivan E, Shaunak S, Simcock P, Matthews T, Wade J, Kennard C. Transient monocular blindness. *J Neurol Neurosurg Psychiatry* 1995;**59**:559.

23 Barr CC, Glaser JS, Blankenship G. Acute disc swelling in juvenile diabetes: clinical profile and natural history of 12 cases. *Arch Ophthalmol* 1980;**98**:2185–92.

24 Pavan PR, Aiello LM, Wafai MZ, Briones JC, Sebastyen JC, Bradbury MJ. Optic disc edema in juvenile-onset diabetes. *Arch Ophthalmol* 1980;**98**:2185–92.

25 Fletcher WA, Imes RK, Goodman D, Hoyt WF. Acute idiopathic blind spot enlargement: a big blind spot syndrome without optic disc edema. *Arch Ophthalmol* 1988;**106**:44–9.

26 Dodson PM, Kritzinger EE. Management of retinal vein occlusion. *BMJ* 1987;**295**: 1434–5.

27 Walters RF, Spalton DJ. Central retinal vein occlusion in people aged 40 years or less: a review of 17 patients. *Br J Ophthalmol* 1990;**74**:30–5.

28 Beck RW, Servais GE, Hayreh SS. Acute ischaemic optic neuropathy. IX. Cup-disc ratio and its role in the pathogenesis of acute ischaemic optic neuropathy. *Ophthalmology* 1987;**94**:1503–8.

29 Beck RW, Corbett JJ, Thompson HS, Sergott RC. Decreased visual acuity from optic disc drusen. *Arch Ophthalmol* 1985;**103**:1155–9.

30 Acheson JF, Saunders MD. Coagulation abnormalities in ischaemic optic neuropathy. *Eye* 1994;**8**:89–92.

31 Maitland CG, Miller NR. Neuroretinitis. *Arch Ophthalmol* 1984;**102**:1146–50.

32 Purvin VA, Chioran G. Recurrent neuroretinitis. *Arch Ophthalmol* 1994;**112**:365–71.

33 Kimmell AS, Folk JC, Thompson HS. The multiple evanescent white dot syndrome with acute blind spot enlargement. *Am J Ophthalmol* 1989;**107**:425–6.

34 Noble KG. Central retinal artery occlusion: the presenting sign in radiation retinopathy. *Arch Ophthalmol* 1994;**112**:1409–10.

35 Merry P, Acheson JF, Asherson RA, Hughes GRV. Management of retinal vein occlusion. *BMJ* 1988;**296**:294.
36 Glacet-Bernard A, Bayam N, Chretien P, Cochard C, Lelong F, Coscas G. Antiphospholipid antibodies in retinal vascular occlusion. A prospective study of 75 patients. *Arch Ophthalmol* 1994;**112**:790–5.
37 Ho AC, Sergott RC, Regillo CD, Savino PJ, Lieb WE, Flaherty PM, Bosley TM. Color Doppler hemodynamics of giant cell arteritis. *Arch Ophthalmol* 1994;**112**:938–945.
38 Williamson TH, Harris A. Ocular blood flow measurement. *Br J Ophthalmol* 1994;**78**: 939–45.
39 Bos PJM, Deutman AF. Acute macular neuroretinopathy. *Am J Ophthalmol* 1975;**80**: 573–84.
40 Smith JL, Hoyt WF, Susac JO. Ocular fundus in acute Leber optic neuropathy. *Arch Ophthalmol* 1973;**90**:349–54.
41 Riordan-Eva P, Sanders MD, Govan GG, Sweeney MG, Da Costa J, Harding AE. The clinical features of Leber's hereditary optic neuropathy defined by the presence of a pathogenic mitochondrial DNA mutation. *Brain* 1995;**118**:319–37.
42 Wakakura M, Yokoe J. Evidence for preserved direct pupillary light response in Leber's hereditary optic neuropathy. *Br J Ophthalmol* 1995;**79**:442–6.
43 Kheterpal S, Good PA, Beale DJ, Kritzinger EE. Imaging of optic disc drusen: a comparative study. *Eye* 1995;**9**:67–9.
44 Beck RW, Cleary PA, Trobe JD, Kaufman DI, Kupersmith MJ, Paty DW, Brown CH, and the Optic Neuritis Study Group. The effect of corticosteroids for acute optic neuritis on the subsequent development of multiple sclerosis. *N Eng J Med* 1993;**329**:1764–9.
45 Beck RW. The optic neuritis treatment trial: three year follow up results. *Arch Ophthalmol* 1995;**113**:136–7.
46 Morrissey SP, Miller DH, Kendall BE, *et al.* The significance of brain magnetic resonance imaging abnormalities at presentation with clinically isolated syndromes suggestive of multiple sclerosis. A 5-year follow-up study. *Brain* 1993;**116**:135–46.
47 Wray SH. Optic neuritis: guidelines. *Curr Opin Neurol* 1995;**8**:72–6.
48 Castillo M. *Neuroradiology companion. Methods, guidelines and imaging fundamentals.* Philadelphia: JB Lippincott, 1995.
49 Moseley I. Imaging the adult brain. *J Neurol Neurosurg Psychiatry* 1995;**58**:7–21.
50 Moseley IF. The plain radiograph in ophthalmology: a wasteful and potentially dangerous anachronism. *J R Soc Med* 1991;**84**:76–80.
51 Morrissey SP, Borruat FX, Miller DH, *et al.* Bilateral simultaneous optic neuropathy in adults: clinical, imaging, serological and genetic studies. *J Neurol Neurosurg Psychiatry* 1995;**58**:70–4.
52 Sibony PA, Krauss HR, Kennerdell JS, *et al.* Optic nerve sheath meningiomas: clinical manifestations. *Ophthalmology* 1984;**91**:1313–26.
53 Spector RH, Carlisle JA. Minimal thyroid ophthalmopathy. *Neurology* 1987;**37**:1803–8.
54 Savino PJ, Glaser JS, Rosenberg MA. A clinical analysis of pseudopapilledema II. Visual field defects. *Arch Ophthalmol* 1979;**97**:71–5.
55 Miller NR. *Walsh and Hoyt's clinical neuro-ophthalmology.* 4th ed. Vol 5, part 2. Baltimore: Williams and Wilkins, 1985:4541–63.

9 Eye movements

S SHAUNAK, E O'SULLIVAN, C KENNARD

The clinical diagnosis of eye movement disorders requires the use of a range of investigations of varying degrees of complexity, from the simple cover-uncover test used at the bedside in the evaluation of diplopia to the magnetic field scleral search coil oculographic technique required to measure accurately abnormalities of torsional eye movements.[1] Before we consider the full range of investigations from the bedside to the laboratory, however, it is essential to understand the use to which the results of these investigations are put; these include clinical diagnosis, the study of pathophysiological mechanisms, or determination of therapeutic response. In the case of diplopia (an awareness of seeing the same object in two different locations in visual space), for example, a systematic approach is required to determine which extraocular muscles are affected, the aetiology, and the appropriate management. At each stage it is essential to have a clear understanding of the anatomy and actions of the extraocular muscles so that appropriate investigations can be undertaken and the results correctly interpreted.

Although disturbances of eye position giving rise to diplopia are probably the most common eye movement disorder encountered by clinical neurologists, evaluation of reflexive and voluntary eye movement and identification of nystagmus or some other spontaneous, involuntary, eye movement can provide important clues to the topographical diagnosis. This is possible because the neural pathways controlling the different types of reflex and voluntary eye movements are fairly well segregated in the neuraxis, at least until they feed into the final common "lower" motor neurons in the brainstem, which are responsible for activation of the extraocular muscles. In humans the various types of eye movement all subserve the same goal; the projection of the image of the object of interest on to the most sensitive part of the retina, the fovea. Rapid conjugate eye movements, saccades, enable changes in the line of sight to bring the image of a new object of interest on to the fovea, and the dysjunctive or vergence eye movements ensure that these images are simultaneously placed on both foveae. There is also a need to stabilise the image of the object of interest on the fovea when the object itself moves, achieved by the smooth pursuit system, or when the subject's head or body moves as occurs during locomotion when the vestibular and optokinetic ocular motor reflexes are activated. It is, therefore, necessary to observe each of these different types of eye movement in any assessment. We will only briefly mention the vestibular and optokinetic reflexes, as they are fully discussed in chapter 10.

The examination of static eye movements

Actions of the extraocular muscles

Each eye is rotated by six muscles: four recti and two obliques (box 9.1). It should be noted that the actions of the extraocular muscles are dependent on the starting position of the eye. Hence the superior rectus, because of the anatomy of its insertion into the sclera, acts as a pure elevator only when the globe is abducted by

---

Box 9.1 Action of the extraocular muscles from the primary position

Muscle	Primary action	Secondary action	Tertiary action
Medial rectus	Adduction	—	—
Lateral rectus	Abduction	—	—
Superior rectus	Elevation	Intorsion	Adduction
Inferior rectus	Depression	Extorsion	Adduction
Superior oblique	Intorsion	Depression	Abduction
Inferior oblique	Extortion	Elevation	Abduction

The superior muscles are intortors of the eye and the inferior muscles are extortors.

23°. With increasing adduction of the eye from this position, the superior rectus acts more as an intortor and less as an elevator. Similarly, the superior oblique acts purely as a depressor only when the eye is adducted, and more as an intortor with increasing abduction of the eye. To assess the function of all the extraocular muscles, eye movements should therefore be examined in the nine cardinal positions of gaze. Assessment should include movements of the eyes together, called *versions*, and of each eye individually, called *ductions*.

Hering's and Sherrington's laws

Sherrington's law states that whenever an agonist receives a neural impulse to contract, an equivalent inhibitory impulse is sent to the motor neurons serving the antagonist muscle of the same eye. Every ocular muscle has a contralateral synergist and these muscles, the yoke muscles, act together to move the two eyes in the same direction (for example, the right lateral rectus and left medial rectus both mediate gaze to the right). When an impulse is sent to a muscle causing it to contract, an equal impulse goes to the contralateral synergist to maintain parallelism of the visual axes (Hering's law of motor correspondence). It should be noted that the fixating eye determines the innervational input to both eyes. This is of importance in the assessment of the cover test, and also in the interpretation of investigations such as the Hess screen test.

Abnormalities of fixation

The subject's eyes should be observed in the primary position while fixing an object that requires visual discrimination. Each eye should then be occluded in turn, and any abnormalities such as latent nystagmus observed. The use of an ophthalmoscope to view one optic disc while the patient fixates with the other eye will magnify any movements seen. The most common intrusions are square wave jerks, which have an amplitude of 0.5–10° with refixation within 250 ms. A high frequency of square wave jerks has been reported in cerebellar disease[2] and parkinsonism plus syndromes,[3] among other conditions (box 9.2).[4-7]

Assessment of diplopia

Diplopia is among the most commonly encountered neuro-ophthalmological symptoms in neurological practice, and usually

Box 9.2   Causes of increased square wave jerk frequency (greater than 15 per minute)

Normal elderly subjects
Cerebellar disease
Progressive supranuclear palsy
Multiple system atrophy
Huntington's disease
Motor neuron disease
Schizophrenia

arises from a disparity in retinal stimulation between the two eyes. If diplopia is present with one eye covered, an optical aberration within the refracting media of the eye is likely to be present, although there are other causes of this phenomenon[8] (box 9.3) If diplopia is alleviated by covering one eye, a systematic approach to evaluation is required. As well as determining the nature of separation of the two images and the direction of maximal separation, enquiries as to the presence of a family history of strabismus, or a childhood history of orthoptic treatment should be made. If the eyes are misaligned, it should be ascertained at an early stage if one is dealing with a *non-comitant* or *comitant* strabismus; the degree of misalignment varies with gaze position in the first, but does not vary with gaze position in the second. Non-comitance suggests a recent paretic or restrictive aetiology. Comitance is characteristic of childhood strabismus, and diplopia in such circumstances is usually due to decompensation of a longstanding *phoria* (a deviation of the visual axes when only one eye is viewing, normally kept in check by fusional mechanisms—that is, a latent deviation). The term *tropia* as used later refers to a deviation of the visual axes when both eyes are viewing, which is not kept in check by fusion (a manifest deviation).

Head posture

Patients with diplopia may adopt a compensatory head posture, and the position of the chin, head, and face should therefore be carefully observed. The purpose of an abnormal head posture is to turn the eyes as far as possible from the field of action of the weak muscle. Hence, if one of the muscles that mediates conjugate gaze

---

Box 9.3   Causes of monocular diplopia

Corneal abnormality
Iris abnormality
Lens abnormality
Foreign body (in aqueous or vitreous humour)
Retinal disease
Occipital cortex pathology
Psychogenic

---

to the left is underacting, the face will also be turned to the left. Underaction of the superior or inferior recti, which act primarily to move the eyes in the vertical plane, is compensated by head flexion or extension respectively. Torsional diplopia usually arises from underaction of the superior or inferior oblique muscles, and patients with this symptom often tilt their head towards the shoulder opposite to that of the weak muscle.

Hirschberg's test

This is a rough objective test to determine the degree of tropia, and is particularly useful in young or uncooperative patients. The corneal reflections should be observed while the patient fixates a light source at a distance of 33 cm with both eyes open, and then while each eye fixates in turn. A decentration of the corneal reflex by 1 mm corresponds to about 7° of ocular deviation. The Krimsky test is a variation of this in which prisms are placed in front of the deviated eye until the corneal reflections are symmetric. It should be noted that a small angle strabismus will displace corneal reflections by a degree that is unlikely to be clinically detected.

Ocular ductions and versions

Ocular ductions and versions should be assessed in the nine cardinal positions of gaze. Ductions may not show minimal muscle weakness that can be overcome by the patient, but versions will often show a subtle paresis. A limitation of movement in a particular direction may be related to paresis of the agonist muscle or tethering of the ipsilateral antagonist muscle. Apparent underaction of a muscle may also arise from the phenomenon termed *inhi-*

257

bition of the contralateral antagonist. This arises when a patient fixes with the paretic eye. In these circumstances the unopposed ipsilateral antagonist of the paretic muscle requires less neural input than normal to move the eye. Consequently, from Hering's law, the contralateral yoke muscle also receives subnormal innervation, and seems to have limited excursion. This most commonly causes confusion between true paresis of a superior oblique muscle and apparent paresis of the contralateral superior rectus. In such a situation, however, ocular ductions will be full in the non-paretic eye, although ocular versions may suggest limitation of movement of the contralateral superior rectus if the paretic eye is fixating.

Identification of the paretic muscle
Cover-uncover test (figure 9.1A)

Cover tests rely on the fact that foveation occurs in an eye that is forced to fixate. If the retinal image was not directed on to the fovea before the eye took up fixation, a movement of redress will be noted as the eye fixates, which gives an indication of the degree of misalignment of the visual axes.

The cover-uncover test should be performed both before and after the correction of any abnormal head posture, and with the eyes in the nine cardinal positions of gaze. A clearly defined fixation target at a distance of 6 m should be used, and the test repeated with a near target at a distance of 33 cm to determine the effect of vergence and accommodation on any response seen. The test is performed by occluding one eye at a time, and initially observing the movements of the uncovered eye. If the *uncovered* eye moves to take up fixation, it can be assumed that under binocular conditions the eye was not aligned with fixation, and a manifest deviation was present (a tropia). Inward movement of the uncovered eye indicates an *exotropia*, and outward movement an *esotropia*. A vertical deviation may be either a *hypotropia* or a *hypertropia*, depending on whether the eye moves up or down respectively. The examiner should determine whether the tropia is comitant or non-comitant by seeing if the magnitude of the deviation varies in the different positions of gaze. If no tropia is present, and the covered eye is noted to move to assume fixation just after it is uncovered, a latent deviation (a heterophoria) is present, and this may also be classified as an exophoria, esophoria, hypophoria, or a hyperphoria depending on the direction of the deviation. The test is then repeated, and the same observations

258

made while covering the other eye. It should be noted that the convention is that if there is a vertical deviation of the eyes, the higher of the two is referred to as hypertropic/hyperphoric, regardless of which eye is actually at fault.

Alternate cover test (figure 9.1B)

The alternate cover test is more dissociating than the cover-uncover test, and should be used to fully dissociate the eyes and show the maximal deviation. While the patient fixates a target the occluder is quickly switched from eye to eye to prevent binocular viewing, allowing sufficient time for the eyes to settle in their new position. The alternate cover test should also be performed in the nine cardinal positions of gaze to determine the direction of gaze

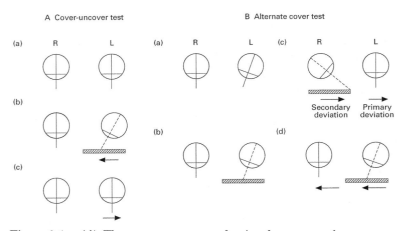

Figure 9.1   *(A) The cover-uncover test, showing the presence of an esophoria. Dotted lines indicate the position of the eye when under cover. (a) At rest the visual axes are aligned correctly. (b) When the cover is placed before the left eye, the eye no longer fixates and moves inwards. (c) On removal of the cover the eye moves outwards to take up fixation, indicating an esophoria. (B) The alternate cover test, showing the presence of an esotropia. (a) At rest, with both eyes viewing, there is a manifest inward deviation of the left eye. (b) A cover placed before the non-fixating left eye causes no movement. (c) When the right eye is occluded, the left eye is forced to fixate, and a movement of redress occurs (the primary deviation). The resulting additional innervation to the contralateral yoke muscle leads to deviation of the sound eye under the cover (the secondary deviation). Note that the secondary deviation is greater than the primary deviation. (d) When the cover is transferred to the left eye both eyes assume their original position*

that elicits the maximal deviation, and the eye in which fixation in that field of gaze causes the greater deviation. It is important that the patient should never be allowed to regain fusion while the occluder is being transferred. The examiner should note the movement of the uncovered eye as the occluder is changed from one eye to the other. Movement of the uncovered eye may indicate either a heterotropia or a heterophoria, and the alternate cover test will not differentiate between these possibilities. The cover-uncover test must therefore be performed first to determine if a tropia is present.

The size of the deviation of the paretic eye when under cover, with the non-paretic eye fixating, is termed the *primary deviation.* When the paretic eye is forced to fixate, additional innervation is required to overcome the paresis. This excessive innervation is also, by Hering's law, equally transmitted to the contralateral synergist, which consequently overacts. This overaction is termed *secondary deviation,* and is greater than the primary deviation. The alternate cover test best shows the difference in size between the primary and secondary deviation, and this finding can be used to identify the weak muscle in a yoke pair by comparing the movements of redress in the two eyes. It should be noted that the movement of redress is equal in both eyes in the case of a comitant strabismus.

Prisms can be used in conjunction with the alternate cover test (prism and cover test) to quantify the deviation by determining the prism strength that nullifies or just reverses the movement of redress. This test measures the total deviation and does not separate tropia from phoria.

The red glass test

This technique allows the patient with diplopia to readily differentiate between the images from each eye. A red filter is placed in front of one eye (by convention the right) so that the subject with diplopia sees two different coloured images. The separation of these images can then be reported by the patient in the nine cardinal positions of gaze, and in head tilts to the right and left. The red image is towards the right (uncrossed) with an esotropia, and towards the left (crossed) with an exotropia. The separation of the two images becomes maximal in the direction of gaze of the paretic muscle, with the image from the paretic eye projected more peripherally.

The Maddox rod test

This technique provides a subjective method of measuring ocular deviations and depends on dissociation of the eyes by presenting a point source of light to one eye and a line image to the other eye. The Maddox rod device consists of small glass rods with a red filter, and has the effect of transforming a point source of light into a line perpendicular to the axes of the cylinder; hence the rods may be oriented according to the desired plane of testing. The test is particularly useful in torsional diplopia where superior or inferior oblique muscle weakness is suspected. In the case of a suspected right superior oblique palsy, for example, the rod is held horizontally before the right eye while the left eye views a white point source of light. The patient will report that the red line is lower than the point source, and relatively intorted, and the separation of the images will be maximal on looking down and to the left. By rotating the rods in their frame until the red line is vertical the amount of cyclotropia (torsional deviation) can be determined. A variation of the test uses both red and white lenses so that the subject can compare the position and orientation of two lines, rather than a line and point source.

The Maddox rod test primarily detects the presence of phorias, because the red lens used produces very dissimilar images and therefore prevents fusional vergence. It should be noted that some patients may be able to fuse the two images in the red glass test, and a phoria can therefore be overlooked. For this reason, the results of the Maddox rod test are usually more reliable. The clinician should be aware that orthophoria (the condition of perfect alignment of the visual axes) is a physiologically unusual state, and normal people often have a small comitant phoria.

Parks-Bielschowsky test for vertical diplopia (figure 9.2)

The Parks-Bielschowsky test is used to ascertain the weak muscle in patients with vertical or torsional diplopia. The first step is to determine with the cover-uncover test whether there is a right or left hypertropia in the primary position and after correction of any abnormal head posture. A right hypertropia, for example, may arise from underaction of the depressors of the right eye (right inferior rectus and superior oblique). Alternatively, the left eye may be hypotropic because of weakness of the elevators of that eye (left inferior oblique and superior rectus). The alternate cover test should then be used to determine whether the amount of vertical

261

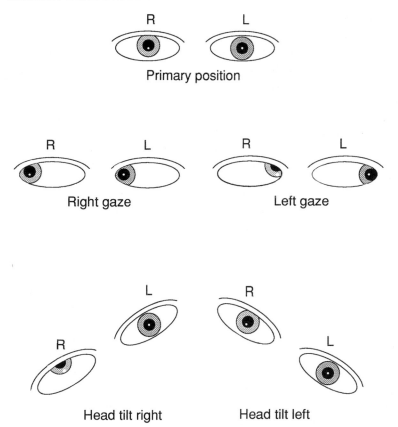

R   L

Primary position

R   L   R   L

Right gaze   Left gaze

L   R

R   L

Head tilt right   Head tilt left

Figure 9.2 *The Parks-Bielschowsky test for vertical diplopia, illustrated for a right fourth nerve palsy. See text for full explanation*

deviation increases in right or left gaze. If the hypertropia increases on left gaze, the right superior oblique or left superior rectus are underacting. Further differentiation between these alternatives is possible by asking the subject to look up and down in left gaze. An increase in hypertropia in gaze downwards implicates the superior oblique as the weak muscle.

Finally, the vertical deviation should be compared with the alternate cover test in right and left head tilt positions. The degree of misalignment will increase when the head is tilted to the side of the paretic muscle if the ipsilateral intortors (superior oblique and superior rectus) are weak, and to the opposite side if the extorting muscles (inferior oblique and inferior rectus) are weak. In practice, an increased misalignment on head tilt is usually indicative of an ipsilateral superior oblique palsy, although the test will help to differentiate this from apparent weakness of the contralateral superior rectus arising from the phenomenon of inhibition of the contralateral antagonist (see earlier). The test is less often positive with palsies of the vertical recti or inferior oblique muscles.

The explanation for the effect lies in the fact that a head tilt to either shoulder induces an ocular counter rolling, which is mediated by the ipsilateral intortors (superior rectus and superior oblique), and the contralateral extortors (inferior rectus and inferior oblique). If, for example, the ipsilateral superior oblique is paretic, the superior rectus on the same side receives excessive innervation to intort the eye, and by virtue of its relatively unopposed primary action elevates the eye.

The Hess screen test

This test is used in the investigation of non-comitant strabismus to assess the paretic element, and depends on the use of mirrors or filters to dissociate the eyes and show the position of the non-fixing eye when the other eye is fixing in specified positions of gaze.[9] The test is invaluable in providing a permanent record of ocular motility that can be used to monitor progress and treatment. Two test objects are presented in the field of view and the patient is required to place them in such a fashion that they seem to be superimposed (the haploscopic principle).

In the Lee's screen adaptation of the test (figure 9.3), the apparatus consists of two glass screens at 90° to each other, which are bisected by a double sided plane mirror. A grid on each screen is marked with dots at 5° intervals, which are connected to form inner and outer fields at displacements of 15° and 30° respectively. The subject fixates with one eye through the mirror the dots on one of the screens which is illuminated, and the examiner uses a pointer to indicate the position of a dot in the field of this eye. The patient is required to place his pointer on the non-illuminated screen, viewed with the other eye, so that it is superimposed over the foveal image of the fixating eye. The blank screen is then briefly illuminated, and the position of the pointer recorded on a chart that is a copy of the grid on the screen. As the innervation of the extraocular muscles of both eyes is determined by the fixating eye, any muscle underaction or overaction in the non-fixating eye

263

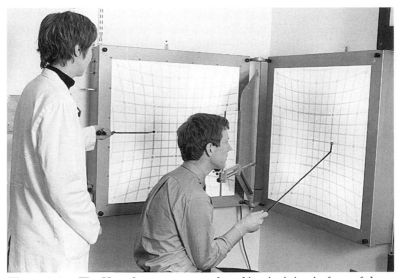

Figure 9.3   *The Hess chart apparatus: the subject is sitting in front of the apparatus and is positioned to test the ocular motility of his right eye. He views the illuminated left screen via the mirror and the orthoptist points to a specific point on the screen. The subject directly views the right screen, which is not illuminated, with his right eye, and places the pointer on the corresponding position. This screen is then illuminated so that the orthoptist may note the location of the pointer in relation to the chart*

can be identified. The procedure is performed in the cardinal positions of gaze, and then repeated with the other eye fixating.

The charts from the two eyes are assessed by comparing the plotted fields with each other and with the normal fields on the chart. A difference in the size of the fields shows non-comitance, which usually indicates the recent onset of paresis. The smaller of the two fields indicates the primarily affected eye. If the fields are displaced but of the same size, comitance is present, and this suggests a longstanding deviation or a non-paretic aetiology.

Each field is then compared with the normal field. The position of the central dot in the smaller field indicates the primary deviation (the result of fixating with the unaffected eye), and its position in the larger field indicates the secondary deviation (the result of fixating with the affected eye). Underaction is identified as inward displacement of the dots, and overaction as outward displacement; maximum displacement will occur in the direction of

264

action of the overacting contralateral synergist. A narrow, symmetric field with restriction in opposite directions implies a mechanical restriction of ocular movement. The outer field should also always be examined; this may show a defect when the central fields appear normal, particularly when a mechanical defect is present, or in cases of slight paresis. Figure 9.4 shows examples of paretic and restrictive Hess charts.

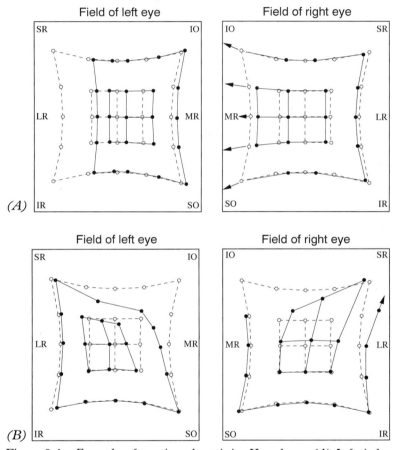

Figure 9.4   *Examples of paretic and restrictive Hess charts. (A) Left sixth nerve palsy. There is underaction of the left lateral rectus, shown by a reduction in size of the inner and outer fields. Note the overaction of the contralateral medial rectus as indicated by the arrows. (B) Left Brown's syndrome, caused by restriction of movement of the superior oblique tendon in the trochlea. There is limitation of elevation of the left eye in adduction, with no abnormality of the lower field, and overaction of the right superior rectus*

265

Secondary changes may occur with time that make determination of the primarily paretic muscle difficult (spread of comitance), and the Hess chart in such circumstances will become increasingly comitant. As well as overaction of the contralateral synergist, overaction of the ipsilateral antagonist due to contracture, and inhibition of the contralateral antagonist will appreciably alter the appearance of the Hess chart. In these circumstances the fact that the overaction of the contralateral synergist to the primarily paretic muscle remains slightly greater than that of the ipsilateral antagonist may help to identify the muscle that was initially paretic.

The Lancaster red-green test

The Lancaster red-green test makes use of the same basic principles, but uses red and green filters to dissociate the eyes.[10] The patient wears reversible goggles with a red filter in front of the right eye and a green filter in front of the left eye, and therefore sees only the image of a red light with the right eye, and the image of a green light with the left eye. The examiner projects the linear image of a red torch on to a screen in the nine cardinal positions of gaze and the patient is asked to superimpose the image of a green torch on to the screen so that the two images seen to him to exactly coincide. If there is a deviation of the visual axes the two images will be separated on the screen. The effect of fixating with either eye can be investigated by either reversing the goggles, or simply by the patient and examiner exchanging torches.

Restrictive muscle disease

Forced duction testing

The forced duction test is used to determine the presence of a mechanical restriction to eye movements. This may occur in, for example, thyroid ophthalmopathy,[11] Brown's superior oblique tendon sheath syndrome,[12] or after orbital blowout fractures (box 9.4). Local or general anaesthesia is required. Two pairs of forceps are applied to diametrically opposed limbal points, and horizontal, oblique, and vertical rotations of the globe are performed. Failure of movement or retraction of the globe into the orbit indicates a restrictive process. Care must be taken that the globe is not inadvertently pushed back into the orbit, as this increases the relative length of the tethered muscle, and may mask a positive result.

An alternative, less invasive, procedure, which may also be used in an uncooperative patient, is to measure intraocular pressures in

Box 9.4 Causes of restrictive ophthalmopathy

Thyroid disease
Brown's syndrome: congenital or acquired
Duane's syndrome
Blowout fractures
Infiltration: for example, metastases, lymphoma, amyloid, orbital myositis, pseudotumour
Caroticocavernous fistula
Extraocular muscle fibrosis
Prolonged muscle weakness with secondary contracture

the primary position and again with gaze in the direction of the limitation of movement. An increase in pressure of greater than 6 mm Hg suggests a mechanical limitation.[13]

The Tensilon test

Myasthenia gravis may mimic any single or combined extraocular muscle palsy, or infranuclear or supranuclear ophthalmoplegia, and must therefore be considered in the differential diagnosis of any puzzling acquired ocular motility disturbance. Although the Tensilon test remains an important tool in the diagnosis of this condition, the clinician must be aware of the limitations and potential pitfalls of the procedure.[14] In particular, it is important that a definite goal or end point be chosen such as a quantifiable change in the degree of ptosis or ocular misalignment (for example, pretest and post-test Hess charts or cover and prism tests).

Bedside examination of dynamic eye movements

After examination of static eye movements the various dynamic eye movement systems, including saccades, pursuit, vestibulo-ocular reflex (VOR), and optokinetic nystagmus (OKN) should be tested, firstly at the bedside and then if necessary by oculography. It should be noted that oculomotor performance may be modulated by the patients' age, attentiveness, and concurrent medication.

Saccades

Voluntary saccade initiation should be assessed by instructing the patient to look from side to side. The patient is then asked to fixate two targets alternately—for example, a pen in one hand and a raised finger in the other—each time they are briefly moved. The distance between the two objects is varied. This generates reflexive saccades, which are tested in both horizontal and vertical planes, and the examiner should observe saccadic variables such as speed of initiation (latency), accuracy, and velocity. Saccadic accuracy can be determined by noting the size and direction of any corrective saccades. Careful observation allows detection of saccades as small as 0.5°. Normal subjects often show a minor degree of saccadic undershoot, which is more often found with larger gaze shifts.

Any slowing of saccades can be accentuated by using an optokinetic striped drum or tape, when the repositioning saccades will appear slowed. This is of particular help when showing slowed adduction in a partial internuclear ophthalmoplegia.[15] Another method to accentuate this abnormality is to use oblique targets. Because the velocity is slowed in one plane the resulting saccade will be L shaped, because the normal vertical component is completed before the abnormal horizontal one.

Other types of saccades can also be generated at the bedside.[16] For example, antisaccades (saccades in the opposite direction to the target) can be tested by holding up both hands on either side of the patient and asking them not to look at the finger that is moved but instead to look in the opposite direction. If the patient repeatedly makes a reflexive saccade to the finger that has moved rather than in the opposite direction a high level of distractibility (impaired ability to suppress reflexive saccades) is shown. Elevated antisaccade error rates are associated with frontal lobe dysfunction, and have been reported in patients with frontal lobe lesions,[17] schizophrenia,[18] Huntington's disease,[19] progressive supranuclear palsy and corticobasal degeneration,[20] and motor neuron disease.[7] Predictive saccades can be tested by alternately raising a finger of one hand and then the other in a predictable regular pattern, and asking the patient to make saccades to the target.

Finally the patient should be observed for any head movements or blinks before making a saccade, as occurs in Huntington's disease[5] and ocular motor apraxia.[21]

Smooth pursuit

Smooth pursuit can be tested by asking the patient to track a small target at a distance of about 1 m while keeping their head still. Assessment of both horizontal and vertical smooth pursuit should be performed. The target should be moved initially at a slow uniform speed and the pursuit eye movements observed to determine whether they are smooth, or broken up by catch up saccades. This is a non-specific sign if present in both directions—for example, due to aging[22] or cerebellar disease[23]—or it may indicate a focal posterior cortical lesion if only present in one direction.[24] The speed should be gradually increased, but at high velocities all smooth pursuit eye movements will be broken up by saccades, even in normal subjects. These saccadic intrusions occur as the smooth pursuit velocity of the eye fails to match that of the target—that is, the pursuit gain (pursuit velocity divided by target velocity) is reduced.

The OKN drum and tape actually stimulate pursuit eye movements rather than optokinetic nystagmus.[1] They are useful in testing for pursuit asymmetries (pursuit which is worse in one direction), and reversed pursuit in which the fast phases are in the direction of the drum rotation, as in congenital nystagmus.[25] If the smooth pursuit gain is reduced to one side, the eyes will deviate less quickly from their primary position, so fewer quick phases are seen when the subject observes an OKN drum.

If a target is tracked by head movements the VOR acts to generate eye movements that would compensate for the head movements. These are in an inappropriate direction and are therefore normally suppressed. Studies in normal subjects[26] and patients[27] have led to the belief that the suppression of the VOR is derived from the smooth pursuit system, and that patients with abnormal smooth pursuit have impaired suppression of the VOR. This may be tested by asking the patient to fixate their thumbnail with their arms outstretched while rotating their head and trunk in harmony.[28] Impaired cancellation of the VOR and hence abnormal pursuit are shown by observing the eye repeatedly moving off fixation due to the VOR, followed by refixation saccades. This is a particularly useful technique for testing pursuit in patients with gaze evoked nystagmus.

Optokinetic nystagmus

As discussed earlier the optokinetic system cannot be tested as part of a clinical examination, because the OKN drum and tape commonly used actually test smooth pursuit and not the optokinetic system.

Vestibular system

The patient should be observed for nystagmus with and without fixation and also after shaking the head for 15 seconds.[29] Frenzel goggles may be useful for studying eye movements without the subject fixating.

If the vestibulo-ocular system is functioning normally passive rotation of the patient's head should result in a slow eye movement so that the eyes deviate in the opposite direction to that of the head movement. This is known as the doll's head (oculocephalic) manoeuvre and should be performed both horizontally and vertically. This technique is not only valuable for assessing vestibular function, but also for differentiating between nuclear and supranuclear gaze palsies, and in the evaluation of brainstem function in comatose patients. It should be noted that the eye movements elicited by this procedure in unconscious patients largely reflect the integrity of the semicircular canals and their central connections, although in conscious patients the effects of visual input on eye movements may influence the response to head rotation.

A rough estimate of any deterioration of vestibular gain (head velocity divided by eye velocity) can be obtained by asking the patient to read a Snellen chart while their head is being passively rotated. If there is an abnormality the visual acuity will show a deterioration compared with the acuity obtained with the head still. With an ophthalmoscope the examiner can observe the patient's optic disc while they fixate a distant object and shake their head from side to side.[30] If the gain of the VOR is unity the examiner will not see any movement of the patient's disc.

Vestibular nystagmus can be elicited by rotating the patient in a swivel chair at a constant velocity. By altering head position horizontal, vertical and torsional nystagmus can be shown. Postrotatory nystagmus will be seen if the chair is suddenly stopped. This will be emphasised if the patient wears Frenzel goggles, so removing fixation and allowing the examiner to estimate the duration of the postrotatory nystagmus.

Caloric stimulation can also be used to test the vestibulo-ocular system. The test is performed with the patient supine. The external auditory meatus is checked to ensure that the tympanic membrane is intact. The head is flexed to 30° to allow maximum stimulation of the horizontal semicircular canals. One to two hundred millilitres of either warm water (44°C) or cold water (30°C) is infused into the patient's ear. The normal response in an awake patient is for a slow-phase response towards the side of the cold water irrigation (or away from the warm water) with the fast phase away from the cold water (or towards the warm water). The test is best performed both with and without fixation to assess the degree of suppression of the nystagmus by fixation. Frenzel goggles can be used to remove fixation.

Oculographic techniques

Although a correct diagnosis of many eye movement disorders can be ascertained by the bedside methods already described, it is only by using oculographic recording techniques that more subtle abnormalities can be detected by the quantitative analysis and evaluation they afford. In particular the development of very precise behavioural paradigms in the laboratory evoking saccadic and pursuit eye movements has shown disturbances previously undetected at the bedside.

The ideal system

When considering the various techniques available it is necessary to be clear about the requirements for an ideal eye movement recording system.[31] These are:

(a) Easy, non-traumatic application, ideally with no contact with the eye.

(b) No interference with normal vision, and a sufficiently large field of vision.

(c) Simultaneous measurement of horizontal, vertical, and torsional eye movements.

(d) High accuracy and repeatability, with a wide linear range of over 90° of eye position.

(e) High resolution allowing detection of eye movements as small as a few seconds of arc.

(f) Good stability with no baseline drift.

(g) Good dynamic measuring range (frequency bandwidth) of zero to a few hundred Hz.

(h) Insensitivity to translational head movements, and thus no need for rigid head fixation.

(i) Insensitivity to surrounding levels of illumination, and to artefacts arising from blinks and electromyographic or electromechanical interference.

271

Unfortunately none of the current techniques fulfil all these criteria, although some of the four main methodologies in current use fulfil most of them.

Electro-oculography

The most commonly used technique and the one that has been available for the longest period is electro-oculography (EOG). As a method to provide a simple visual record of an eye movement disorder EOG is the simplest and cheapest. If high resolution analysis of eye movements, particularly saccades is required, however, this technique has numerous disadvantages. It relies on the fact that the globe acts as an electrostatic dipole, with the cornea 0.4–1.0 mV positive with respect to the posterior pole. Electrodes are placed on the skin on either side of the eye and the magnitude of the potential recorded depends on the proximity of the cornea to the electrode.[32] A major disadvantage is the variability of the corneoretinal potential, particularly in relation to ambient illumination.[33] This results in drifting of the baseline, and it is, therefore, necessary to dark adapt the subject for 15–20 minutes before testing. There is also a rather high baseline noise level due both to electromagnetic interference and periorbital muscle activity.[34] This necessitates the use of low pass filtering with a differential amplifier and great care with the placement of the electrodes. Its sensitivity is at best 0.5° and more usually only 1–2°.

There are advantages to EOC over other techniques. There is a large measurement range of up to ±60° horizontally and ±40° vertically although the vertical movement recordings are subject to error and only provide qualitative assessment; the analogue output is linear over a range of ±30°[34]; there are no limitations of the fields of vision and the subjects can wear their spectacles; and recordings can be made with the eyelids closed, which is useful during vestibular and caloric testing.

Infrared limbus reflection oculography (figure 9.5)

The second technique that is being increasingly used both for routine eye movement assessment and research is the infrared limbus reflection (IRLR) technique. The eye is diffusely illuminated with infrared, which is differentially reflected by the iris and the sclera back to photocells positioned near the limbus.[35] As the sclera reflects better than the iris the output from the photocells will be directly proportional to the position of the eye. The posi-

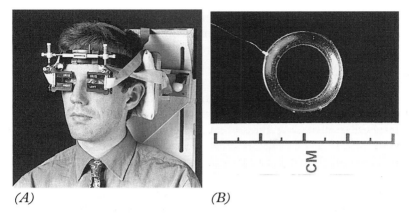

(A)   *(B)*

Figure 9.5   *Laboratory equipment used to record eye movements. (A) A subject wearing the headset used for infrared oculography. (IRIS IR light tracker, Skalar, Delft, Netherlands). (B) The magnetic scleral search coil*

tioning of the infrared emitters and the photocells is crucial for accurate and linear recordings.[36] The other problem is fixation of the head, which is necessary if the recorded eye movement is to be an accurate representation of direction of gaze. Infrared oculography systems are generally linear within a horizontal range of ±15°, and a vertical range of ±10°, although satisfactory vertical recording can be difficult.[37] It has been claimed that sensitivity for this technique is of the order of 3 minutes of arc, but in practice it is not quite so impressive.

High speed video recorders

A third technique is high speed television recording, which with the rapid advances in technology, and therefore of temporal resolution, is likely to become increasingly used for oculography. These systems usually locate the pupil centre using software algorithms for each frame.[38] Currently the spatial resolution is very good in both horizontal and vertical axes, and is highly suitable for recording two dimensional scanpaths, but temporal resolution is still inadequate for full analysis of saccadic metrics.

Magnetic field scleral search coil technique

Finally, probably the most accurate system is the magnetic field scleral search coil (MFSSC) method.[39] The subject is seated so that the head is located in an alternating magnetic field. The sub-

273

ject wears a ring shaped contact lens in which is embedded a coil of wire. An alternating current is thereby induced in the wire, which is proportional to the sine of the angle between the planes of the search coil and the direction of the magnetic field. Both horizontal and vertical eye position may be measured simultaneously, and with appropriate windings of the wire coil so may torsional eye movements. The method has low noise levels and high sensitivity in the order of a few seconds of arc,[39 40] and its linear range is ±20°, greater if a sine function correction is used.

There are, however, two main disadvantages of the method. Firstly, the subject has to wear a scleral contact lens held to the eye by suction.[41] Although topical local anaesthetic is used, some subjects find the insertion and removal of the coil unpleasant. As the coil can only be left in place for up to 30 minutes this can limit the number of tests performed. The second main disadvantage is cost. Most complete systems are expensive as are the coils, which usually last for only about five subjects.

It becomes apparent that none of the currently available techniques meets the full set of ideal criteria discussed earlier. The method chosen rather depends on the clinician's requirements. If, for example, a record of a patient's nystagmus is required, then a straightforward video recording would be appropriate, perhaps with an EOG chart record. For recording slow eye movements such as VOR or OKN the use of EOG is adequate, but if a detailed analysis of saccadic metrics is required IRLR or MFSSC would be more appropriate. The cheapest method is EOG and MFSSC is the most expensive. If large eccentric eye movements are to be recorded then EOG is best, as it is for recording patients with their eyes closed, required in testing vestibular function, or when unconscious.

Although it is possible to perform some quantification of eye movement records directly from the chart records, the analogue signal produced by the oculographic equipment is usually digitised and the data analysis proceeds off line at a later date with interactive computer programs.

Laboratory investigation of dynamic eye movements

Saccades

Essentially when saccadic eye movements are investigated in the laboratory, the same paradigms described earlier are tested. A

274

range of more behaviourally demanding saccadic paradigms such as the antisaccade, predictive saccade, and remembered saccade tasks may be used in the laboratory, and may show a dissociation in performance in different patient groups.[16] The measurement of saccades in the laboratory also allows both more controlled presentation of the stimuli and more accurate measurement of the variables mentioned. The beginning and end of a saccade are defined arbitrarily, often when the eye velocity rises above or falls below 20°/s respectively.

Rapid refixation gaze movements are largely achieved by a saccade that covers about 90% of the required distance (primary saccade), followed by a series of secondary saccades until the target is foveated. Accuracy of the primary saccade is expressed as saccadic gain. This is the value of the primary saccadic amplitude divided by the target amplitude, so that a perfectly accurate primary saccade has a gain of 1.0. Often the gain of the primary saccade and also the gain of the final eye position (FEP) after the secondary saccades are recorded. Figure 9.6 shows an example of a laboratory recording of performance in a saccadic task.

The peak velocities of saccades show a unique feature; there is a progressive exponential increase in velocity with saccadic amplitude until it saturates at about 20–30°. This consistent relation between saccadic amplitude and peak velocity is known as the main sequence (figure 9.7).[42] Clinical laboratories should derive their own normative values for saccadic variables, as these vary depending on the precise details of the test procedures and the oculographic equipment.

Smooth pursuit (figure 9.8)

Laboratory evaluation of smooth pursuit uses many different types of stimulus presentation, some of which cannot be tested at the bedside. Usually the stimulus is a small bright spot of light, the position of which is controlled by mirror galvanometers, and which is projected on to a screen. Alternatively a spot on a computer screen may be used although this method does not allow testing of such a large range of movements.

The most commonly used pursuit stimuli are either constant velocity (ramp stimulus) or sinusoidal waveforms. A range of different velocities or frequencies are tested. Interactive computer programs allow the analysis of smooth pursuit to calculate such pursuit variables as velocity gain (eye velocity/target velocity). The

275

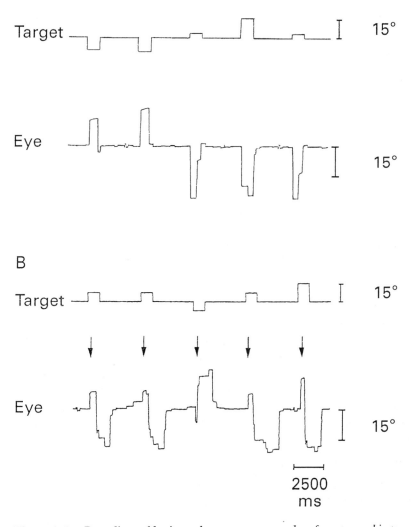

Figure 9.6   *Recordings of horizontal eye movements taken from two subjects performing the antisaccade task (magnetic field scleral search coil technique). Upward displacements indicate movement of the eye or target to the right, and downward displacements movements to the left. (A) Control subject. The subject is performing the paradigm correctly, and making saccades in the opposite direction to the target. (B) Subject with frontal lobe dysfunction. The arrows denote the onset of reflexive saccades in the same direction as the target, which are corrected in all cases by saccades in the opposite direction*

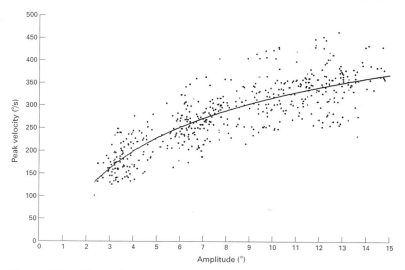

Figure 9.7   *The main sequence: a graph of the peak velocity of saccades from 11 normal subjects plotted as a function of their amplitude*

maximum gain averaged from a series of cycles or the gain averaged as the eye passes the primary position is measured. For sinusoidal targets both gain and phase can be measured. The gain is calculated from peak eye velocity/peak target velocity. The gain is known to be dependent on the peak acceleration of the target.[43] These stimuli mainly test the maintenance of pursuit, although another aspect of the pursuit system of interest is pursuit initiation.

Optokinetic nystagmus

Adequate assessment of the optokinetic system requires a stimulus that fills the patient's field of vision and induces the sense of self rotation (circularvection). One method is to rotate the patient at a constant velocity in the light for more than a minute. This allows the VOR to decay and so the nystagmus is solely due to visual input. Another method is to sit the patient inside a large optokinetic drum. The eye movements stimulated are conjugate eye movements of constant velocity in the direction of the stimulus, interspersed with quick phases in the opposite dlrection. The way in which the patient is instructed determines the type of

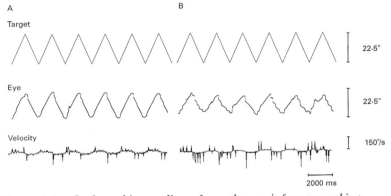

Figure 9.8   *Oculographic recordings of smooth pursuit from two subjects tracking a target moving horizontally at a constant velocity of 20°/s (magnetic field scleral search coil technique). (A) Tracing from a normal subject showing accurate tracking. (B) Tracing from a patient with motor neuron disease showing poor tracking with frequent catch up saccades*

response. If the patient is asked to follow the stripes *look nystagmus*, which consists of prolonged slow phases with large corrective saccades, is seen. If the subject is asked to stare ahead at the stripes *stare nystagnus* is induced, which is characterised by smaller and more frequent quick phases.

Both the smooth pursuit system and the optokinetic system contribute to the response. During the initial few seconds smooth pursuit constitutes the more important component. When the visual stimulus ceases the response should continue. This is known as optokinetic after-nystagmus (OKAN). The optokinetic system acts as a velocity storage mechanism during the presence of the stimuli and when this is no longer visible the nystagmus continues in the same direction for a few seconds with a declining slow phase velocity.

When studying OKN the nystagmus seen in the presence and absence of visual stimuli should be studied. This is most easily done by turning out the lights after a period of optokinetic stimulation, often after the drum has rotated at 60°/s for 60 seconds. The velocity gain (eye velocity/target velocity) and the symmetry of the response are measured for both OKN and OKAN. The time constant of the slow phase eye movements of the OKAN can also be measured.

Box 9.5 Clinical and investigative approach to eye movement abnormalities

Bedside assessment   Laboratory investigation

Static eye movements (diplopia)

Ocular ductions and versions   Hess screen test
Hirschberg/Krimsky test   Red glass test
Cover-uncover test   Lancaster red-green test
Alternate cover test   Maddox rod test
Parks-Bielschowsky test   Tensilon test
                                  Forced ductions

Dynamic eye movements

Saccades: EOG, IRLR, MFSSC, high
                                     speed video
                                  Variables studied:
  Fixation stability   Primary saccade gain
  Latency, accuracy, velocity   FEP gain
  Distractibility   Latency, velocity
    (for example, antisaccades)   Distractibility
Smooth pursuit: EOG, IRLR, MFSSC, high
  Saccadic intrusions   speed video
  Symmetry/asymmetry   Variables studied:
  Vestibulo-ocular reflex   Velocity gain
    suppression   Saccadic intrusions
                                    Phase

Vestibulo-ocular reflex:
  Doll's head manoeuvre   See chapter 10
  Caloric stimulation
Optokinetic nystagmus:
  OKN drum   Full field visual stimulation
  (actually tests smooth pursuit; see text)

See text for abbreviations.

Because of the great variability in the measurement of a subject's OKAN eye velocity and time constant, repeated measures are needed.[45] Alternatively the build up of the slow phase velocity of the OKAN can be monitored by briefly turning out the lights during frequent, two second periods of darkness during the stimulation.[46] To prevent contamination of the data by smooth pursuit the first one second of each two second period should be discarded.

Conclusion

The intention of this review has been to provide the clinician with an overview of the clinical assessment and appropriate investigation of a patient presenting with a disturbance of eye movements (box 9.5). Because many neurological conditions may cause abnormalities of ocular motility, a rational approach to this situation remains of great importance to the practising neurologist. Although a variety of specialised investigations are available, an appreciation of the basic anatomical and physiological principles involved is necessary, both for an adequate bedside assessment and for such investigations to be appropriately employed and interpreted. These findings must of course be viewed in conjunction with the general neurological examination and the results of other appropriate investigations, such as neuroimaging, discussion of which is beyond the remit of this review.

1 Leigh RJ, Zee DS. *The neurology of eye movement.* 2nd ed. Philadelphia: FA Davis, 1991.
2 Sharpe JA, Herishanu YO, White OB. Cerebral square wave jerks. *Neurology* 1982;32: 57–62.
3 Rascol O, Sabatini U, Simonetta-Moreau M, *et al.* Square wave jerks in parkinsonian syndromes. *J Neurol Neurosurg Psychiatry* 1991;54:599–602.
4 Elidan J, Gay I, Lev S. Square wave jerks—incidence, characteristics and significance. *J Otolaryngol* 1984;13:375–81.
5 Leigh R, Newman S, Folstein S, *et al.* Abnormal ocular motor control in Huntington's chorea. *Neurology* 1983;33:1268–75.
6 Ross D, Ochs A, Hill M, *et al.* Erratic eye tracking in schizophrenic patients as revealed by high-resolution techniques. *Biol Psychiatry* 1988;24:675–88.
7 Shaunak S, Orrell R, O'Sullivan E, *et al.* Oculomotor function in amyotrophic lateral sclerosis: evidence for frontal impairment. *Ann Neurol* 1995;38:38–44.
8 Smith JL. Monocular diplopia [editorial comment]. *Journal of Clinical Neuroophthalmology* 1986;6:184–5.
9 Mein J, Trimble R. *Diagnosis and management of ocular motility disorders.* 2nd ed. Oxford: Blackwell, 1991.
10 Lancaster WB. Detecting, measuring, plotting and interpreting ocular deviations. *Arch Ophthalmol* 1939;22:867–80.
11 de Waard R, Koorneef L, Verbeeten G. Motility disturbances in Graves' ophthalmopathy. *Doc Ophthalmol* 1983;56:41–7.
12 Moore AT, Morin JD. Bilateral acquired inflammatory Brown's syndrome. *J Pediatr Ophthalmol Strabismus* 1985;22:26–30.
13 Zappia RJ, Winkelman JZ, Gay AJ. Intraocular presure changes in normal subjects and the adhesive muscle syndrome. *Am J Ophthalmol* 1971;71:880–3.
14 Moorthy G, Behrens M, Drachman D, *et al.* Ocular pseudomyasthenia or ocular myasthenia 'plus': a warning to clinicians. *Neurology* 1989;39:1150–4.

15 Smith JL, David NJ. Internuclear ophthalmoplegia. Two new clinical signs. *Neurology* 1964;**14**:307–9.

16 Kennard C, Crawford TJ, Henderson L. A pathophysiological approach to saccadic eye movements in neurological and psychiatric disease. *J Neurol Neurosurg Psychiatry* 1994;**57**: 881–5.

17 Guitton D, Buchtal H, Douglas R. Frontal lobe lesions in man cause difficulties in suppressing reflexive glances and in generating goal directed saccades. *Exp Brain Res* 1985;**58**:455–74.

18 Fukushima J, Fukushima K, Chiba T, *et al*. Disturbances of voluntary control of saccadic eye movements in schizophrenic patients. *Biol Psychiatry* 1988;**23**:670–7.

19 Lasker A, Zee D, Hain T, *et al*. Saccades in Huntington's disease: initiation defects and distractibility. *Neurology* 1987;**37**:364–70.

20 Vidailhet M, Rivaud S, Gouidet-Khouja N, *et al*. Eye movements in parkinsonian syndromes. *Ann Neurol* 1994;**35**:420–6.

21 Zee DS, Yee RD, Singer HS. Congenital ocular motor apraxia. *Brain* 1977;**100**:581–99.

22 Zackon D, Sharpe J. Smooth pursuit in senescence. *Acta Otolaryngol (Stockh)* 1987; **104**:297–8.

23 Pierrot-Deseilligny C, Amarenco P, Roullet E, Marteau R. Vermal infarct with pursuit eye movement disorders. *J Neurol Neurosurg Psychiatry* 1990;**53**:519–21.

24 Morrow MJ, Sharpe JA. Cerebral hemispheric localisation of smooth pursuit asymmetry. *Neurology* 1990;**40**:284–92.

25 Halmagyi GM, Gresty MA, Leech J. Reversed optokinetic nystagmus (OKN): mechanism and clinical significance. *Ann Neurol* 1979;**6**:80–3.

26 Barnes GR, Benson AJ, Prior ARJ. Visual-vestibular interaction in the control of eye movement. *Aviat Space Environ Med* 1978;**49**:557–64.

27 Halmagyi GM, Gresty MA. Clinical signs of visual-vestibular interaction. *J Neurol Neurosurg Psychiatry* 1979;**42**:934–9.

28 Dichgans J, Von Reutern GM, Rommelt U. Impaired suppression of vestibular nystagmus by fixation in cerebellar and noncerebellar patients. *Archiv für Psychiatrie und Nervenkrankheiten* 1978;**226**:183–99.

29 Hai TC, Fetter M, Zee DS. Head shaking nystagmus in patients with unilateral peripheral vestibular lesions. *Am J Otolaryngol* 1987;**8**:36–47.

30 Zee DS. Ophthalmoloscopy in examination of patients with vestibular disorders. *Ann Neurol* 1978;**3**:373–74.

31 Lueck CJ, Kennard C. Oculography and techniques for eye movement recording. *Bull Soc Belge Ophthalmol* 1989;**237**:485–502.

32 Shackel B. Eye movement recording by electrooculography. In: Venables PH, Martion I, eds. *A manual of psychophysiological methods.* Amsterdam: North Holland Publishing, 1967:300–34.

33 Arden FH, Kelsey JH. Changes produced by light in the standing potential of the human eye. *J Physiol* 1962;**161**:189–204.

34 Young LR, Sheena D. Survey of eye movement recording methods. *Behaviour Research Methods and Instrumentation* 1975;**7**:397–429.

35 Stark L, Vossius G, Young LR. Predictive control of eye tracking movements. *Institute of Radioengineering Transactions on Human Factors in Electronics* 1962;**3**:52–7

36 Truong DM, Feldon SE. Sources of artefact in infrared recording of eye movements. *Invest Ophthalmol Vis Sci* 1987;**28**:1018–22.

37 Gauthier GM, Volle M. Two-dimensional eye movement monitor for clinical and laboratory recordings. *Electroencephologr Clin Neurophysiol* 1975;**39**:285–91.

38 Barbur JL, Thomson WD, Forsyth PM. A new system for the simultaneous measurement of pupil size and three-dimensional eye movements. *Clin Vis Sci* 1987;**2**:131–42.

39 Robinson DA. A method of measuring eye movement using a scleral coil in a magnetic field. *Institute of Radioengineering Transactions of Biomedical Electronics* 1963;**10**:137–45.

40 Remmel RS. An inexpensive eye movement monitor using the scleral search coil technique. *Institute of Radioengineering Transactions Biomedical Engineering* 1984;**31**:388–90.

41 Collewijn H, Van der Mark F, Jansen TC. Precise recording of human eye movements. *Vision Res* 1975;**15**:447–50.

42 Boghen D, Troost BT, Daroff RB, *et al*. Velocity characteristics of normal human saccades. *Invest Ophthalmol Vis Sci* 1974;**13**:619–23.

43 Lisberger SG, Evinger C, Johanson GW, Fuchs AF. Relationship between eye acceleration and retinal image velocity during foveal smooth pursuit in man and monkey. *J Neurophysiol*

1981;**46**:229–49.
44 Thurston SE, Leigh RJ, Crawford TJ *et al.* Two distinct deficits of vision tracking caused by unilateral lesions of cerebral cortex in humans. *Ann Neurol* 1988;**23**:266–73.
45 Tijssen MAJ, Straathof CSM, Hain TC, Zee DS. Optokinetic afternystagmus in humans: normal values of amplitude, time constant and asymmetry. *Ann Otol Rhinol Laryngol* 1989;**98**:741–6.
46 Segal BN, Liben S. Modulation of human velocity storage sampled during intermittently-illuminated optokinetic stimulation. *Exp Brain Res* 1985;**59**:515–23.

10 Investigations of disorders of balance

P RUDGE, A M BRONSTEIN

To maintain balance in the upright position, a complex and not altogether successful series of neurological mechanisms have evolved. These comprise visual, proprioceptive, and vestibular systems, all of which interact, and information which is analysed by the cerebellum, cerebral cortex, and basal ganglia. As a result of this analysis appropriate motor outputs occur in an attempt to maintain posture and gait. Dysfunction of any part can result in imbalance or a feeling of spatial disorientation.

In this article we consider tests primarily of the vestibular system, which help to determine what abnormalities account for a patient's symptoms. We will not consider in any detail research techniques or analyses that are of little value in the clinical assessment of the patient at the present time. As in all branches of medicine it is essential to obtain an accurate history and to do a thorough general and neurological examination of any patient complaining of impaired balance before embarking on extensive investigation; a complaint of imbalance may signify a wide range of possible diseases including disorders of the cardiovascular and musculoskeletal systems, as well as dysfunction of the nervous system.

Clinical investigation of the vestibular system

The vestibular system comprises two main components; one concerned with detection of angular acceleration (semicircular canals) and one concerned with detection of linear acceleration (otoliths).

283

The semicircular canals comprise three pairs of accelerometers arranged roughly in three orthogonal planes, one set on each side of the head. In humans and other erect primates, the vertical canals are large compared with those in quadrupeds, a point of some relevance in that we have greater ability to assess the horizontal than the vertical canals.[1] Whereas the adequate stimulus is acceleration, because of the nature of flow of fluids through narrow tubes of large radius of curvature, the VIIIth nerve carries velocity (first integral) information to the vestibular nuclei.[2] Further integration to position occurs at a central level and this information is fed to various motor nuclei in the brain stem and cord as well as to the cerebellum and cerebral cortex.[2]

Clinical assessment of the integrity of the vestibulospinal connections is not entirely satisfactory. Traditionally this is determined by studying stance and gait with and without fixation. Acute failure of vestibular input from one side results in the patient falling to that side, a situation made worse by removal of fixation. Similarly, when such patients walk they usually veer to the side of the lesion; again this is accentuated by eye closure. Various clinical tests with eponymous titles have been devised in an attempt to increase the accuracy in determining the side of a unilateral lesion. For example, in Unterburger's test the patient is instructed to march on the spot with the eyes closed; in the case of a unilateral lesion the patient rotates to the side of the lesion. Although these clinical tests may be indicative of abnormality, their ability to predict the side of a unilateral lesion is poor, especially in chronic, progressive, or partially compensated lesions. Removal of proprioceptive cues can also be useful in assessing patients especially those with total vestibular failure. If such patients are placed on a rubber mattress and then fixation is removed they will fall as proprioceptive cues function poorly under these circumstances. Attempts have been made to improve the sensitivity and specificity of stance assessment by the development of various mechanical platforms (see posturography).

Of particular concern to the neurologist are the connections to the extraocular muscle nuclei which permit the vestibulo-ocular reflex (VOR). This reflex functions in the three cardinal planes. Stimulation or inhibition of complementary pairs of canals results in appropriate movement of the eyes ensuring adequate foveation during head movement. The system has a wide dynamic range sufficient to stabilise a retinal image on the fovea through most

284

movements.[3] This is necessary as the only other mechanism available for image stabilisation is the pursuit optokinetic system, which functions poorly above 1 Hz.

The other major part of the vestibular system is that involved in gravity detection. This system comprises two end organs (saccule and utricle) which detect linear acceleration (including gravity) by virtue of the otoconia that rest on hair cells of the macula. Each macula can signal acceleration in many directions because of the multiple orientation of hair cells in the end organ.[2] Connections of these linear accelerometers are less well determined than those from semicircular canals but there are connections to the neurons innervating somatic and eye muscles.

Clinical assessment of the VOR

The most useful reflexes clinically to assess the vestibular system are the vestibulo-ocular ones. In the main, these involve activation of the semicircular canals (VOR in the three cardinal planes) by variants of the doll's head manoeuvre. However, it is difficult clinically to assess canal function in isolation because of the presence of pursuit-optokinetic eye movements in the light and excitation of cervical receptors. Normal neck-eye reflexes are weak and contamination from them can be avoided by using a swivel office chair to rotate the whole patient in the horizontal plane; this is also of value in cases of neck rigidity or poor patient cooperation. Despite these limitations VOR examination is useful in cases of ophthalmoplegia to see if restriction of gaze can be overridden by a rotation of the head in the appropriate plane. For example, in Steele-Richardson syndrome the ophthalmoplegia is initially supranuclear leaving the final common pathway via the extraocular motor nuclei intact; pursuit and especially saccadic movements are limited due to the disconnection of cortical pathways in the mesencephalon and brain stem. Proof that the ophthalmoplegia is indeed supranuclear is obtained by showing full range of movement, or improvement of movement, by the VOR. This is most easily done by getting the subject to fixate an earthbound target and rotating the head in a sinusoidal fashion up and down (the direction in which limitation first occurs) and showing improvement in the excursion of the eye. Clearly, pursuit may play a part in this improvement but the VOR is the most important factor. Information is fed from the vestibular nuclei and lower brain stem to the mesencephalic nuclei responsible for vertical gaze.

285

Clinically, some information on VOR function can be obtained by turning the patient's head while observing the optic disc during funduscopy.[4] The patient must be instructed to maintain fixation on an object across the room. Normally, the disc remains steady in space but if, say, the right labyrinth is hypoactive, the disc will seem to jerk during turning of the head (chin) to the right. When the vestibular loss is profound, this jerky eye movement in response to turns of the head can be seen by the naked eye. In this case it is best to instruct the patient to fixate on the examiner's nose.

Assessment of otolith function clinically is even less easily done. Counter rolling of the eyes can be seen when the head is rotated to the ear down on one shoulder; the eyes slowly deviate in the opposite sense and then there is a rotatory quick phase causing torsional nystagmus. This response is, however, mainly dependent on the vertical semicircular canals rather than the otoliths. Skew deviation of the eyes (vertical divergence of the eyes) without nystagmus is thought to reflect tonic otolith pathway imbalance. It can be seen with utricular nerve lesion[5] or with lesions of the mesencephalon, especially those involving the interstitial nucleus of Cajal[6] and medulla; this type of tonic rotation may be suspected from a head tilt, or the eye covering test, or seen from tilting of the optic disc.

A further important finding that can be made on the VOR in a clinical setting is assessment of VOR suppression (VORS). In a normal subject the VOR enables fixation to be maintained during head motion. However, if a subject is rotated through large angles, the VOR is interrupted by repetitive saccadic movements in the opposite sense to the slow movement; this is vestibular nystagmus. The VORS is easily tested by getting the subject to fixate a long spatula gripped in the teeth while oscillating the head in the horizontal or vertical plane,[7] or more simply by fixating their thumbs with arms outstretched while rotating at the waist or on a swivel chair. No nystagmus is seen in the normal subject until the frequency of oscillation approaches 1 Hz or the peak velocity is greater than 60°/s. Similarly, in peripheral disturbances the VORS is intact. In many patients with cerebellar and brain stem lesions VORS is absent—that is, nystagmus is even seen during slow head movements. There is usually a good correlation between VORS and pursuit; absent pursuit usually results in absent VORS. Using electronystagmography (ENG) and other methods of eye movement recording it is possible to obtain an accurate measure of the VORS (see laboratory assessment).

Clinical assessment of spontaneous nystagmus

One of the cardinal signs of abnormal vestibular function is nystagmus but not all nystagmus signifies vestibular abnormality. To differentiate between types of nystagmus may require an analog or digital recording of the wave form of the movement and an assessment of the effect of the removal of fixation on the nystagmus.

Vestibular nystagmus is caused by an imbalance between the paired vestibular structures (end organ, VIIIth nerve, or relevant brain stem nuclei). Briefly, reduction of vestibular activity on one side of the brain stem causes a slow drift of the eyes to the side of that reduction. This slow movement, which is essentially linear—that is, constant velocity—is followed by a rapid saccadic movement in the opposite direction. Repetition of this results in saw tooth vestibular nystagmus. The nystagmus is called first degree if present only when gaze is directed towards the fast phase, second degree if present in the primary position, or third degree if present when the eyes are deviated in the direction of the slow phase (Alexander's law).[8] Removal of fixation typically enhances the nystagmus if the lesion is peripheral and the eyes drift markedly towards the deranged side (figure 10.1). This can be seen clinically with infrared apparatus or Frenzel's glasses; these have high dioptre convergence lenses which allow a magnified view of the eye of the patient, without the patient being able to fixate due to the blur produced by the lenses. Alternatively, low amplitude nystagmus can be detected with fundoscopy (which makes the nystagmus seem reversed).[4] In some patients vigorous head shaking may generate a nystagmus that is not clinically apparent. The "head shaking" test (20–30 full cycles at around 2 Hz followed by Frenzel's glasses observation) is claimed to be a useful addition to the clinical vestibular examination; there is a fair correlation with caloric test findings.[9 10]

The wave form of nystagmus is not always saw toothed with a linear (constant velocity) slow phase; with gaze paretic nystagmus the slow phase has a roughly exponential decline interrupted by repeated fast phases (figure 10.2). This form of nystagmus is due to a failure of integration of the burst of actitivity arising from the saccadic generators in the paramedian pontine reticular formation (PPRF).[11] This results in insufficient tonic holding activity to

287

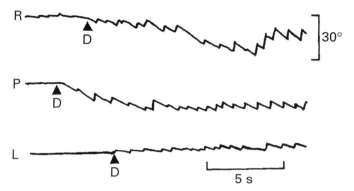

Figure 10.1 *ENG of vestibular nystagmus due to left peripheral lesion. Note nystagmus is only apparent with eyes deviated to right (R) in presence of fixation but when light is extinguished at D, nystagmus is apparent in primary (P) and on left (L) gaze. The nystagmus is saw toothed—that is, has a linear slow phase, its magnitude increases with deviation of the eyes in the direction of fast phase, and it is always in the same direction. In all figures for horizontal recordings up deflection is to the right*

maintain the eyes in the eccentric position against the orbital elastic forces tending to return the eye to the orbital midposition. Failure of integration most commonly occurs in lesions of the brain stem or cerebellum but can also be seen if there is a failure of faithful transmission of activity through the final common pathway to the extraocular muscles—for example, myasthenia gravis—or if the muscles themselves are unable to contract effectively—for example, ocular myopathy. This form of nystagmus occurs in a

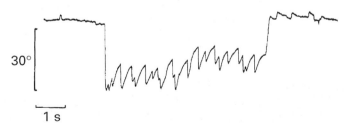

Figure 10.2 *ENG of gaze paretic nystagmus in cerebellar lesion. Note exponential decline of slow phase and some rebound nystagmus when eyes return to midline*

wide variety of CNS conditions, many of which are associated with imbalance. At the clinical level, bidirectional nystagmus in the horizontal plane is nearly always associated with central dysfunction (figure 10.3). An exception is congenital nystagmus (see oculography).

Acquired nystagmus in the vertical plane occurs less often than horizontal nystagmus and is almost always an indication of a central disorder. Further, it is invariably accompanied by imbalance. Vertical upbeat nystagmus, especially if present in the primary position, indicates a lesion in the floor of the IVth ventricle or ventral to the aqueduct, or possibly within the superior cerebellar vermis; it is often seen in patients with bilateral internuclear

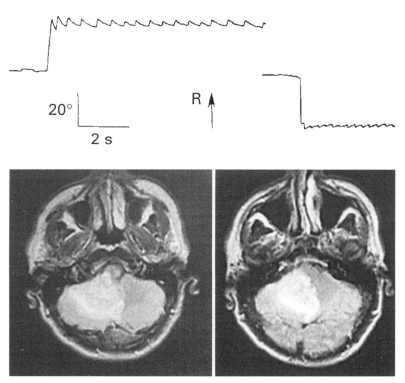

Figure 10.3 *ENG of gaze paretic nystagmus to right and vestibular to left (above) in patient with a right sided brain stem glioma shown in the MRI (below)*

ophthalmoplegia (figure 10.4).[12] Down beat nystagmus is seen with lesions at the foramen magnum—for example, Arnold-Chiari malformation—or with cerebellar atrophy.[13] However, no cause is apparent in probably 40% of all cases; of note is the rarity of this type of nystagmus in patients with multiple sclerosis or intra-axial tumours (box 10.1). Characteristically, vertical nystagmus is altered by position[14] and down beat nystagmus is increased in amplitude if the eyes are deviated 30° to the left or right of the midline. Convergence can also modify vertical nystagmus. Down beat nystagmus has been associated with syringomyelia but this is not entirely true. In patients with cerebellar ectopia and a syrinx in whom there is nystagmus (about 30% of the total) the nystagmus is often torsional with the fast phase usually directed towards the side of greater sensory loss in the limbs—that is, clockwise fast phase from the examiner's viewpoint is associated with left sided sensory loss. Torsional nystagmus is not confined to syringomyelia; it is also typically found in lesions of the medial vestibular nucleus (figure 10.5), as in Wallenberg's syndrome, and lesions of the cerebellum.[15]

There are some rarer types of nystagmus, all of which are often associated with imbalance. Of these, rebound nystagmus is the most frequent.[16] If gaze-paretic nystagmus is induced on looking in one direction, and the eyes are kept deviated for a prolonged period, the nystagmus sometimes diminishes and ceases. When the eyes are returned to the midline a nystagmus in the reverse direction is seen for a short period, even though nystagmus in the primary position was not initially present (figure 10.2). Such nys-

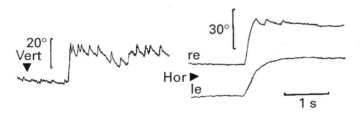

Figure 10.4   *ENG of internuclear ophthalmoplegia showing up beat nystagmus. On the left the vertical trace (Vert) shows gaze paretic up beat nystagmus on looking upwards. On the right the horizontal eye movement record (Hor) for left (le) and right (re) eyes at rapid paper speed shows slow adduction velocity in the left eye and gaze paretic nystagmus in the right eye*

Box 10.1   Causes of down beat nystagmus[13 70]

Diagnosis	%
Cerebellar ectopia	27
Cerebellar degeneration	
Generic	18
Acquired	10
Tumour	2
Multiple sclerosis	1
Undiagnosed	42

tagmus is typical of cerebellar lesions. Pendular nystagmus is nystagmus in which there is no clear distinction between the fast and slow phase. It may be symmetric—that is, identical in each eye or highly asymmetric differing in amplitude, direction, or both in either eye. On occasion complex trajectories are followed—for example, elliptical or figure of eight. This type of nystagmus occurs in patients with longstanding visual failure and in lesions of the brain stem especially those involving the central tegmental tract.[17 18] In neurological practice it is most often seen in multiple sclerosis, in which it is often associated with an internuclear ophthalmoplegia. Although some workers consider that impaired visual acuity is important in the generation of pendular nystagmus[19] this has not been our experience. Convergence retraction nystagmus due to lesions in the region of the quadrigeminal plate and posterior commissure can readily be seen clinically, especially using an optokinetic drum rotated downwards; it is difficult to record without video filming. Periodic alternating nystagmus—that is, nystagmus in which the direction spontaneously and repeatedly reverses despite eye position being constant—is found in various cerebellar disorders and can readily be seen; it is clearly shown by prolonged recordings of horizontal eye movement. Finally seesaw nystagmus, in which one eye elevates and intorts and the other is depressed and extorts repeatedly, indicates a lesion in the region of the peduncular fossa and is probably due to damage in the interstitial nucleus of the medial longitudinal fasiculus and the adjacent nucleus of Cajal.[6] It is readily seen clinically but recordings are necessary to delineate it fully.

291

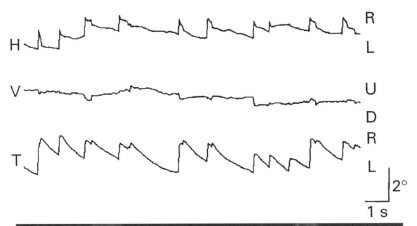

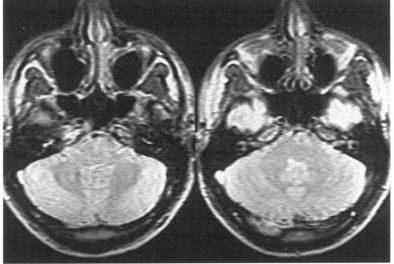

Figure 10.5   *Horizontal (H), vertical (V), and torsional (T) eye movement recordings (scleral search coil technique) of a patient with predominantly torsional right beating nystagmus (top) due to a left sided lesion on the floor of the IVth ventricle (bottom). The lesion is likely to have involved the left medial vestibular nucleus*

Clinical assessment of induced nystagmus

Because many patients with imbalance do not have nystagmus, techniques for inducing nystagmus are commonly used in the clinic. The most valuable methods are optokinetic, rotational, caloric, and positional stimuli.

292

Optokinetic nystagmus

Optokinetic nystagmus can be assessed at the bedside with a small striped drum rotated in front of the patient. This is basically a pursuit task and not surprisingly correlates well with other pursuit measures. It is possible to measure optokinetic responses with a small drum, or with a large visual field rotating about the patient using various special techniques such as electronystagmography (ENG, see later). A common abnormality is a directional preponderance—that is, a greater response in one direction. Typically a right directional preponderance correlates with abnormal pursuit to the right (for example, a right cerebellar or parietal lesion results in greater optokinetic nystagmus towards the right). In normal subjects the eyes deviate in the direction of the fast phase of optokinetic nystagmus but in certain disorders of the basal ganglia the converse happens—that is, deviation is in the direction of the slow phase.[20]

Nystagmus induced by stimulation of the semicircular canals

Two clinical methods are available to stimulate the semicircular canals: caloric testing and rotational stimuli. Because much information can be obtained from clinical assessment of the caloric tests they will be considered next. Complex assessment of rotational stimuli—for example, ENG—will be considered in a later section.

Caloric testing

This test depends primarily on convection set up in the relevant canal by thermal stimulation. In the clinical setting the test is most commonly used to measure horizontal canal function. The usual method is that described by Fitzgerald and Hallpike in their classic paper[21] in which the horizontal canal is put in the vertical plane with its ampulla uppermost by lying the patient horizontally on the back and flexing the neck to 30°. One external meatus is irrigated with water at 7° above or below body temperature for 40 seconds, with the flow rate being greater than 6 ml/s. This stimulus sets up a convection current which flows up if hot water is used and stimulates the hair cells; conversely the cold stimulus causes movement of endolymph away from the ampulla and reduces the firing rate of the cells.[22] Thermal stimulation of hair cells without any convection would also cause similar effects on the hair cell firing rate but in fact this probably only accounts for a small proportion

293

of the alteration[23] (although it accounts for all of it in conditions of zero gravity such as space travel).[24] The interested clinician can prove to himself the importance of convection by doing a caloric test on a colleague and repeatedly turning the subject prone and supine and showing that the nystagmus reverses as the ampulla changes from being inferior to being superior.

The nystagmic response is used to assess the effect of canal irrigation. The eyes are viewed in the light while the subject fixates a spot on the ceiling. During and after completion of irrigation nystagmus is induced to the side opposite the irrigated ear in the case of cold irrigation and vice versa for warm irrigation. The test is carried out sequentially using the left and right ear alternately and leaving about five minutes between irrigations. This interval is not sufficient for all the thermal gradient to disappear but is reasonably satisfactory.[25] Several variables can be assessed of which duration of the nystagmus and slow phase velocity are the two most common. Only duration can be used as a clinical measure without special equipment such as ENG. There is no doubt that slow phase velocity is more physiologically meaningful, but interestingly, not more clinically useful. This is because the variance of duration of nystagmus is less than that of slow phase velocity.[26]

Three types of abnormality are seen with horizontal canal irrigation. Firstly, there may be an underfunctioning of one canal, conventionally called "canal paresis" (CP). In our laboratory, a 9% difference in the duration of nystagmus between the two sides is significant.* This typically occurs in peripheral lesions and a total failure of function of one horizontal canal is nearly always due to end organ or VIIIth nerve damage. Secondly, there may be a bias of the nystagmus, such that the duration in one direction, say the left (with right cold and left hot irrigation), is greater than that to the opposite side. This is known as "directional preponderance" (DP) and can be seen in peripheral disorders as well as with lesions at any level of the nervous system. It does, however, show that there is a vestibular bias in one direction and if there is

---

*
$$CP = \frac{f\,(\text{Lcold} + \text{Lhot}) - f\,(\text{Rcold} + \text{Rhot})}{f\,(\text{Lcold} + \text{Lhot} + \text{Rcold} + \text{Rhot})} \times 100$$

$$DP = \frac{f\,(\text{L beating nystagmus} - \text{R beating nystagmus})}{f\,(\text{sum all nystagmus})} \times 100$$

a canal paresis as well it indicates that this is not fully compensated. Finally, there may be hypofunction of both horizontal canals—for example, after aminoglycoside antibiotic treatment. The advantage of caloric testing of horizontal canals is that the function of a single canal can be assessed, a situation that applies to no other test routinely available. The primary disadvantages of caloric testing are that the stimulus intensity varies in different subjects—for example, because of differences in meatal diameter, and that water irrigation cannot be used if there is a defect of the tympanic membrane.

Caloric testing can also be used to assess the function of the vertical canals but in this case only pairs of canals, either anterior or posterior, are studied. These canals are set deeper in the petrous temporal bone than the horizontal canals and therefore longer duration and more intense thermal stimuli are required. Both ears are irrigated simultaneously with either cold (20°C) or hot (47°C) water for 60 seconds with the head in the usual position for caloric testing. The cold stimulus causes slow downward deviation of the eyes with upbeat nystagmus and the hot stimulus the reverse. It is essential to perform horizontal irrigation first to ensure that there is no underfunctioning of the horizontal canal; if there is, reduction of duration of irrigation of the relatively "normal" ear is necessary to avoid oblique nystagmus. Bilateral, bithermal caloric testing is particularly useful in patients with ophthalmoplegias to determine if the paresis of the eye movements is nuclear or supranuclear—for example, Steele-Richardson syndrome.[26] As will be noted from the temperature of water used for this type of testing the cold stimulus is of greater magnitude. Unfortunately it is not possible to raise the temperature of the hot stimulus above 47°C and even that is very uncomfortable indeed.

During caloric testing it is possible to assess visual suppression (VORS) of nystagmus without contamination from other reflex eye movements.[27 28] A practicable method is to perform each irrigation with fixation and when the nystagmus ceases, to extinguish the fixation spot and view the eyes in the dark with an infrared viewer, or to use Frenzel's glasses. In a normal subject or patients with a peripheral lesion, the nystagmus will again be seen and its duration without fixation gives a measure of the visual suppression. In the case of central lesions, especially those involving cerebellar connections, visual suppression is reduced or absent so that there is pronounced nystagmus with fixation but when the nystagmus stops, removal of fixation does not result in a recurrence of it. The duration of nystagmus is never greater with fixation than without.

Rotational responses

It is possible to obtain a general clinical impression of the degree of symmetry of vestibular ocular function by conducting the doll's head manoeuvre with careful examination of the eye, directly or during ophthalmoscopy,[4] or by manually rotating the subject at a roughly constant velocity on an office swivel chair and observing the postrotational response. The last is essentially the original Barany test, in which subjects are rotated at about 90 or 120°/s (one revolution every three or four seconds) for 30 seconds in one direction and then stopped facing the examiner to time the duration of the observed nystagmus. By comparing the postrotational response in the two directions an idea of symmetry can be obtained. Although now superseded by recording techniques and motorised equipment, this procedure is occasionally used even in well equipped centres when a rapid assessment of vertical semicircular canal function is required. In this case the patient should be rotated with the head extended so that the face is directed towards the ceiling; horizontal rotation of the chair then stimulates the vertical canals. Of course in this case the nystagmus seen is torsional and because its amplitude is usually low the clinician should examine the subject's eyes closely under bright illumination. Asymmetries in the duration of the nystagmus should be 15–20% or more to be of relevance.

Positional nystagmus

Nystagmus may readily be induced or, if already present, modified by changes in position of the head. The conventional method is the Hallpike manoeuvre. In this the patient sits on a couch and the examiner firmly grasps the head, which is turned 60° towards one shoulder. The patient is instructed to keep the eyes open and to fixate the examiner's forehead. The patient's head is rapidly lowered to below the level of the couch and the eyes observed for any nystagmus. After an interval of 30 seconds, if nystagmus is not found, or after the nystagmus ceases (the test may have to be terminated if the nystagmus lasts longer than two minutes) the patient is returned to the sitting position. Again, any nystagmus is noted. The test is repeated if nystagmus is found to see if there is any adaptation. After this the test is performed with the opposite ear dependent. The variables noted are latency to onset of nystagmus, its duration and adaptation, its direction, and finally, associated symptoms. Broadly two types of nystagmus are seen: benign positional nystagmus and central positional nystagmus (box 10.2).

Typical benign positional nystagmus indicates a peripheral lesion in which debris from the otolith apparatus accumulate on the cupula of the posterior semicircular canal. Two theories have been proposed to account for the nystagmus and both depend on inversion of the posterior canal resulting in either displacement of the cupula of that canal because the debris alter its specific gravity (cupulolithiasis)[29] or the passage of debris down that canal acts as a plunger (canal lithiasis).[30][31] Occasionally what seems to be bilateral benign positional nystagmus occurs. Recently, benign positional nystagmus arising in the horizontal canal system has been reported. It is elicited by brisk turning of the head to one side while in the supine position.[32]

Typical central positional nystagmus occurs in a wide variety of lesions, especially those involving the vestibulocerebellum. Of note is the fact that spontaneous vertical nystagmus, either upwards or downwards, can often be modified by positional testing using the conventional Hallpike manoeuvre or by placing the subject supine or prone. If the nystagmus is increased in the prone position it is usually decreased lying supine. Nystagmus induced by canal stimulation can also be profoundly modified by alteration of position of the head, due to otolith/semicircular canal interaction.[14][33][34]

Box 10.2   Positional nystagmus

	Benign	Central
Direction	To dependent ear (torsional)	Any
Vertigo	++	+
Latent interval	+	−
Adaptation	+	−
Fatigue	+	−

Laboratory assessment of patients

Oculography and electronystagmography

The techniques currently available for recording and the analysis of eye movement have been presented in chapter 9 (also Shaunak *et al*[35]). Box 10.3 presents a summary of the main advantages and disadvantages of these systems. From the point of view of the investigation of the patient with a balance disorder, in whom an investigation of vestibular responses is required, the technique generally recommended is ENG as it allows recording over a wide range of amplitudes; ENG, also called electro-oculography (EOG), is the cheapest system and one not requiring a great deal of technical or scientific support. It is mainly used for investigation of horizontal eye movements and therefore for assessment of horizontal semicircular canal function. It can produce some reasonable recordings in the vertical plane but it is totally insensitive to torsional movements—that is, those occurring around the visual axis. Thus the recording of abnormalities of eye movements in these planes, related to dysfunction in the vertical canal system or the otoliths, requires the use of more complex techniques such as video-oculography or the more invasive scleral search coil system. Fortunately the most common abnormality affecting the vertical canal/otolith system is benign paroxysmal positional vertigo (BPPV), which does not require eye movement recordings for its diagnosis (see positional nystagmus).

It is important to consider when referral for eye movement recording is necessary (box 10.4).

(1) Recordings may be required when the abnormality seen during clinical examination of the eye movement is ambiguous. For example, the presence of square wave jerks superimposed on the slow phase eye movement of smooth pursuit can give the impression that pursuit is abnormal. As square wave jerks may be seen in anxious but otherwise neurologically normal patients, the suspicion of broken pursuit may lead incorrectly to the thought that there is structural brainstem/cerebellar damage. Similarly the presence of a mild internuclear ophthalmoplegia can be difficult to detect clinically and separate eye recordings may be necessary to show the difference in velocity between adduction and abduction movements (figure 10.4).

(2) Recording of eye movements can be used to characterise the waveform of a nystagmus or other types of ocular oscillation. A

Box 10.3   Eye movement recording techniques

	Electro-oculography (EOG/ENG)	*Infrared oculography (IRO)*	*Scleral search coil (SCC)*	*Video-oculography (VOG)*
Signal source	Corneoretinal potential	Limbus infrared light reflection	Contact lens mounted search coil	Iris/pupil image processing
Advantages	Non-invasive Simple/inexpensive Prolonged recordings Good linearity	Non-invasive Intermediate price Good resolution (10')	Excellent resolution (5') Torsional recordings	Non-invasive Torsional recordings Good resolution (10')
Disadvantages	Low resolution (1°) Noise/drift	Poor linearity	Invasive Expensive	Expensive Low temporal resolution

---

Box 10.4   Indications for eye movement recordings to investigate imbalance

- Assessment of eye movements in the dark
  Is there vestibular nystagmus?
  Vestibular function (for example, rotational test)

- Nystagmus wave form
  Vestibular v gaze paretic
  Acquired or congenital

- Confirmation/detection of subtle abnormalities of diagnostic value (for example, abnormal pursuit, subclinical INO)

- Research, quantification, and follow up

---

good example of the value of oculography is the recognition of congenital nystagmus. Congenital nystagmus, a condition with no neurological consequences, can show various wave forms but some of them are pathognomonic and this will be of importance when a patient who is not aware of having nystagmus develops a neurological problem. Occasionally patients with congenital nystagmus develop visual symptoms in later life and the finding of a nystagmus in these patients is of concern.[36] In cases like this eye movement recordings have the value of ruling out structural brainstem cerebellar disease and the positive confirmation of a congenital nystagmus (figure 10.6). Oculography is also useful in characterising the wave form of acquired nystagmus, especially in separating gaze evoked from vestibular nystagmus (see clinical assessment of spontaneous nystagmus).

(3) Non-nystagmic oscillations can be accurately diagnosed with oculography. For example, flutter (horizontal saccades without intersaccadic interval) or opsoclonus (polydirectional saccades without intersaccadic interval) can be separated from other saccadic oscillations in which there is a saccadic interval (for example, square wave jerks). The duration of the saccadic interval may help to decide if the movements are voluntary as in this case the intersaccadic interval exceeds 150 ms.

(4) Eye movement recordings may be required to see if there is any nystagmus in the dark in patients in whom no nystagmus is

300

Congenital nystagmus

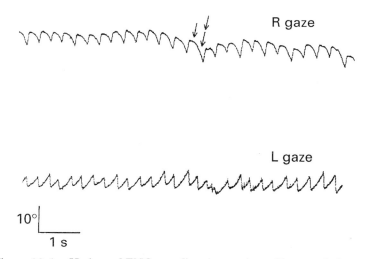

Figure 10.6   *Horizontal ENG recordings in a patient with congenital nystagmus. The nystagmus shows increasing velocity slow phase waveforms (arrows). Compare these slow phase waveforms with those of peripheral vestibular origin (which are rectilinear figures 10.1 and 10.7) and those of brainstem-cerebellar origin (which are frequently velocity decreasing figures 10.2, 10.3, and 10.5)*

seen in the light (figure 10.7). This is typically found in patients with peripheral vestibular dysfunction (figures 10.1 and 10.7). Alternatives to eye movement recordings for observation of nystagmus in the absence of optic fixation are Frenzel's glasses, infrared viewers, or an infrared camera attached to a video recorder.

(5) Eye movement recordings are necessary when quantification of eye movement performance or abnormalities is required for research or in follow up of individual patients. In degenerative akinetic rigid or cerebellar syndromes successive eye recordings can show progressive abnormalities.

(6) The most common reason for eye movement recording is the investigation of vestibular function without interference from visually guided eye movements as detailed in the next section.

301

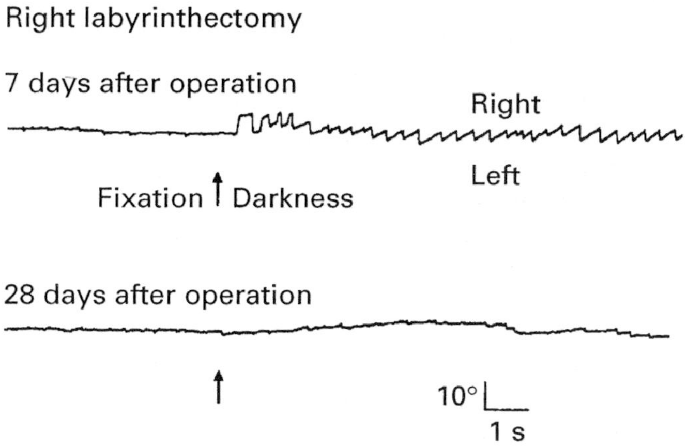

Right labyrinthectomy

7 days after operation

Right

Left

Fixation ↑ Darkness

28 days after operation

↑   10° └__
                     1 s

Figure 10.7   *Horizontal eye movement recordings (engs) in a patient with a right sided labyrinthectomy. Top: nystagmus in the presence of fixation is almost entirely suppressed by fixation, as early as seven days postoperatively. Bottom: the process of vestibular compensation accounts for the fact that 28 days after the operation the nystagmus had almost entirely disappeared even in the dark. Visual suppression and vestibular compensation explain the lack of clinical findings in peripheral vestibular disorders and underline the need for special investigations in many of these patients*

Examination of vestibular function

Caloric response

Much information can be obtained by direct observation of the eyes with the caloric test. Many centres have resorted to eye movement recording techniques so that technical staff can carry out the test, to save medical time, and to quantify the response. The interpretation of the caloric abnormality in terms of canal paresis or directional preponderance is the same but usually based on slow phase eye velocity rather than on nystagmus duration.

Rotational testing

To obtain reliable and quantitative information on vestibular function a motorised chair or turntable and a light tight room are required. Two variables are used to define rotational stimuli: the waveform of the stimulus, whether sinusoidal, trapezoidal, or square wave (impulsive), and the peak velocity reached during the rotation.

The rotational test described in the clinical section is based on the original Barany stimulus and represents a velocity step—that is, impulsive stimulus. The constant velocity rotation is maintained until the nystagmic response disappears (40–60 s) and then the patient is stopped with a similar sudden deceleration. After the induced nystagmus has ceased, the patient is rotated in the opposite direction so that two sets of right beating responses (right start and stop from the left) and left beating responses (left start and stop from the right) are collected. The actual stimulus variables used vary (40–90°/s) but are a compromise between the highest velocity necessary to detect abnormalities and the emetic potential of this test. Responses can be expressed in terms of duration, peak slow phase velocity achieved, time constant of decay of the initial peak velocity—that is, time to decay to about a third of the induced velocity, or by a combination of these. Some machines are produced commercially that enable a printout of these variables. Understandably, different workers prefer to use the technique with which they have the most experience and there is, therefore, no consensus on the ideal "rotational stimulus".

If the stimulus is sinusoidal it is important that a range, rather than a single, frequency is tested to achieve a thorough investigation of the vestibular ocular system.[37] In our experience, sinusoidal testing in a patient with considerable loss of vestibular function can lead to gross underestimation of the degree of vestibular loss. As discussed in the clinical section, a useful addition to the sinusoidal rotational test is to determine suppression of the VOR by visual fixation (VORS). This is investigated by attaching a visual target to the rotating chair so that the subjects fixate an object that moves with them during the oscillation. The threshold of frequency or velocity at which subjects are no longer able effectively to suppress a vestibular nystagmus or the ratio of one of the nystagmus variables—for example, slow phase velocity achieved by the stimulus with and without fixation—is an extremely useful addition to vestibular examination.[27 28]

Two types of abnormality are encountered during rotational investigation in patients with a balance disorder. The first is asymmetry of the response: directional preponderance which, as discussed earlier, simply indicates a dynamic asymmetry in the peripheral or central vestibular system. As these rotational responses are induced by stimulation of one canal at the same time as inhibition of the opposite one it is not possible to establish with certainty which labyrinth is primarily responsible. The second type of abnormality is less common and comprises changes in magnitude of the induced response. A reduction of the induced response is the commonest finding. Clinicians often do not consider the possibility of bilateral loss of vestibular function in the differential diagnosis of a patient with a balance or gait disorder. In our recent review of bilateral vestibular failure in a neurological hospital, in addition to well known and usually suspected causes of bilateral vestibular loss such as meningitis or antibiotic ototoxicity, many patients had vestibular failure which was idiopathic or associated with cerebellar system degenerations or peripheral/cranial neuropathies.[38] The converse of vestibular failure—enhanced responses—also occurs. Bilaterally enhanced vestibular responses can be seen usually in the course of cerebellar disease perhaps because of disinhibition of the vestibular system.[39-41] This leads to short lasting but high velocity responses to rotational or caloric stimuli. It is important to remember that patients with bilateral abnormalities of the VOR, either in the form of diminished or enhanced vestibular responses, may have visual symptoms (oscillopsia) particularly during head movement. Thus patients with unusual visual symptoms related to head or body motion, especially if associated with unsteadiness, should also be investigated from a vestibular point of view.[42]

"Full" or "routine" ENG

Because balance depends on the interaction of vestibular, visual, and proprioceptive signals it is customary to extend the neuro-otological examination to areas other than the purely vestibular. This is particularly true in terms of investigation of smooth pursuit, saccades, and optokinetic nystagmus by means of oculography. Although a detailed description of these abnormalities has been presented in chapter 9 it should be noted here that any significant finding on investigation of oculomotor functions would suggest a central, rather than a peripheral vestibular disorder. The same can be said about the important visual/vestibular interaction assessed during VORS. Similarly, the diagnosis of peripheral vestibular disorder implies that saccades, pursuit, optokinetic nystagmus, and VORS will be normal on clinical and/or elecronystagmographic investigation. Box 10.5 gives a brief summary highlighting the criteria that can be used to distinguish between peripheral and central vestibular disorders.

304

Box 10.5 Differences between central and peripheral vestibular disorders

	Peripheral (Labyrinthine/VIIIth nerve only)	Central (CNS)
CNS symptons/ examination	Normal	Abnormal
Auditory symptoms/ examination	Frequently abnormal	Usually normal
Vertigo:		
Acute lesion	++++	–/+++
Chronic lesion	+/–	+/–
Oscillopsia	Rare (head movement induced)	Common (usually spontaneous)
Unsteadiness:		
Acute	++++	++++
Chronic	+/–	+++
Nystagmus:		
Acute	++	+/+++
Chronic	+/–	+/+++
Trajectory	Horizontal or horizontal with a torsional component	Any direction
Amplitude	+	+++
Wave form	Rectilinear	Frequently exponential
Effect of fixation removal	Appears/enhances	Variable
Eye movements Pursuit, OKN, Saccades, INO	Normal	Usually abnormal

Techniques being developed

Posturography

The recording of postural sway is not a widely accepted or routine part of the examination of the patient with a balance disorder. Body sway is normally assessed indirectly by recording the movement of the centre of foot pressure while the patient stands on a force transducing platform. Other motion transducers (for example, accelerometers) and EMG recordings of the lower limbs and trunk, can be added. In its simplest form, recordings of body sway for periods between 20 and 60 seconds with eyes open and closed provide objective quantification of the Romberg test but add no extra information to the clinical observation of that test. Patients with unilateral or even bilateral vestibular disorders are often normal both clinically and quantitatively on the Romberg test.[43] It has been reported that if the recordings separate lateral and anterior/posterior components of sway and include frequency analysis of sway with power spectrum techniques, the information obtained can be useful to distinguish the various forms of cerebellar ataxia.[44] In the form described, often termed static posturography, there is general agreement that the technique is of no practical value in the diagnosis of balance disorders.[45] When one or more motion stimuli are applied to the subject standing on a force plate the procedure is called dynamic posturography. Such stimuli can be visual,[46-48] vestibular (for example, galvanic),[49] somatosensory, or combined—for instance, by rotational or translational displacements of the platform.[50 51] The most popular but expensive commercial system used combines disorienting somatosensory and visual stimuli, by means of coupling the movements of the supporting surface or of the visual surround to the patient's own body sway.[52] This effectively reduces the efficiency of the somatosensory or visual loops, respectively, in postural control. It is claimed that when all stimulus combinations are studied different patterns of abnormal postural control can be detected which indicate the primary source of disorder. In this way, if a patient cannot balance in the absence of visual input, or with conflicting visual input, and when the somatosensory input has been made unreliable, a "vestibular pattern" is diagnosed. This, as well as many other claims, has not been supported by rigorous clinical studies.[45] The use of posturography is therefore debatable. Although clearly of research interest in a specialised environment, we recommend a critical view of claims by manufacturers.

Otolith function

Some patients attending balance disorder clinics report symptoms of unsteadiness which suggest involvement of otolith rather than semicircular canal function.[34] This may include a sense of bobbing up and down, being carried upwards or downwards in a lift, or lateral and sagittal pulsions. Certain disorders of head and eye coordination—for instance, the ocular tilt reaction combining head tilt and ocular skew deviation—are thought to be due to interruption of central graviceptive otolith pathways.[53] Similarly, positional nystagmus particularly of the central type, as mentioned earlier, is reduced or modified by tilt of the head with respect to the gravity vector, and is therefore interpreted as under otolith control.[33] Despite all this clinical evidence, reliable and simple tests of otolith function in humans are lacking. This is due to the difficulties in delivering the appropriate stimuli (whole body tilt or linear accelerations) which require large motion devices and simultaneously recording a meaningful response (ocular torsion), which requires eye coils or video-oculography.[33] Perhaps the only technique which does not require extraordinary equipment to investigate otolith function is that described by Gresty and Bronstein.[54] In this procedure the subject's head is placed eccentrically in front of the axis of rotation of a conventional rotating chair while horizontal eye movements are recorded with standard techniques. The rationale is that in this position the head experiences not only angular acceleration but also a tangential component along the interaural axis which gives rise to stimulation of the utricular macula.[55] The enhanced VOR elicited in this position has been proved in experimental animals to be due to otolith stimulation.[56] Although clinical abnormalities can be detected,[57] full evaluation in the clinical setting has not been undertaken.

Assessment of the "visual vertical" in which subjects have to set a line vertical in an otherwise totally darkened room is sensitive to acute peripheral or central vestibular deficits, but it is not proved that the abnormalities are specific to the otolith system.[34 53] Indeed, semicircular canal, visual, or proprioceptive stimuli induce profound modifications of the settings of the visual vertical in normal subjects.[58 59] The simplicity of the procedure, the inexpensive techniques involved, and clear abnormalities in some cases make this technique an attractive one for the clinician, even if the meaning of the abnormalities is not entirely clear.

Self generated rotational stimuli

In subjects with good neck mobility the head can be rotated about the shoulders either passively by the examiner, or actively by the patient, to stimulate the semicircular canals. Eye movements can be recorded and therefore vestibulo-ocular reflex measurements can be obtained with relatively simple equipment. Halmagyi et al [60] have used high velocity head displacements while recording eye movements with a scleral search coil system and have shown that profound unilateral lesions—for example, vestibular neurectomy—show a clear hypoactivity of the vestibulo-ocular reflex during rotation towards the damaged side. The sensitivity of this technique with less complex or less invasive eye recording methods, as well as its general use in the balance disorder clinic, has not been established. Self generated head movements can be particularly useful for the assessment of the vertical canal system but here again there is the difficulty of having to resort to complex eye movement recording devices to measure torsion or vertical eye motion accurately.

Perceptual studies of vestibular function

Before eye movement recordings became widely available a great deal of the clinical and research assessment of the vestibular system relied on psychophysical estimates.[61] In the past 30 or 40 years such studies became overshadowed by vestibulo-ocular investigations but more recently interest in psychophysical assessment has again emerged, not least because of the relatively poor correlation of patient symptoms and vestibulo-ocular findings.[62 63] The simplest assessment is to enquire about the type and intensity of the sensation during irrigation of the external canals in the caloric test. Often, patients describe sensations during the caloric test that are identical to their own symptoms during dizzy spells, thereby indicating a likely vestibular origin for their symptoms. This can be particularly useful in patients with severe ocular myopathies or with congenital nystagmus in whom vestibulo-ocular function cannot be established. More refined techniques are also currently being developed which allow assessment of symmetry of function in the vestibular system.[63-65]

Sound evoked vestibulocollic responses

Colebatch and coworkers[66-68] have further described the phenomenon originally discovered by Bickford et al,[69] that repeated clicks delivered through headphones are able to stimulate the vestibular apparatus and generate a short latency (6–12 ms) inhibitory potential in muscles of the neck under continuous activation. Although this technique is also under development it has the advantage that, together with the caloric test and galvanic stimulation of the ear, it can stimulate the vestibular system on either side of the head independently. The click evoked vestibular cervical potentials seem to be promising in identification of patients with the Tullio phenomenon (sound induced vestibular symptoms).[68] The technology required for this procedure is currently available in most EEG departments—that is, a click generator and an averager as used for instance for auditory brain stem evoked responses.

Conclusions

We have considered the consequences of vestibular dysfunction in causing imbalance and discussed various methods of assessment of the vestibular system. Inevitably these methods are heavily dependent on the vestibulo-ocular connections both at the clinical and at the investigational level. In figures 10.8 and 10.9 we produced algorithms that are of some use in investigating these connections. At the outset we stated that the neuro-otological examination could not be considered in isolation and in this respect we have not considered two areas. Firstly, because of the close association of the auditory and vestibular systems, full auditory function assessment is essential. In particular, middle ear and petrous bone pathology should be sought by expert ear, nose, and throat surgeons. Secondly, imaging of the VIIIth nerve system has been revolutionised by MRI, which is an essential part of the full neuro-otological assessment. Both these areas are omitted from the discussion, not because they have little importance, but because they are not part of the remit of this article.

Finally, even after exhaustive documentation of the clinical and investigative findings a large proportion of patients remain undiagnosed. Clear cut diagnoses such as Ménière's disease or tumours of the cerebellopontine angle are relatively easy to make but in our experience a substantial proportion of patients referred to a specialist neuro-otological clinic remain without a specific diagnosis or are given a diagnosis such as vestibular neuronitis that implies an anatomical and aetiological precision that is not often justified. Hopefully this unsatisfactory situation will improve with developments in imaging, neurophysiological techniques, and further understanding of symptomatology.

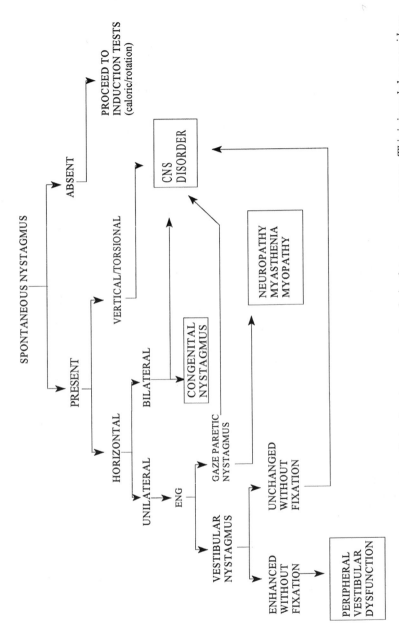

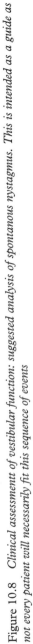

Figure 10.8   *Clinical assessment of vestibular function: suggested analysis of spontanous nystagmus. This is intended as a guide as not every patient will necessarily fit this sequence of events*

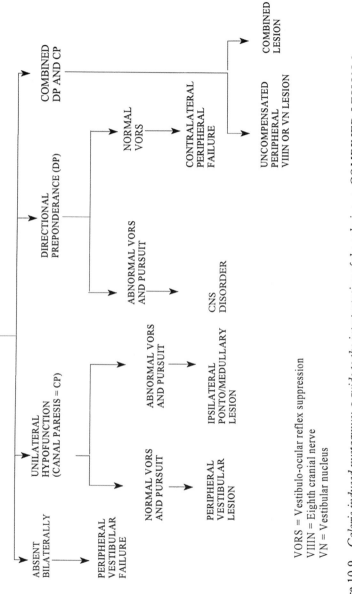

CALORIC TEST

Figure 10.9 *Caloric induced nystagmus: a guide to the interpretation of the caloric test: COMBINED LESION denotes CENTRAL and PERIPHERAL LESION*

VORS = Vestibulo-ocular reflex suppression
VIIIN = Eighth cranial nerve
VN = Vestibular nucleus

1 Spoor F, Wood B, Zonneveld F. Implications of early hominid labyrinthine morphology for evolution of human bipedal locomotion. *Nature* 1994;369:645–8.

2 Wilson VJ, Jones GM. *Mammalian vestibular physiology*. New York: Plenum Press, 1975:365.

3 Donaghy M. The cat's vestibulo-ocular reflex. *J Physiol* 1980;300:337–51.

4 Zee DS. Ophthalmoscopy in examination of patients with vestibular disorders. *Ann Neurol* 1978;3:373–4.

5 Halmagyi GM, Gresty MA, Gibson WPR. Ocular tilt reaction with peripheral vestibular lesion. *Ann Neurol* 1979;6:80–3.

6 Halmagyi GM, Aw ST, Demaene I, Curthoys IS, Todd MJ. Jerk-waveform see-saw nystagmus due to unilateral meso-diencephalic lesion. *Brain* 1994;117:789–803.

7 Halmagyi GM, Gresty MA. Clinical signs of visual-vestibular interaction. *J Neurol Neurosurg Psychiatry* 1979;42:934–9.

8 Alexander G. Die Ohrenkrankheiten im Kindesalter. In: Pfaundler M, Schlossmann A, eds. *Handbuch der Kinderheilkunde*. Band VI. Leipzig: Vogel, 1912:84–5.

9 Hain TC, Spindler J. Head-shaking nystagmus. In: Sharpe JA, Barber HO, eds. *The vestibulo-ocular reflex and vertigo*. New York: Raven Press, 1993: 217–28.

10 Takahashi S, Fetter M, Koenig E, Dichgans J. The clinical significance of head-shaking nystagmus in the dizzy patient. *Acta Otolaryngol (Stockh)* 1990;109:8–14.

11 Leigh RJ, Zee DS. *The neurology of eye movements*. 2nd ed. Philadelphia: FA Davis, 1991:89–93

12 Fisher A, Gresty MA, Chambers B, Rudge P. Primary position upbeating nystagmus. *Brain* 1983;106:949–64.

13 Halmagyi GM, Rudge P, Gresty MA, Sanders MD. Downbeating nystagmus. A review of 62 cases. *Arch Neurol* 1983;40:777–84.

14 Gresty MA, Barratt HJ, Rudge P, Page NGR. Analysis of downbeat nystagmus: otolith vs semicircular canal influences. *Arch Neurol* 1986;43:52–5.

15 Lopez L, Bronstein AM, Gresty MA, Rudge P, du Boulay EPGH. Torsional nystagmus. A neuro-otological and MRI study of thirty-five cases. *Brain* 1992;115:1107–24.

16 Hood JD, Kayan A, Leech J. Rebound nystagmus. *Brain* 1973;96:507–26.

17 Gresty MA, Ell JJ, Findley LJ. Acquired pendular nystagmus: its characteristics, localising value and pathophysiology. *J Neurol Neurosurg Psychiatry* 1982;45:431–39.

18 Lopez L, Gresty MA, Bronstein AM, du Boulay EPGH, Rudge P. Acquired pendular nystagmus: ocular motor and MRI findings. *Brain* 1996;119:465–72.

19 Barton JJS, Cox TA. Acquired pendular nystagmus in multiple sclerosis: clinical observations and the role of optic neuropathy. *J Neurol Neurosurg Psychiatry* 1993;56:262–7.

20 Dix MR, Harrison MJG, Lewis PD. Progressive supranuclear palsy. *J Neurol Sci* 1971;13:237–56.

21 Fitzgerald G, Hallpike CS. Observations on the directional preponderance of caloric nystagmus resulting from cerebral lesions. *Brain* 1942;65:115–37.

22 Barany R. Untersuchungen uber den vom Vestibularapparat des Ohres reflecktorisch ausgelosten rhythmischen Nystagmus und seine Begleiterscheinungen. *Monatsschr Ohrenheilk Laryngol Rhinol* 1906;40:193–212.

23 Hood JD. Evidence of direct thermal action upon the vestibular receptors in the caloric test. *Acta Otolaryngol (Stockh)* 1989;107:161–5.

24 Scherer H, Clark AM. The caloric vestibular reaction in space. *Acta Otolaryngol (Stockh)* 1985;100:328–36.

25 Hood JD. Persistence of response in the caloric test. *Aerospace Medicine* 1973;44:444–9.

26 Sills AW, Baloh RW, Honrubia V. Caloric testing. II Results in normal subjects. *Ann Otorhinolaryngol* 1972;86 (suppl 43):7–23.

27 Demanez JP, Ledoux A. Automatic fixation mechanisms and vestibular stimulation. *Adv Otorhinolaryngol* 1970;17:90–8.

28 Hood JD, Korres S. Vestibular suppression in peripheral and central vestibular disorders. *Brain* 1979;102:785–804.

29 Schuknecht HF. Cupulolithiasis. *Arch Otolaryngol* 1969;90:765–78.

30 Parnes LS, McClure JA. Free-floating endolymph particles: a new operative finding during posterior semicircular canal occlusion. *Laryngoscope* 1992;102:988–92.

31 Brandt T, Steddin S, Daroff RB. Therapy for benign paroxysmal positioning vertigo, revisited. *Neurology* 1994;44:796–800.

32 Baloh RW, Jacobson K, Honrubia V. Horizontal semicirular canal variant of benign positional vertigo. *Neurology* 1993;43:2542–9.

33 Gresty MA, Bronstein AM. Testing otolith function. Review article. *Br J Audiol* 1992;**26**:125–36.
34 Gresty MA, Bronstein AM, Brandt T, Dieterich M. Neurology of otolith function: peripheral and central disorders. *Brain* 1992;**115**:647–73.
35 Shaunak S, O'Sullivan E, Kennard C. Eye movements. *J Neurol Neurosurg Psychiatry* 1996;**60**:115–25.
36 Gresty MA, Bronstein AM, Page NGR, Rudge P. Congenital-type nystagmus emerging in later life. *Neurology* 1991;**41**:653–6.
37 Baloh RW, Hess K, Honrubia V, Yee RD. Low and high frequency sinusoidal rotational testing in patients with peripheral vestibular lesions. *Acta Otolaryngol (Stockh)* 1984;(suppl 406):189–93.
38 Rinne T, Bronstein AM, Rudge P, Gresty MA, Luxon LM. Bilateral loss of vestibular function. *Acta Otolaryngol (Stockh)* 1995;suppl 520:247–50.
39 Baloh RW, Yee RD, Kimm J, Honrubia V. The vestibulo-ocular reflex in patients with lesions of the vestibulocerebellum. *Exp Neurol* 1981;**72**:141–52.
40 Stell R, Bronstein AM, Plant GT, Harding AE. Ataxia telangiectasia: a reappraisal of the ocular motor features and their value in the diagnosis of atypical cases. *Mov Disord* 1989;**4**:320–9.
41 Thurston SE, Leigh RJ, Abel LA, Dell'Osso LF. Hyperactive vestibulo-ocular reflex in cerebellar degeneration: pathogenesis and treatment. *Neurology* 1987;**37**:53–7.
42 Bronstein AM, Gresty MA, Mossman SS. Pendular pseudonystagmus arising as a combination of head tremor and vestibular failure. *Neurology* 1992;**42**:1527–31.
43 Bles W, De Jong JMBV. Uni- and bilateral loss of vestibular function. In: Bles W, Brandt T, eds. *Disorders of posture and gait.* Amsterdam: Elsevier, 1986:127–39.
44 Diener HC, Dichgans J, Bacher M, Gompf B. Quantification of postural sway in normals and patients with cerebellar diseases. *Electroencephalogr Clin Neurophysiol* 1984;**57**:134–42.
45 Furman JMR, Baloh RW, Barin K, *et al.* Assessment: posturography. *Neurology* 1993;**43**:1261–4.
46 Bronstein AM, Hood JD, Gresty MA, Panagi C. Visual control of balance in cerebellar and Parkinsonian syndromes. *Brain* 1990;**113**:767–79.
47 Dichgans J, Mauritz KH, Allum JHJ, Brandt T. Postural sway in normals and atactic patients: analysis of the stabilizing and destabilizing effects of vision. *Agressologie* 1976;**17**:15–24.
48 Bronstein AM. Visual vertigo syndrome: clinical and posturography findings. *J Neurol Neurosurg Psychiatry* 1995;**59**:472–6.
49 Pastor MA, Day BL, Marsden CD. Vestibular induced postural responses in Parkinson's disease. *Brain* 1993;**116**:1177–90.
50 Nashner L, Peters JF. Dynamic posturography in the diagnosis and management of dizziness and balance disorders. *Neurol Clin* 1990;**8**:331–49.
51 Allum JHJ, Keshner EA, Honegger F, Pfaltz CR. Indicators of the influence a peripheral-vestibular deficit has on vestibulo-spinal reflex responses controlling postural stability. *Acta Otolaryngol (Stockh)* 1988;**106**:252–63.
52 EquiTest System NeuroCom International, Inc. *Disorders of posture and gait.* Stuttgart: Georg Thieme Verlag, 1990:466–7.
53 Brandt T, Dieterich M. Pathological eye-head co-ordination in roll: tonic ocular tilt reaction in mesencephalic and medullary lesions. *Brain* 1987;**110**:649–66.
54 Gresty MA, Bronstein AM. Otolith stimulation evokes compensatory reflex eye movements of high velocity when linear motion of the head is combined with concurrent angular motion. *Neurosci Lett* 1986;**65**:149–54.
55 Gresty MA, Bronstein AM, Barratt HJ. Eye movement responses to combined linear and angular head movement. *Exp Brain Res* 1987;**65**:377–84.
56 Takeda N, Igarashi M, Koizuka I, Chae S, Matsunaga T. Recovery of the otolith-ocular reflex after unilateral deafferentation of the otolith organs in squirrel monkeys. *Acta Otolaryngol (Stockh)* 1990;**110**:25–30.
57 Barratt HJ, Bronstein AM, Gresty MA. Testing the vestibular-ocular reflexes: abnormalities of the otolith contribution in patients with neuro-otological disease. *J Neurol Neurosurg Psychiatry* 1987;**50**:1029–35.
58 Haustein W, Mittelstaedt H. Evaluation of retinal orientation and gaze direction in the perception of the vertical. *Vision Res* 1990;**30**:255–62.
59 Mittelstaedt H. The information processing structure of the subjective vertical. A cybernetic bridge between its psychophysics and its neurobiology. In: Marko H, Hauske G,

Struppler A, eds. *Processing structures for perception and action.* Germany: VCH Verlag, 1988:217–63.

60 Halmagyi GM, Curthoys IS, Cremer PD, *et al.* The human horizontal vestibulo-ocular reflex in response to high-acceleration stimulation before and after unilateral vestibular neurectomy. *Exp Brain Res* 1990;**479**:490.

61 Guedry FE. Psychophysics of vestibular sensation. In: Kornhuber HH, ed. *Handbook of sensory physiology.* 6th ed. New York: Springer-Verlag, 1974:1–154.

62 Brookes GB, Faldon M, Kanayama R, Nakamura T, Gresty MA. Recovery from unilateral vestibular nerve section in human subjects evaluated by physiological, psychological and questionnaire assessments. *Acta Otolaryngol (Stockh) (suppl)* 1994;**513**:40–8.

63 Kanayama R, Bronstein AM, Gresty MA, Brookes GB, Faldon ME, Nakamura T. Perceptual studies in patients with vestibular neurectomy. *Acta Otolaryngol (Stockh)* 1995;suppl 520:408–11.

64 Metcalfe T, Gresty MA. Self-controlled reorienting movements in response to rotational displacements in normal subjects and patients with labrinthine diseases. *Ann NY Acad Sci* 1992;**656**;695–8.

65 Bloomberg JG, Jones GM, Segal B. Adaptive modification of vestibularly perceived rotation. *Exp Brain Res* 1991;**84**:47–56.

66 Colebatch JG, Halmagyi GM. Vestibular evoked potentials in human neck muscles before and after unilateral vestibular deafferrentation. *Neurology* 1992;**42**:1635–6.

67 Colebatch JG, Rothwell JC. Vestibular-evoked EMG responses in human neck muscles. *J Physiol* 1993;**473**:18P.

68 Colebatch JG, Rothwell JC, Bronstein AM, Ludman H. Click-evoked vestibular activation in the Tullio phenomenon. *J Neurol Neurosurg Psychiatry.* 1994;**57**:1538–40.

69 Bickford RG, Jacobsen JL, Cody DJR. Nature of average evoked potentials to sound and other stimuli. *Ann NY Acad Sci* 1964;**112**:204–23.

11 Investigation of peripheral neuropathy

J G MCLEOD

Peripheral neuropathy is a common condition that is associated with many systemic diseases. Its exact prevalence in the community is not known although epidemiological studies have established the frequency of certain subtypes—for example, Guillain-Barré syndrome,[1] diabetic neuropathy,[2] and Charcot-Marie-Tooth disease.[3] Because of the numerous causes (well over 100) of peripheral neuropathy and the likelihood of finding an underlying treatable condition, it is important to take a systematic approach to the diagnosis. Diagnostic algorithms for evaluation of neuropathies have been published.[4 5] Although it used to be believed that in more than half the cases a cause was not found,[6] several large series have shown that after intensive investigation only about 20% of cases remain undiagnosed and these tend to have a relatively good prognosis.[7-9]

Pathological types of peripheral neuropathy

There are three major pathological processes that affect the peripheral nervous system: axonal degeneration, segmental demyelination, and neuronopathy. It is important in the investigation of a peripheral neuropathy to be able to recognise the underlying pathological nature of the condition as it influences subsequent management. *Axonal degeneration* is the most common pathology seen in systemic, metabolic, toxic, and nutritional disorders. It characteristically has a predilection for large diameter and long fibres—distal axonopathy or dying back neuropathy.

315

Segmental demyelination is primary destruction of the myelin sheath leaving the axon intact although, axonal degeneration may also be present in demyelinating neuropathies and secondary segmental demyelination may be seen in axonal degeneration. Electrophysiological studies are helpful in differentiating primary demyelination from axonal degeneration. *Neuronopathies* are those conditions in which the cell bodies of axons—anterior horn cells or dorsal root ganglia—are primarily affected.

Clinical evaluation

The most important parts of the investigation of suspected peripheral neuropathy are the taking of an accurate history and the performance of a careful clinical examination. Sensory symptoms are usually the presenting features of neuropathy and include numbness, tingling, pins and needles in the hands and feet, burning sensations, pain in the extremities, sensations of walking on cotton wool, band like sensations around the wrists or ankles, unsteadiness on the feet, or stumbling. Motor symptoms are usually those of weakness and patients may find it difficult to turn keys in locks, unfasten buttons, and remove the tops of bottles and jars. In the early stages of peripheral neuropathy, weakness is usually distal; however, early proximal weakness is a feature of inflammatory neuropathies and porphyric neuropathy. Autonomic symptoms, particularly postural hypotension, impotence, sphincter disturbances, diarrhoea, constipation, and dryness or excessive sweating of the extremities point to damage of small myelinated and unmyelinated fibres. In the history, attention should be paid to recent upper respiratory tract or other infections, alcohol and drug intake, diet, possible exposure to industrial and environmental toxins, family history, and symptoms of systemic diseases. It is important to note the tempo of the disease—acute, subacute, or insidious onset; rapid or slow progression; progressive, stepwise, or relapsing and remitting course. Some of the more common causes of peripheral neuropathy with acute onset are shown in box 11.1.

Signs are usually those of distal muscle wasting and weakness, and sensory impairment, predominantly over distal regions and often in a glove and stocking distribution. In distal axonopathies, particularly in diabetes, there may be loss of sensation over the ventral regions of the trunk due to distal degeneration of the inter-

Box 11.1 Clinical types of peripheral neuropathy

Acute onset:
- Guillain-Barré syndrome
- Porphyria
- Toxic (for example, arsenic, nitrofurantoin)
- Serum sickness (postimmunisation)
- Diphtheria
- Malignancy
- Critical illness polyneuropathy
- Diabetes, uraemia (rarely)

Predominantly motor:
- Guillain-Barré syndrome
- Porphyria
- Diphtheria
- Lead
- Charcot-Marie-Tooth disease
- Diabetes (diabetic amyotrophy)

Predominantly sensory:
- Leprosy
- Diabetes (distal sensory polyneuropathy)
- Vitamin B12 or thiamine deficiency
- Malignancy
- Hereditary sensory and autonomic neuropthy
- Primary or familial amyloidosis
- Uraemia
- Lyme disease
- Sjögren's syndrome

Radicular:
- Diabetic truncal neuropathy
- Lyme disease
- Sjögren's syndrome

Painful neuropathies
- Alcohol, nutritional deficiencies
- Diabetes (acute painful neuropathy)
- Hereditary sensory and autosomal neuropathy (HSAN type 1)
- Arsenic
- Cryoglobulinaemia
- Lyme disease
- Paraneoplastic sensory neuropathy
- Vasculitic neuropathies

costal nerves. A truncal neuropathy, with a dermatomal distribution of dysaesthesia and sensory loss, may also be seen in diabetes[10] as well as in Lyme disease[11] and Sjögren's syndrome[12] (box 11.1). In conditions that affect predominantly small fibres (amyloid neuropathy, Tangier disease, and some cases of diabetic neuropathy) there may be dissociated loss of sensation with loss of pain and temperature sensation and preservation of tactile sensation. Reflexes are usually depressed or absent but in mild cases, in small fibre neuropathies, and when peripheral neuropathy is associated with pyramidal tract lesions, reflexes may be preserved. Careful general examination should seek evidence of pes cavus or other skeletal deformities, enlarged nerves, skin lesions, arthritis, dry mucous membranes, and enlargement of liver, spleen, and lymph glands.

The clinical features of the neuropathy may indicate the underlying cause and enable the most appropriate investigations to be undertaken (box 11.1). Mononeuropathy is usually due to direct compression or entrapment but may be the first manifestation of diabetic or vasculitic neuropathy. Mononeuritis multiplex (multiple mononeuropathy) is caused by vasculitis, leprosy, sarcoidosis, and some other conditions (box 11.2).

Laboratory investigations

General laboratory tests and nerve conduction studies will be performed as the first stage of investigation in all patients unless the diagnosis is clinically obvious—for example, diabetic or alcoholic neuropathy; subsequent investigation will depend on the results of these initial studies.

General laboratory tests

Basic laboratory investigations that should be performed on all patients with peripheral neuropathy of undetermined aetiology include urinalysis, haemoglobin, white cell count, platelets, erythrocyte sedimentation rate, fasting blood glucose, serum electrolytes, serum proteins, serum protein electrophoresis and immunoelectrophoresis, serum creatinine, liver function tests, chest radiographs, and electrophysiological studies (see later). If these do not provide a diagnosis, other special investigations may include thyroid function tests, serum vitamin E levels, serum cholesterol and triglycerides, cryoglobulins, urinary heavy metals

---

Box 11.2   Causes of mononeuritis multiplex

Vascular:
- Diabetes
- Polyarteritis nodosa
- Rheumatoid arthritis
- Systemic lupus erythematosus
- Wegener's granulomatosis
- Sjögren's syndrome
- Non-systemic vasculitis

Inflammatory:
- Leprosy
- Sarcoidosis
- Lyme disease

Infiltrations:
- Malignancy
- Amyloidosis

Immune reactions:
- Immunisation, foreign serum and proteins

Trauma:
- Multiple nerve injuries

---

and porphyrins, antinuclear antibodies, rheumatoid factor, Sjögren's syndrome (SS) antibodies, (SS-A (anti-Ro) and SS-B (anti-La)), serology for Lyme disease and HIV, antiganglioside GM1 antibodies, Schirmer's test, and screening for occult malignancy with endoscopic and radiological examinations including skeletal surveys (see box 11.3).

Nerve conduction studies

Nerve conduction studies play a key part in confirming the presence of peripheral neuropathy and in establishing its cause. They assist in determining whether the patient has a mononeuropathy, mononeuritis multiplex, or a generalised peripheral neuropathy, and if so, whether it is symmetric or asymmetric, whether both sensory and motor fibres are affected, and whether the underlying pathology is that of axonal degeneration or segmental demyelination as there is a correlation between the conduction velocity and the underlying pathological process.[13-17] Box 11.4

319

Box 11.3   General laboratory investigations

Condition	Investigations
Metabolic:	
Diabetes	Urinalysis, fasting blood glucose, glucose tolerance test
Hypoglycaemia	Fasting blood glucose, serum insulin, or C peptide concentrations
Uraemia	Blood urea, serum creatine, urinalysis
Porphyria	Urinary porphyrins, antinuclear antibodies, porphobilinogen, total faecal porphyrins, erythrocyte porphobilinogen deaminase
Hypothyroidism	Serum free thyroxine, serum thyroid stimulating hormone
Acromegaly	Serum growth hormone concentrations
Deficiencies:	
B1 (thiamine)	Erythrocyte transketolase activity + enhancement with thiamine pyrophosphate
Vitamin B6 (pyridoxine)	Erythrocyte aspartate amino transferase + enhancement with pyridoxal-5-phosphate
Vitamin B12	Serum B12, Schilling test
Vitamin E	Serum vitamin E
Toxic:	
Arsenic, lead, mercury, thallium	24 hour urinary heavy metals
Paraproteinaemias, dysproteinaemias:	
Multiple myeloma, Waldenstrom's macroglobulinaemia, cryoglobulinaemia, monoclonal gammopathy of uncertain significance (MGUS)	Hb, WCC, platelets, ESR, plasma immunoelectrophoresis, urinary Bence Jones protein, radiological skeletal survey, bone marrow biopsy, plasma cryoglobulins

Box 11.3 General laboratory investigations—cont

Connective tissue disorders:

Systemic lupus erythematosus, mixed connective tissue disease, scleroderma, rheumatoid arthritis, polyarteritis nodosa, Sjögren's syndrome, Wegener's granulomatosis

Hb, WCC, platelets, ESR, serum immunoelectrophoresis, antinuclear antibodies, antidouble stranded DNA antibodies, rheumatoid factor, serum complement (C3, C4, CH50), antineutrophil cytoplasmic antibodies (ANCA)

Sjögren's syndrome

All above + anti-Sjögren's syndrome antibodies, Schirmer's test, lip biopsy

Inflammatory neuropathies:

Acute inflammatory neuropathy

HIV, blood glucose, urinary porphyrins, Epstein-Barr virus, *Campylobacter* infections, cytomegalovirus, mycoplasma

Chronic inflammatory demyelinating polyradiculoneuropathy

ESR, serum immunoelectrophoresis, anti-ganglioside GM1 antibodies, antinuclear antibodies, antineutrophil cytoplasmic antibodies

Infections:

HIV

HIV serology

Lyme disease

Lyme serology

Leprosy

Lepromin tests; skin, nasal scrapings; skin, nerve biopsy

Hereditary neuropathies with known biochemical abnormalities:

Primary amyloid neuropathy

Rectal, liver, renal, abdominal fat, nerve biopsy; serum immunoelectrophoresis; urinary Bence Jones protein

Familial amyloid polyneuropathy

Serum, tissue transthyretin

Metachromatic leukodystrophy

Blood leucocyte, skin fibroblast arylsulphatase

Krabbe's disease (globoid cell leukodystrophy)

Blood leucocyte, skin fibroblast α-galactosidase

A-β lipoproteinaemia (Bassen-Kornzweig disease)

Acanthocytes in blood, serum cholesterol, plasma low density and very low density lipoproteins

An-α lipoproteinaemia (Tangier disease)

Serum cholesterol
Plasma high density lipoproteins

Refsum's disease

Serum phytanic acid. α Oxidation of phytanic acid in skin fibroblasts

ESR = erythrocyte sedimentation rate; Hb = haemoglobin; WCC = white cell count.

Box 11.4 Demyelinating neuropathies

Inflammatory neuropathies:
- Guillain-Barré syndrome
- Chronic inflammatory demyelinating polyradiculoneuropathy
- Motor neuropathy with multifocal conduction block
- Chronic inflammatory neuropathy associated with paraproteinaemia
- Inflammatory neuropathy associated with HIV infection

Hereditary neuropathies:
- HMSN type I
- HMSN type III
- Refsum's syndrome
- Metachromatic leukodystrophy
- Krabbe's disease

Metabolic neuropathies:
- Diabetes (sometimes)
- Uraemia (sometimes)

Toxic neuropathies:
- Perhexiline maleate
- Amiodorone
- Hexacarbons

Infections:
- Diphtheria

Malignancy:
- Some acute or subacute neuropathies associated with lymphoma, carcinoma

---

shows the causes of segmental demyelination and conduction velocities in the demyelinating range.

Nerve conduction studies should be performed on nerves that are clinically unaffected as well as those that are clinically affected. In general, several nerves should be studied in upper and lower limbs—for example, motor and sensory conduction in median and ulnar nerves, motor conduction in common peroneal and posterior tibial nerves, and sensory conduction in sural nerves. In some cases it may be appropriate to perform sensory conduction on radial, tibial, and saphenous nerves and to record mixed nerve action potentials in ulnar and common peroneal nerves. Every clinical neurophysiology laboratory should have established its own control values. The age of the patient needs to be taken into account because nerve conduction velocities in full term infants are about half the adult values but increase to the adult range at 3 to 5 years of age; there is also a reduction in conduction velocity after the age of 40. Temperature of the limbs must be controlled or a temperature correction applied because the conduction velocity changes by 2·4 m/s/1°C from 29 to 38°C.[18-19]

Motor conduction velocities should be recorded from surface electrodes to measure the amplitudes of the muscle action potential after stimulation at distal and proximal sites; reduced amplitude of the muscle action potential at distal stimulation sites is indicative of axonal degeneration, or, rarely, demyelination in distal motor fibres. A significant reduction in the amplitude of the muscle action potential on moving the stimulating electrode from a distal to a more proximal site is supportive evidence of conduction block.[20] Conduction block is suspected if there is greater than 20% reduction in amplitude (provided there is less than a 15% change in duration of the muscle action potential between proximal and distal sites of stimulation[21] as dispersion and polyphasic action potentials can cause phase cancellation).[22] Abrupt change in area, or amplitude, or both over a short segment of nerve, rather than a gradual reduction over a longer distance, is strong evidence of conduction block.[22] Further evidence of demyelination is temporal dispersion (increased duration of the muscle action potential), prolonged distal latencies, and reduction in conduction velocity to less than 80% of the lower limit of normal in two or more motor nerves.[21 23]

In axonal degeneration there is normal or only mild slowing of conduction due to fall out of the damaged large diameter fibres, the remaining intact fibres having normal conduction velocities. Other evidence of axonal degeneration is a reduced muscle action potential and electromyographic evidence of denervation. It should be noted that mild degrees of slowing of conduction do not exclude the possibility of underlying segmental demyelination in peripheral nerves.[15 17] Sensory conduction is usually impaired, with reduced amplitudes of action potentials in both axonal degeneration and segmental demyelination. Although sensory action potentials are difficult to record over long distances in diseased nerves, slowed conduction and dispersion of the action potentials can be recorded in segmental demyelination with appropriate

323

techniques. Because motor and sensory conduction are routinely measured only in large diameter fibres with standard nerve conduction techniques, they may be normal in small fibre neuropathies.

F waves

F waves are late waves that can be recorded from muscles after supramaximal stimulation of the nerve and result from antidromic nerve impulses causing anterior horn cells to backfire.[24] They provide a measure of conduction over the whole length of the motor nerve and are therefore a useful way of recording conduction in proximal segments.[19]

H reflex

The H reflex measures the conduction through afferent and efferent fibres in the monosynaptic reflex arc. It is most easily recorded from the calf muscles. It is usually absent when the F wave and other nerve conduction studies are abnormal.[19]

Needle electromyography

When muscles are denervated, spontaneous fibrillation, positive sharp waves, and a reduced interference pattern are recorded on needle electromyography. Electromyography is useful in confirming the presence of axonal degeneration in the Guillain-Barré syndrome.[25] It should be borne in mind that denervation potentials may not appear until three weeks after the onset of axonal degeneration.

Somatosensory evoked potentials

Somatosensory potentials may be useful in detecting abnormalities of conduction in proximal segments when conventional nerve conduction studies are normal.[25] Walsh et al[26] found them more useful than the F waves in the Guillain-Barré syndrome although others have had a different experience.[27]

Examination of CSF

A lumbar puncture with CSF examination is unrewarding in most cases of axonal neuropathy but should be performed in demyelinating neuropathies. In the Guillain-Barré syndrome the CSF protein rises during the first week. The white cell count varies with the time of lumbar puncture and is raised in about 10%

of cases.[28][29] An increased white cell count raises the possibility of HIV infection or Lyme disease.[28][30] CSF protein is also raised in chronic inflammatory demyelinating polyradiculoneuropathy (CIDP) and may help to distinguish this condition from hereditary demyelinating neuropathies. A high CSF protein suggests inflammatory causes and demyelination of spinal roots or both. In my experience, oligoclonal bands IgG are present in the CSF of about 6% of cases of Guillain-Barré syndrome, and 16% of cases of CIDP.

Quantitative sensory testing (QST)

QST is the use of psychophysical methods for measuring abnormalities of the different modalities of sensation. With these techniques, quantitative values for thresholds of vibration, touch—pressure, and warm and cold sensation may be obtained on individuals and compared with control values. These investigations are not routinely employed in the investigation of peripheral neuropathy but are useful in detecting early sensory abnormalities in people exposed to occupational and environmental toxins, in controlled clinical trials, and in epidemiological studies.[31]

Autonomic function studies

Autonomic dysfunction is a common complication of peripheral neuropathies although often it is mild and of little relevance. In some conditions, however, there may be profound disturbance of autonomic function including orthostatic hypotension, impairment of blood pressure, heart rate and bladder control, and impotence. Diseases that primarily affect small fibres in peripheral nerves or cause acute demyelination of small myelinated fibres are those most likely to cause autonomic dysfunction. These include acute dysautonomia, familial and primary amyloidosis, Guillain-Barré syndrome, diabetes, porphyria, Chagas' disease, and some hereditary sensory and autonomic neuropathies.[32-35] There are many available tests from which to select; tests of both sympathetic and parasympathetic function should be included and it is generally necessary to find abnormalities in two or more of these tests to confirm the presence of autonomic dysfunction.[33] Tests of autonomic function that can be readily undertaken in the clinical neurophysiology laboratory are heart rate variation with respiration, Valsalva ratio, heart rate response to standing or tilting,

325

blood pressure response to sustained handgrip, and the sympathetic skin response.[34] Autonomic function studies, together with quantitative sensory testing and sural nerve biopsy, are the most useful ways of confirming a diagnosis of small fibre neuropathy.[36]

Molecular genetics

There are now several hereditary neuropathies in which the gene locus has been identified and the number is rapidly increasing with advances in recombinant DNA technology. The types of genetic analysis available to the clinician fall into two groups: linkage studies for conditions in which the region of the gene on the chromosome has been identified but the defective gene has not been cloned, and mutation analysis or positional cloning in those conditions in which the gene has been cloned.[37-39]

Box 11.5 shows the hereditary peripheral neuropathies in which the gene has been identified.

Sural nerve biopsy

Nerve biopsy is a valuable method for establishing a cause of peripheral neuropathy in specific circumstances.[5 40 41] It should not be performed simply to establish the presence of peripheral neuropathy as clinical evaluation and nerve conduction studies are nearly always adequate for this purpose. It should be undertaken only where the biopsy can be evaluated by a laboratory experienced in the techniques of light and electron microscopy, teased fibre studies, and the use of immunohistochemical methods of staining. Biopsies should only be undertaken after full clinical and electrophysiological assessment and when other laboratory investigations have been completed. It is usually performed on the sural nerve but sometimes the radial sensory nerve is more appropriate. Whole nerve or fascicular biopsies are undertaken in different centres. Although not required in those cases where the diagnosis is certain from family history or from other investigations, nerve biopsy may confirm a diagnosis of chronic inflammatory demyelinating polyradiculoneuropathy (CIDP),[42 43] hereditary motor and sensory neuropathy (HMSN),[44-48] hereditary sensory and autonomic neuropathy (HSAN),[49] primary and familial amyloid neuropathy,[50-53] vasculitis,[54-57] sarcoidosis,[58] giant axonal neuropathy,[59 60] hereditary liability to pressure palsies (tomaculous neuropathy),[61] and hexacarbon (n-hexane and methyl n-butyl ketone) neuropathy.[62] Specific appearances may be seen in the

Box 11.5 Genetic tests for hereditary neuropathies

Disease	Chromosome location	Gene product	Genetic defect
CMT Ia (HMSN Ia)	17p11.2–12	PMP22	Duplication Point mutation
CMT Ib (HMSN Ib)	1q21.2, 23	Po	Point mutation
CMT X (HMSN-X)	Xq13	Connexin-32	Point mutation
Hereditary liability to pressure palsies (tomaculous neuropathy)	17p.11.2, 12	PMP22	Deletion Point mutation
Familial amyloid polyneuropathy, (most types)	18q11.2, 12.1	Transthyretin, Apo A1 + two unidentified genes on chromosomes 9 and 11	Point mutations

nerve biopsy in IgM κ paraproteinaemic neuropathy,[63] metachromatic leukodystrophy,[64-66] Krabbe's disease,[66 67] Fabry's disease,[68 69] and Friedreich's ataxia.[70] In some cases of vasculitis, sarcoidosis, amyloidosis, sensory perineuritis, and chronic inflammatory neuropathy, the biopsy is essential for diagnosis.

In general, nerve biopsy is of little diagnostic value in metabolic disorders and alcoholic and nutritional neuropathies, in which the appearances are non-specific. There is a case for performing biopsies in patients with chronic neuropathies of undetermined cause when all other investigations have been completed. The morphometry of peripheral nerves is related to age and every laboratory should have its own established control values for different age groups.

Application of investigations to specific types of peripheral neuropathy

Hereditary neuropathies

Charcot-Marie-Tooth disease (hereditary motor and sensory neuropathy, peroneal muscular atrophy)

Charcot-Marie-Tooth disease (CMT) is a genetically heterogeneous disorder. There are four major types: HMSN I (CMT 1a and 1b), HMSN II (CMT 2), X linked (CMT-X), and HMSN III (Déjèrine-Sottas disease).[3] HMSN I and II are usually dominant although some autosomal recessive cases have been described. Déjèrine-Sottas disease (HMSN III) is autosomal recessive.

Nerve conduction studies—Nerve conduction studies are of considerable value in the initial categorisation of Charcot-Marie-Tooth disease into different subtypes. Although there is some overlap, motor conduction velocities in both HMSN Ia and Ib are greatly slowed (median motor conduction velocity <38 m/s) and sensory conduction is impaired. By contrast, there is only mildly impaired or normal motor conduction velocity in HMSN II.[3 44-46 71-74] Bradley et al[45] suggested that there was also an intermediate type of Charcot-Marie-Tooth disease with intermediate conduction velocities (25–45 m/s) and intermediate changes on nerve biopsy. It is likely that some of these cases were CMT-X as slow conduction velocities are found in affected males with CMT-X (<40 m/s) and intermediate range motor conduction velocities (>40 m/s) in affected or obligate female carriers.[75] In HMSN III (Déjèrine-Sottas disease) motor conduction velocities are typically grossly slowed (<12 m/s).[47 48 71] It may be a genetically heterogeneous condition.[76]

Sural nerve biopsy—Sural nerve biopsy is helpful in distinguishing the different types of HMSN when they are not clearly separated on the basis of electrophysiological studies.[44–48 71] In HMSN Ia and Ib there is a reduction in the density of fibres, onion bulb formations, evidence of segmental demyelination on light and electron microscopy and teased nerve fibres, and in most myelinated fibres the myelin sheath is of appropriate diameter for the axon. In HMSN II there is a reduction in the density of myelinated fibres but no evidence of demyelination. In HMSN III onion bulbs are prominent and the myelin sheath is abnormally thin relative to the axon diameter (figure 11.1).

Genetic studies—Most cases of HMSN I are type Ia, which is linked to chromosome 17.[77–79] There is usually a duplication on 17p11.2–12[79–81] in which region the PMP22 gene is located. In some cases of the disease, a point mutation of the coding region of PMP22 has been demonstrated where an identical mutation also occurs in the trembler mouse.[81–84] Duplication in this region has also been shown in nine out of 10 sporadic cases that had been considered to be recessive.[85] It has been suggested that overdosage of PMP22 caused by the DNA duplication is the mechanism for producing the HMSN Ia phenotype. A deletion in the same region that is duplicated in HMSN Ia is found in hereditary neuropathy with liability to pressure palsies.[86 87] In this condition there are irregular sausage shaped swellings of the myelin sheath (figure 11.2). It has been shown that the gene involved is also PMP22. A frame shift or null mutation was found, indicating that underdosage of PMP22 is the cause.[88]

The gene mutation in HMSN Ib has been located near the Duffy locus on chromosome 1 where HMSN Ib was originally mapped by linkage analysis.[89 90] A point mutation in the gene for Po (1q21.2q23) was subsequently found when Po was mapped to this region.[91]

HMSN type II is genetically heterogeneous; the gene for one of the forms of autosomal dominant HMSN II (CMT 2) has been localised to chromosome 1p36.[92]

The gap junction protein connexin-32 has been identified for the gene mutation in CMT X (Xq13).[93]

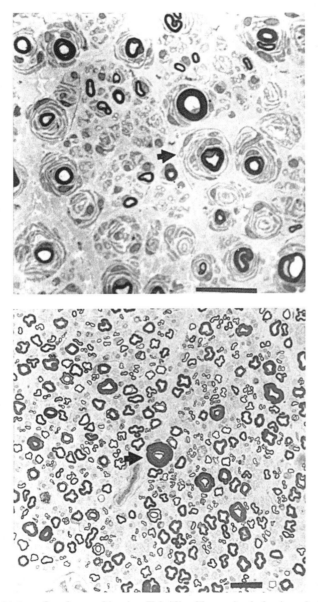

Figure 11.1   *Sural nerve biopsies. Toluidine blue stained plastic embedded sections. Top: Charcot-Marie-Tooth type 1 (HMSN I). Onion bulbs (arrow) are plentiful around well myelinated fibres. Bottom: tomaculous neuropathy. Fibres with abnormally thick myelin sheaths (arrow) are present; Bar = 25 μm*

Déjèrine-Sottas disease (HMSN III) now seems to be a hetero-geneous disorder. Cases have been reported with mutations of PMP22 and Po genes.[94][95]

Amyloid neuropathy

Peripheral neuropathy is a feature of primary amyloidosis and several types of familial amyloid polyneuropathy. Dysaesthesiae, loss of pain and temperature sensation in the extremities, and autonomic dysfunction (postural hypotension, impotence, impaired sweating, bladder disturbance) are characteristic fea-tures. Distal sensory loss, predominantly of pain and temperature sense, are found on examination. Nerve conduction studies and electromyography are consistent with axonal neuropathy. Autonomic function studies are abnormal. Sural nerve biopsy is usually diagnostic and shows amyloid deposits in blood vessels and endoneurium on Congo red staining and there is selective loss of small myelinated and unmyelinated fibres. The diagnosis of amyloidosis may also be established by abdominal fat, rectum, kidney, and liver biopsy.[50-53] A high proportion of patients with pri-mary amyloidosis have monoclonal proteins on immunoelec-trophoresis of urine and blood, and some have multiple myeloma. Immunohistochemical staining of tissue amyloid identifies protein specific types—AL in primary amyloidosis and AF in familial types. The amyloid in familial polyneuropathy is not derived from immunoglobulin and therefore abnormal immunoglobulins are not present in the serum. In most, but not all, types of familial polyneuropathy (Portuguese, Indian, German and Jewish, and Appalachian types), there is a prealbumin (transthyretin) fraction in the serum and a point mutation in the transthyretin gene (chro-mosome 18q.11.2, q12.1). The Finnish type of amyloidosis has been located on 9q33 and the Iowa type on 11q33-q24. The Van Allen type is due to a genetic defect of apolipoprotein A1.[37][53]

Hereditary disorders of lipid metabolism

Metachromatic leukodystrophy—Metachromatic leukodystrophy is associated with peripheral neuropathy that may sometimes be a presenting feature in adult cases. Nerve conduction studies are consistent with the segmental demyelination that is seen on sural nerve biopsy together with metachromatic granular inclusions in Schwann cells.[64-66] Diagnosis may be established in the laboratory by determination of reduced arylsulphatase concentrations in blood leucocytes and skin fibroblasts, and by the finding of intracellular deposits of metachromatic material on microscopic examination of urinary sediment.[66] There is a mutation of the gene encoding for arylsulphatase A on chromosome 22q-13qter.[38]

Krabbe's disease (globoid cell leukodystrophy)—This disease is autosomal recessive, affects children in the first year of life, and is associated with peripheral neuropathy. Nerve biopsy shows loss of myelinated fibres, and inclusions in Schwann cells and macrophages that are diagnostic.[66 67] Assay of the enzyme galactosylceramide β galactosidase in leucocytes, serum, or cultured fibroblasts will establish the diagnosis without the need for biopsy.[66]

A-β lipoproteinaemia (Bassen-Kornzweig disease)—Peripheral neuropathy is associated with a progressive ataxia resembling Friedreich's ataxia.[45] There is moderate slowing of motor conduction, and nerve biopsy shows segmental demyelination and loss of large diameter fibres. The diagnosis can be confirmed by laboratory investigations which show acanthocytes in the peripheral blood, low serum cholesterol and low density and very low density lipoproteins. Genetic testing is not available.

An-α lipoproteinaemia (Tangier disease)—Peripheral neuropathy is usually present. The presence of large orange tonsils is characteristic. Sural nerve biopsy shows reduced numbers of myelinated and unmyelinated fibres and lipid droplets may be seen in Schwann cells.[96] Plasma high density lipoproteins are greatly reduced.

Fabry's disease—This is associated with a painful neuropathy and a selective loss of small myelinated and unmyelinated fibres may be seen in the sural nerve biopsy.[68 69] It is an X linked recessive disorder. Glycolipid granules may be seen in perineurial and endothelial cells in peripheral nerve.[68] There is a deficiency of the enzyme ceramidetrihexsosidase that results in the accumulation of ceramidetrihexaside in tissues. Diagnosis may be established by enzyme assay of α galactosidase which is reduced on leucocyte and skin fibroblast preparations.[97]

Refsum's disease—Refsum's disease is a rare autosomal recessive disorder characterised by demyelinating hypertrophic neuropathy, retinitis pigmentosa, ataxia, ichthyosis, and deafness. Motor nerve conduction is very slow due to demyelination; onion bulb formation may be seen on sural nerve biopsies. There is impaired α oxidation of phytanic acid α hydrolyase causing an accumulation of phytanic acid in the tissues.[98] Diagnosis is made from the clinical picture and by increased serum phytanic acid and defective α oxidation of phytanic acid by skin fibroblasts.

Friedreich's ataxia—Friedreich's ataxia is associated with a sensory neuropathy. Electrophysiological studies typically show small or absent sensory potentials and normal motor conduction and on sural nerve biopsy there is a selective loss of large diameter fibres.[70] Other spinocerebellar degenerations may be associated with a mild neuropathy affecting myelinated fibres of all diameters.[99]

Inflammatory neuropathies

Guillain-Barré syndrome

In the first instance, a clinical diagnosis of peripheral neuropathy must be established and other conditions such as transverse myelitis, spinal cord compression, botulism (pure motor features), and myasthenia gravis (pure motor features) must be excluded. Other causes of acute neuropathy (toxins, drugs, nutritional deficiencies, porphyria, Lyme disease, acute neuropathy of the critically ill, vasculitis, and malignancy) are eliminated by clinical evaluation and appropriate tests. Antecedent precipitating factors (for example, immunisation, *Campylobacter*, Epstein-Barr virus, and mycoplasma infections) should be sought. The CSF may show the typical abnormalities of increased protein and low white cell count; a high white cell count raises the suspicion of HIV, Lyme disease, and other infections.[28 30 100] Nerve conduction studies are essential for diagnosis but may be normal in the early stages in which case recording of F waves and somatosensory evoked potentials should be undertaken to seek evidence of impairment of proximal conduction. Three or more nerves should be studied in upper and lower limbs as the peripheral nerve demyelination may be asymmetric and patchy.[25] Serial studies should be undertaken if the diagnosis is in doubt. Electromyography should be performed after two or three weeks if recovery is slow, or muscle wasting has developed, to ascertain the extent of axonal degeneration. Nerve conduction studies should be repeated if recovery is delayed; persistent slowing of conduction, conduction block, and dispersion should raise the suspicion of chronic inflammatory demyelinating

333

polyneuropathy with acute onset but it should be borne in mind that electrophysiological evidence of demyelination may persist in typical Guillain-Barré syndrome for many weeks.

Chronic inflammatory demyelinating polyradiculoneuropathy (CIDP)

Typically the onset is subacute, the peak of disability being reached later than four weeks. However, it may have a more rapid onset. The diagnosis is confirmed by evidence of demyelination from nerve conduction studies.[42 43 101] These may help differentiate it from the demyelination seen in hereditary demyelinating neuropathies HMSN types I and III and Refsum's syndrome in which the conduction velocities are uniformly slow in all nerves and conduction block and dispersion of the action potential are uncommon.[102] Protein in CSF is usually increased.[42 43 101] Other types of demyelinating neuropathy (paraproteinaemic, vasculitic, leprosy, Lyme disease, HIV infections) must be excluded by appropriate investigations. If there is doubt about the diagnosis, confirmation should be obtained from sural nerve biopsy as the patient is likely to be committed to a long course of immunotherapy with its attendant risks.[103] The progress can be monitored by nerve conduction studies although the changes of improvement or deterioration will lag behind those of the clinical features.

Paraproteinemic neuropathies

Paraproteins may be found on immunoelectrophoresis during the investigation of patients with peripheral neuropathy, and the finding should arouse suspicion of multiple myeloma, Waldenstrom macroglobulinaemia, cryoglobulinaemia, primary amyloidosis, and other dysproteinaemias. Bone marrow aspiration, examination for urinary Bence Jones protein, and radiological skeletal survey should be performed; if these investigations are normal it is likely that the patient has a benign monoclonal gammopathy, or monoclonal gammopathy of undetermined relevance.[104]

Benign monoclonal gammopathy—There is an association between benign monoclonal paraproteins in the blood and peripheral neuropathy.[105] IgM paraproteins are particularly associated with a chronic demyelinating sensorimotor neuropathy, tending to occur in older people and being accompanied by a postural tremor.[62] Sural nerve biopsy often shows demyelination with widely spaced myelin lamellae being seen on electron microscopy, particularly in the presence of IgM κ.[62] IgA and IgG proteins may also be associated with demyelinating neuropathies. The relation between paraproteinaemia and CIDP is uncertain.[106 107]

Multifocal motor neuropathy with persistent conduction block

This is a rare condition in which there is an asymmetric chronic demyelinating neuropathy affecting predominantly motor nerves and clear electrical evidence of conduction block. It presents with asymmetric weakness and wasting with a motor neuron disease-like picture and increased antiganglioside GM1 antibodies in about 80% of cases.[108 109] Motor nerve conduction studies show conduction block and slowing localised to sharply circumscribed areas in nerve trunks.[110] Sensory conduction is normal, at least in the early stages of the disease, and sural nerve biopsy shows only minor changes.[108 111 112] Biopsy of affected segments of nerves show subperineurial oedema, onion bulb formations, and demyelinated and remyelinated axons.[113] The relation of this condition to CIDP is unclear.

Vasculitic neuropathy

Vasculitic neuropathies (polyarteritis nodosa, Churg-Strauss syndrome, Waldenstrom's macroglobulinaemia, rheumatoid arthritis, mixed connective tissue diseases, Sjögren's syndrome, non-systemic vasculitis, systemic lupus erythematosus) classically present as mononeuritis multiplex although about half the patients have a clinical picture of asymmetric or symmetric generalised sensorimotor polyneuropathy.[54] In most cases there will be evidence of systemic disease and raised erythrocyte sedimentation rate; the presence of increased titres of antinuclear antibodies and rheumatoid factor will confirm the diagnosis. Nerve conduction studies are consistent with an axonal neuropathy. Nerve biopsy usually shows pathological changes of vasculitis in small vessels in the endoneurium and perineurium and acute severe axonal degeneration. Non-systemic vasculitic neuropathy is being increasingly recognised; up to 30% of all vasculitic neuropathies fall into this group.[54-57] Some cases may have increased erythrocyte sedimentation rate and antinuclear antibody titres but in most there are no serological markers and diagnosis can be made only on sural nerve biopsy.

Sjögren's syndrome

Sjögren's syndrome is often difficult to diagnose in the early stages as it may present as a symmetric or asymmetric predominantly sensory neuropathy in which there is evidence of vasculitis on sural biopsy[57 114 115] before systemic symptoms of dry eyes, arthritis, and other manifestations of the disease become obvious and before titres of autoantibodies to Ro(SS-A) and La(SS-B) become raised. Another manifestation of Sjögren's syndrome may be an ataxic sensory neuronopathy in which the primary pathology is dorsal root ganglionitis.[115 116]

Infections

HIV infections

Symptomatic neuropathy affects about 5% to 10% of patients infected with HIV. Acute inflammatory polyneuropathy of the Guillain-Barré type most often occurs at the time of seroconversion.[100 117] The CSF cell count may be raised.[100 117] Subacute multifocal neuropathy of a demyelinating type with inflammatory pathology is the most common pattern of neuropathy before the onset of cellular immunosuppression.[117] The CSF may be normal or show increased protein or white cell count. At the late stage of HIV infections an acute lumbrosacral polyradiculopathy or multifocal neuropathy may be caused by cytomegalovirus infection. It is important to diagnose cytomegalovirus neuropathy as it is treatable.[117 118]

Leprosy

Leprosy should be considered in mononeuropathy or multiple mononeuropathy with predominantly sensory symptoms in patients who live or have lived in endemic regions. Nerve biopsy is useful in the diagnosis and nerve conduction studies are helpful in identifying affected nerves.[117 119]

Summary

The clinical evaluation is the most important step in the investigation of suspected peripheral neuropathy. Clues to the underlying cause may be obtained from the clinical pattern of presentation—acute onset, predominantly motor or sensory, radicular, painful, or mononeuritis multiplex. Most cases will require nerve conduction studies and general laboratory tests but further specific investigations will depend on the clinical picture and the suspected cause. Nerve biopsy may be diagnostic in certain conditions. An increasing number of hereditary neuropathies may be diagnosed by DNA tests.

1 Alter M. The epidemiology of Guillain-Barré syndrome. *Ann Neurol* 1990; 27(suppl):S7–12.
2 Melton LJ, Dyck PJ. Epidemiology. In: Dyck PJ, Thomas PK, Asbury AK, Winegrad AI, Porte D, eds. *Diabetic neuropathy*. Philadelphia: WB Saunders,1987:27–35.
3 Dyck PJ, Chance PF, Lebo RV, Carney JA. Hereditary motor and sensory neuropathies. In: Dyck PJ, Thomas PK, Griffin JW, Low P, Poduslo JF, eds. *Peripheral neuropathy*. 3rd ed. Philadelphia: WB Saunders, 1993:1094–136.
4 Asbury AK, Gilliatt RW. The clinical approach to neuropathy. In: Asbury AK, Gilliatt RW, eds. *Peripheral nerve disorders*. London: Butterworths, 1984:12.
5 Schaumburg HH, Berger AR, Thomas PK. *Disorders of the peripheral nerves*. 2nd ed. Philadelphia: FA Davis, 1992:26–32.
6 Miller H. Polyneuritis. *BMJ* 1966;2:1219–25.
7 Dyck PJ, Oviatt RF, Lambert EH. Intensive evaluation of referred unclassified neuropathies yields improved diagnosis. *Ann Neurol* 1981;10:222–6.
8 McLeod JG, Tuck RR, Pollard JD, Cameron JC, Walsh JC. Chronic polyneuropathy of undetermined cause. *J Neurol Neurosurg Psychiatry* 1984;47:530–5.
9 Notermans NC, Wokke JHJ, Franssen H, *et al*. Chronic idiopathic polyneuropathy presenting in middle or old age: a clinical and electrophysiological study of 75 patients. *J Neurol Neurosurg Psychiatry* 1993;56:1066–71.
10 Stewart JD. Diabetic truncal neuropathy: topography of the sensory deficit. *Ann Neurol* 1989;25:233–8.
11 Pachner AR, Steere AC. The triad of neurologic manifestations of Lyme disease: meningitis, cranial neuritis and radiculoneuritis. *Neurology* 1985;35:47–53.
12 Malinow K, Yannakakis GD, Glusman SM, *et al*. Subacute sensory neuronopathy secondary to dorsal root ganglionitis in primary Sjögren's syndrome. *Ann Neurol* 1986;20:535–7.
13 Gilliatt RW. Nerve conduction in human and experimental neuropathies. *Proceedings of the Royal Society of Medicine* 1966;59:989–93.
14 Thomas PK. The morphological basis for alterations in nerve conduction in peripheral neuropathy. *Proceedings of the Royal Society of Medicine* 1971;64:295–8.
15 McLeod JG, Prineas JW, Walsh JC. The relationship of conduction velocity to pathology in peripheral nerves: a study of the sural nerve in 90 patients. In: Desmed JE, ed. *New developments in electromyography and clinical neurophysiology*. Vol 2. Basel: Karger, 1973:248–58.
16 Behse F, Buchthal F. Sensory action potentials and biopsy of the sural nerve in neuropathy. *Brain* 1978;101:473–93.
17 Logigian EL, Kelly JJ, Adelman S. Nerve conduction and biopsy correlation in over 100 consecutive patients with suspected polyneuropathy. *Muscle Nerve* 1994;17:101–20.
18 Daube JR. Nerve conduction studies. In: Aminoff M, ed. *Electrodiagnosis in clinical neurology*. 3rd ed. New York: Churchill Livingstone, 1992:283–326.
19 Kimura J. Nerve conduction studies and electromyography. In: Dyck PJ, Thomas PK, Low PA, Griffin JW, Poduslo JF, eds. *Peripheral neuropathy*. 3rd ed. Philadelphia: WB Saunders, 1993:598–644.
20 Cornblath DR, Sumner AJ, Daube G, Gilliatt RW, Brown WF, Parry GJ, *et al*. Conduction block in clinical practice. *Muscle Nerve* 1991;14:869–71.
21 Cornblath DR. Electrophysiology in Guillain-Barré syndrome. *Ann Neurol* 1990;27(suppl):S17–20.
22 Asbury AK, Cornblath DR. Assessment of current diagnostic criteria for Guillain-Barré syndrome. *Ann Neurol* 1990;27(suppl):S21–4.
23 Sumner AJ. Electrophysiology of the inflammatory demyelinating polyneuropathies. In: McLeod JG, ed. *Inflammatory neuropathies. Baillière's clinical neurology 3:1*. London: Baillière Tindall, 1994:25–44.
24 McLeod JG, Wray SH. An experimental study of the F-wave in the baboon. *J Neurol Neurosurg Psychiatry* 1966;29:196–200.
25 McLeod JG. Electrophysiological studies in the Guillain-Barré syndrome. *Ann Neurol* 1981;9(suppl):20–7.

26 Walsh JC, Yiannikas C, McLeod JG. Abnormalities of proximal conduction in acute idiopathic polyneuritis: comparison of short latency evoked potentials and F-waves. *J Neurol Neurosurg Psychiatry* 1984;47:197–200.
27 Olney K, Aminoff MJ. Electrodiagnostic features of the Guillain-Barré syndrome. The relative sensitivity of different techniques. *Neurology* 1990;40:471–5.
28 Hughes RAC. *Guillain-Barré syndrome*. Heidelberg: Springer Verlag, 1990.
29 McLeod JG, Walsh JC, Prineas JW, Pollard JD. Acute idiopathic polyneuritis. A clinical and electrophysiological study. *J Neurol Sci* 1976;27:145–62.
30 Ropper AH, Wijdicks EFM, Truax BT. *Guillain-Barré syndrome*. Philadelphia: FA Davis, 1991.
31 Dyck PJ, Karnes J, O'Brien PC, Zimmerman IR. Detection thresholds of cutaneous sensation in humans. In: Dyck PJ, Thomas PK, Griffin JW, Low PA, Poduslo JF, eds. *Peripheral neuropathy* 3rd ed. Philadelphia: WB Saunders, 1993:706–28.
32 McLeod JG, Tuck RR. Disorders of the autonomic nervous system: part I. Pathophysiology and clinical features. *Ann Neurol* 1987;21:419–23.
33 McLeod JG, Tuck RR. Disorders of the autonomic nervous system: part II. Investigation and treatment. *Ann Neurol* 1987;21:519–29.
34 McLeod JG. Autonomic dysfunction in peripheral nerve disease. *J Clin Neurophysiol* 1993;10:51–60.
35 Low PA, McLeod JG. The autonomic neuropathies. In: Low PA, ed. *Clinical autonomic disorders*. Boston: Little Brown, 1993:395–421.
36 Stewart JD, Low PA. Small-fiber neuropathy. In: Low PA, ed. *Clinical autonomic disorders*. Boston: Little Brown, 1993:653–66.
37 Harding AE. The DNA laboratory and neurological practice. *J Neurol Neurosurg Psychiatry* 1993;56:229–33.
38 Martin JB. Molecular genetics in neurology. *Ann Neurol* 1993;34:757–73.
39 MacMillan JC, Harper PS. Clinical genetics in neurological disease. *J Neurol Neurosurg Psychiatry* 1994;57:7–15.
40 McLeod JG, Walsh JC, Little JM. Sural nerve biopsy. *Med J Aust* 1969;1:1092–6.
41 Dyck PJ, Gianni C, Lais A. Pathologic alterations of nerve. In: Dyck PJ, Thomas PK, Griffin JW, Low PA, Poduslo JF, eds. *Peripheral neuropathy*. 3rd ed. Philadelphia: WB Saunders, 1993:514–95.
42 Dyck PJ, Lais AC, Ohta M, Bastron JA, Okazaki H, Groover RV. Chronic inflammatory polyradiculoneuropathy. *Mayo Clin Proc* 1975;50:621–37.
43 Prineas JW, McLeod JG. Chronic relapsing polyneuritis. *J Neurol Sci* 1976;27:427–58.
44 Buchthal F, Behse F. Peroneal muscular atrophy and related disorders I. Clinical manifestations as related to nerve biopsy findings, nerve conduction and electromyography. *Brain* 1977;100:41–66.
45 Bradley WG, Madrid R, Davis CJF. The peroneal muscular atrophy syndrome—clinical, genetic, electrophysiological and nerve biopsy findings part 3. Clinical, electrophysiological and pathological correlations. *J Neurol Sci* 1977;32:123–36.
46 Low PA, McLeod JG, Prineas JW. Hypertrophic Charcot-Marie-Tooth disease. Light and electron microscope studies of the sural nerve. *J Neurol Sci* 1978;35:93–115.
47 Dyck PJ, Lambert EH, Sanders K, O'Brien PC. Severe hypomyelination and marked abnormality of conduction in Déjèrine Sottas hypertrophic neuropathy: myelin thickness and compound action potential of sural nerve *in vitro*. *Mayo Clin Proc* 1971;46:432–43.
48 Ouvrier RA, McLeod JG, Conchin TE. The hypertrophic forms of hereditary motor and sensory neuropathy. A study of hypertrophic Charcot-Marie-Tooth disease (HMSN type I) and Déjèrine Sottas disease (HMSN type III) in childhood. *Brain* 1987;110:121–48.
49 Dyck PJ. Neuronal atrophy and degeneration predominantly affecting peripheral sensory and autonomic neurons. In: Dyck PJ, Thomas PK, Griffin JW, Low PA, Poduslo JF, eds. *Peripheral neuropathy*. 3rd ed. Philadelphia: WB Saunders, 1993:1065–93.
50 Dyck PJ, Lambert EH. Dissociated sensation in amyloidosis: compound action potential, quantitative histologic and teased-fiber and electron microscopic studies of sural nerve biopsies. *Arch Neurol* 1969;20:490–507.
51 Thomas PK, King RHM. Peripheral nerve changes in amyloid neuropathy. *Brain* 1974;97:395–406.
52 Hersch MI, McLeod JG. Peripheral neuropathy associated with amyloidosis. In: Vinken PJ, Bruyn GW, Klavans HL, eds. *Handbook of clinical neurology*. Amsterdam: Elsevier, 1987;57:429–44.
53 Kyle RA, Dyck PJ. Amyloidosis and neuropathy. In: Dyck PJ, Thomas PK, Griffin JW,

Low PA, Poduslo JF, eds. *Peripheral neuropathy.* 3rd ed. Philadelphia: WB Saunders, 1993:1294–309.

54 Hawke SHB, Davies L, Pamphlett R, Guo Y-P, Pollard JD, McLeod JG. Vasculitic neuropathy: a clinical and pathological study. *Brain* 1991;114:2175–90.

55 Dyck PJ, Benstead TJ, Conn DL, Stevens JC, Windebank AJ, Low PA. Non-systemic vasculitic neuropathy. *Brain* 1987;110:843–53.

56 Said G, Lacroix-Ciaudo C, Fujimura H, Blas C, Faux N. The peripheral neuropathy of necrotizing arteritis: a clinicopathological study. *Ann Neurol* 1988;23:461–5.

57 Davies L. Vasculitic neuropathy. In: McLeod JG, ed. *Inflammatory neuropathies. Baillière's clinical neurology 3:1.* London: Baillière Tindall, 1994:193–210.

58 Gainsborough N, Hall SM, Hughes RAC, Leibowitz S. Sarcoid neuropathy. *J Neurol* 1991;238:177–80.

59 Asbury AK, Gale MK, Cox SC, Baringer JR, Berg BO. Giant axonal neuropathy: a unique case with segmental neurofilamentous masses. *Acta Neuropathol (Berl)* 1972;20:237–47.

60 Prineas JW, Ouvrier RA, Wright RG, Walsh JC, McLeod JG. Giant axonal neuropathy—generalised disorder of cytoplasmic microfilament formation. *J Neuropathol Exp Neurol* 1976;35:458–70.

61 Meier C, Moll C. Hereditary neuropathy with liability to pressure palsies. Report of two families and review of the literature. *J Neurol* 1982;228:73–95.

62 Korobkin R, Asbury AK, Sumner AJ, Nielsen SL. Glue-sniffing neuropathy. *Arch Neurol* 1975;32:158–62.

63 Smith IS, Kahn SN, Lacey BW, *et al.* Chronic demyelinating neuropathy associated with benign IgM paraproteinaemia. *Brain* 1983;106:169–95.

64 Webster H de F. Schwann cell alterations in metachromatic leukodystrophy. Preliminary phase and electron microscopic observations. *J Neuropathol Exp Neurol* 1962;21:524–54.

65 Thomas PK, King RHM, Kocen RS, Brett EM. Comparative ultrastructural observations on peripheral nerve abnormalities in the late infantile, juvenile and late onset forms of metachromatic leukodystrophy. *Acta Neuropathol (Berl)* 1977;39:237–45.

66 Thomas PK. Other inherited neuropathies. In: Dyck PJ, Thomas PK, Griffin JW, Low PA, Poduslo JF. *Peripheral neuropathy.* 3rd ed. Philadelphia: WB Saunders, 1993:1194–218.

67 Dunn HG, Lake BD, Dolman CL, Wilson J. The neuropathy of Krabbe's infantile cerebral sclerosis. *Brain* 1969;92:329–44.

68 Kocen RS, Thomas PK. Peripheral nerve involvement in Fabry disease. *Arch Neurol* 1970;22:81–8.

69 Ohnishi A, Dyck PJ. Loss of small peripheral sensory neurons in Fabry disease. Histologic and morphometric evaluation of cutaneous nerves, spinal ganglia, and posterior columns. *Arch Neurol* 1974;31:120–7.

70 McLeod JG. An electrophysiological and pathological study of the peripheral nerves in Friedreich's ataxia. *J Neurol Sci* 1971;12:333–49.

71 Dyck PJ, Lambert EH. Lower motor and primary sensory neuron disease with peroneal muscular atrophy I. Neurologic, genetic and electrophysiological findings in hereditary polyneuropathies. *Arch Neurol* 1968;18:603–18.

72 Dyck PJ, Lambert EH. Lower motor and primary sensory neuron disease with peroneal muscular atrophy. II Neurologic, genetic and electrophysiologic findings in various neuronal degenerations. *Arch Neurol* 1968;18:619–25.

73 Thomas PK, Calne DB. Motor nerve conduction velocity in peroneal muscular atrophy: evidence for genetic heterogeneity. *J Neurol Neurosurg Psychiatry* 1974;37:68–75.

74 Brust JCM, Lovelace RE, Devi S. Clinical features of Charcot-Marie-Tooth syndrome. *Acta Neurol Scand* 1978;58(suppl 68):1–142.

75 Nicholson GA, Nash JA. Intermediate nerve conduction velocities define X-linked Charcot-Marie-Tooth neuropathies. *Neurology* 1993;43:2558–64.

76 Harding AE, Thomas PK. The clinical features of hereditary motor and sensory neuropathies type I and II. *Brain* 1980;103:259–80.

77 Vance J, Nicholson GA, Yamaoka L. Linkage of Charcot-Marie-Tooth disease Type Ia to chromosome 17. *Exp Neurol* 1989;104:186–9.

78 Chance PF, Lupski JR. Inherited neuropathies: Charcot-Marie-Tooth disease and related disorders. In: Harding AE, ed. *Genetics in neurology. Baillière's clinical neurology 3:2.* London: Baillière Tindall, 1994:373–85.

79 MacMillan JC, Upadyaya M, Harper PS. Charcot-Marie-Tooth disease type Ia (CMT

Ia). Evidence for trisomy of the region p11.2 of chromosome 17 in South Wales families. *J Med Genet* 1992;29:12–3.

80 Lupski JR, de Oca-Luna RM, Slaugenhaupt S, *et al.* DNA duplication associated with Charcot-Marie-Tooth disease type Ia. *Cell* 1991;66:219–32.

81 Matsunami N, Smith B, Ballard L, *et al.* Peripheral myelin protein -22 gene maps in the duplication in chromosome 17p11.22 associated with Charcot-Marie-Tooth IA. *Nature Genet* 1992;1:176–9.

82 Patel PI, Roa VB, Welcher AA, *et al.* The gene for the peripheral myelin protein PMP-22 is a candidate for Charcot-Marie-Tooth disease type Ia. *Nature Genet* 1992;1:157–65.

83 Roa BB, Garcia CA, Suter U, *et al.* Charcot-Marie-Tooth disease type Ia: association with a spontaneous point mutation in the PMP22 gene. *New Engl J Med* 1993;329:96–101.

84 Valentijn LJ, Baas F, Wolteman RA, *et al.* Identical point mutation of the peripheral myelin protein-22 in Trembler-J mouse and Charcot-Marie-Tooth disease type 1A. *Nature Genet* 1992;2:288–91.

85 Hoogendijk JE, Hensels GW, Gabreels-Festen AA. De novo mutation in hereditary sensory and motor neuropathy type I. *Lancet* 1992;339:1081–2.

86 Verhaale D, Lofgren A, Nelis E, Dehaene I, Theys P, Lammens N, *et al.* Deletion in the CMT Ia locus on chromosome 17p11.2 in hereditary neuropathy with liability to pressure palsies. *Ann Neurol* 1994;35:704–8.

87 Reisecker F, Lebelhuber F, Lexner R, Radner G, Rosenkranz W, Wagner K. A sporadic form of hereditary neuropathy with liability to pressure palsies: clinical electrodiagnostic and molecular genetic findings. *Neurology* 1994;44:753–6.

88 Nicholson GA, Valentijn LJ, Cheryson AK, *et al.* Frameshift mutation in the PMP22 gene in hereditary neuropathy with a liability to pressure palsies. *Nature Genet* 1994;6:263–6.

89 Bird TD, Ott J, Giblett ER. Evidence for linkage of Charcot-Marie-Tooth to the Duffy locus on chromosome 1. *Am J Hum Genet* 1982;34:388–94.

90 Stebbins NB, Conneally PM. Linkage of dominantly inherited Charcot-Marie-Tooth neuropathy to Duffy locus in an Indiana family. *Am J Hum Genet* 1982;34:195A.

91 Hayasaka K, Ohnishi A, Takoda G, Fukushima Y, Murai Y. Mutation of the myelin Po gene in Charcot-Marie-Tooth neuropathy type 1. *Biochem Biophys Res Commun* 1993;194:1317–22.

92 Denton PH, Ben Othmane K, Loeb D, *et al.* Genetic heterogeneity of Charcot-Marie-Tooth Type 2 disease and mapping of the Charcot-Marie-Tooth 2a locus on chromosome 1p36. *Muscle Nerve* 1994;1(suppl):S229.

93 Bergoffen J, Scherer SS, Wang S, *et al.* Connexin mutations in X-linked Charcot-Marie-Tooth. *Science* 1993;262:2039–42.

94 Roa BB, Dyck PJ, Marks HG, Chance PF, Lupski JR. Déjèrine-Sottas syndrome associated with point mutation in the peripheral nerve myelin protein 22 (PMP22) gene. *Nature Genet* 1993;5:269–73.

95 Hayasaka K, Himoro M, Sawaishi Y, *et al.* De novo mutation in the myelin Po gene in Déjèrine-Sottas disease (hereditary motor and sensory neuropathy type III). *Nature Genet* 1993;5:266–8.

96 Dyck PJ, Ellefson RD, Yao JK, Herbert PN. Adult-onset of Tangier disease 1. Morphometric and pathologic studies suggesting delayed degradation of neutral lipids after fiber degeneration. *J Neuropathol Exp Neurol* 1978;37:119–37.

97 Brady RO. Fabry disease. In: Dyck PJ, Thomas PK, Griffin JW, Low PA, Poduslo JF, eds. *Peripheral neuropathy.* 3rd ed. Philadelphia: WB Saunders, 1993;1169–78.

98 Skjeldal OH, Stokke O, Refsum S. Phytanic acid storage disease. Clinical, genetic and biochemical aspects. In: Dyck PJ, Thomas PK, Griffin JW, Low PA, Poduslo JN, eds. *Peripheral neuropathy.* 3rd ed. Philadelphia: WB Saunders, 1993:1149–60.

99 McLeod JG, Evans WA. Peripheral neuropathy in spinocerebellar degenerations. *Muscle Nerve* 1981;4:51–61.

100 Cornblath DR, McArthur JC, Parry GJG, Griffin JW. Peripheral neuropathies in human immunodeficiency virus infections. In: Dyck PJ, Thomas PK, Griffin JW, Low PA, Poduslo AN, eds. *Peripheral neuropathy.* 3rd ed. Philadelphia: WB Saunders, 1993:1343–53.

101 McCombe PA, Pollard JD, McLeod JG. Chronic inflammatory demyelinating polyradiculoneuropathy. *Brain* 1987;110:1617–30.

102 Lewis RA, Sumner AJ. The electrodiagnostic distinctions between chronic familial and acquired demyelinative neuropathies. *Neurology* 1982;32:592–6.

103 Pollard JD. Chronic inflammatory demyelinating polyradiculoneuropathy. In: McLeod JG, ed. *Inflammatory neuropathies. Baillière's clinical neurology 1:1.* London: Baillière Tindall, 1994:107–27.

104 Kyle 1978. Monoclonal gammopathy of undetermined significance—natural history of 241 cases. *Am J Med* 1978;**64**:814–26.

105 Kahn SN, Riches PG, Kohn J. Paraproteinaemia in neurological disease: incidence, association, and classification of monoclonal immunoglobulins. *J Clin Pathol* 1980;**33**:617–21.

106 Bleasel AF, Hawke SHB, Pollard JD, McLeod JG. IgM monoclonal paraproteinaemia and peripheral neuropathy. *J Neurol Neurosurg Psychiatry* 1993;**56**:52–7.

107 Thomas PK, Willison HJ. Paraproteinaemic neuropathy. In: McLeod JG, ed. *Inflammatory neuropathies. Baillière's clinical neurology 3:1.* London: Baillière Tindall, 1994:129–47.

108 Pestronk A, Cornblath DR, Ilyas AA, *et al*. A treatable multifocal motor neuropathy with antibodies to GM1 ganglioside. *Ann Neurol* 1988;**24**:73–8.

109 Pestronk A, Chaudhry V, Feldman EL, *et al*. Lower motor neuron syndromes defined by patterns of weakness, nerve conduction abnormalities and high titres of antiglycolipid antibodies. *Ann Neurol* 1990;**27**:315–26.

110 Krarup C, Stewart MB, Sumner AJ, Pestronk A, Lipton SA. A syndrome of asymmetric limb weakness with motor conduction block. *Neurology* 1990;**40**:118–27.

111 Lange DJ, Trojaborg W, Latov N, *et al*. Multifocal motor neuropathy with conduction block: Is it a distinct clinical entity? *Neurology* 1992;**42**:497–505.

112 Prineas JW. Pathology of inflammatory demyelinating neuropathies. In: McLeod JG, ed. *Inflammatory neuropathies. Baillière's clinical neurology 3:1.* London: Baillière Tindall, 1994:1–24.

113 Kaji R, Oka N, Tsuji T, Mezaki T, Nishio T, Akiguchi I, Kimura J. Pathological findings at the site of conduction block in multifocal motor neuropathy. *Ann Neurol* 1993;**33**:152–8.

114 Mellgren S, Conn DL, Stevens JC, Dyck PJ. Peripheral neuropathy in primary Sjögren's syndrome. *Neurology* 1989;**39**:390–4.

115 Gemignani F, Marbini A, Pavesi G, *et al*. Peripheral neuropathy associated with primary Sjögren's syndrome. *J Neurol Neurosurg Psychiatry* 1994;**57**:983–6.

116 Griffin JW, Cornblath DR, Alexander E. Ataxic sensory neuropathy and dorsal root ganglionitis associated with Sjögren's syndrome. *Ann Neurol* 1990;**27**:304–15.

117 Said G. Inflammatory neuropathies associated with known infections (HIV, leprosy, Chagas' disease, Lyme disease). In: McLeod JG, ed. *Inflammatory neuropathies. Baillière's clinical neurology 3:1.* London: Baillière Tindall, 1994:149–72.

118 So YT, Olney RK. Acute lumbosacral polyradiculopathy in acquired immunodeficiency syndrome: Experience in 23 patients. *Ann Neurol* 1994;**35**:53–8.

119 Sabin TD, Swift TR, Jacobson RR. Leprosy. In: Dyck PJ, Thomas PK, Griffin JW, Low PA, Poduslo AN, eds. *Peripheral neuropathy*. 3rd ed. Philadelphia: WB Saunders, 1993:1354–79.

12 Investigation of muscle disease

F L MASTAGLIA, N G LAING

Various pathological processes, some genetically determined and others acquired, may affect the function of the skeletal muscles and may manifest in different ways. Some, such as the congenital myopathies, produce weakness and hypotonia at birth whereas others do not cause functional abnormalities until childhood, adolescence, or adult life. With the application of modern molecular biological techniques major advances have taken place in the identification of the genetic mutations responsible for many of the hereditary muscle diseases and new mutations in nuclear or mitochondrial DNA are being reported on a regular basis.[1 2] These discoveries have had a major impact on the diagnostic approach to patients with these disorders and have led to the definition of new categories of myopathy such as the *dystrophinopathies*, encompassing the Duchenne and Becker forms of muscular dystrophy, the *sarcoglycanopathies*, which include many cases of limb-girdle muscular dystrophy, and the *channelopathies* comprising the periodic paralyses and myotonic syndromes.

This review focuses on the modern approach to the clinical and laboratory investigation of patients with muscle diseases with particular emphasis on the application of molecular techniques in diagnosis.

Clinical evaluation

The investigation of a patient with muscle disease should always commence with a detailed history which, in the case of known

342

hereditary disorders, may provide an immediate indication of the nature of the patient's condition. Moreover, a history of heavy alcohol consumption or administration of drugs with known myotoxic actions (box 12.1) may point to a toxic and therefore potentially reversible aetiology for the patient's symptoms.[3-5] A history of a thyroidectomy or parathyroidectomy, or symptoms of hypothyroidism or hyperthyroidism, should alert the physician to the possibility of an endocrine cause whereas a history of chronic diarrhoea, diuretic treatment, purgative misuse, or excessive consumption of liquorice or other preparations containing gly-

---

Box 12.1   Drug induced muscle disorders

Myalgia:
Suxamethonium, danazol, clofibrate, salbutamol, lithium, captopril, colchicine, procainamide, metolazone, cytotoxics, zidovudine, isoetherine, zimeldine, labetalol, pindolol, cimetidine, penicillamine, gold, enalapril, rifampicin, L-tryptophan, nifedipine

Myotonia:
Diazacholesterol, β blockers*, β agonists* (fenoterol, ritodrine), clofibrate†, diuretics† (frusemide, ethacrynic acid, mersalyl, acetazolamide)

Necrotising myopathy:
Alcohol, gemfibrozil, lovastatin, simvastatin, clofibrate, ε-aminocaproic acid, cyclosporin, zidovudine, cocaine, emetine

Mitochondrial myopathy:
Zidovudine

Inflammatory myopathy:
D-penicillamine, L-tryptophan, others rarely

Autophagic myopathy:
Chloroquine, vincristine, colchicine, amiodarone, perhexiline

Type 2 atrophy:
Corticosteroids

Localised myopathy:
Intramuscular antibiotics, narcotics

*May exacerbate myotonia. †May cause myotonia in animals.

343

cyrrhizinic acid such as snuff, chewing tobacco, and certain traditional Chinese medicines, should suggest the possibility of hypokalaemic myopathy. A history of malignancy, of a systemic connective tissue disease, other autoimmune disease, or immunodeficiency state may indicate a predisposition to an inflammatory myopathy.

When muscle pain is a feature, hypothyroid, osteomalacic, or other metabolic myopathy, parasitic infestation (for example, trichinosis), or a toxic myopathy or neuromyopathy should be considered, (box 12.2), although in many patients no specific aetiology will be found even with complete investigation. Myalgia, muscle weakness, or fatigue developing after an acute viral infec-

---

Box 12.2 Disorders in which muscle pain may be a prominent feature

Inflammatory
Viral myositis
Pyomyositis

Parasitic myositis

Polymyositis/dermatomyositis
Granulomatous myositis
Interstitial myositis
Localised nodular myositis
Vasculitis
Eosinophilic fasciitis

Toxic
Acute alcoholic myopathy
Acute/subacute drug induced
 myopathies
Myopathies due to
 envenomation

Endocrine
Hypothyroidism
Osteomalacia
Hyperparathyroidism

Hereditary
Disorders of glycogen metabolism
Carnitine palmityl transferase
 deficiency
Myoadenylate deaminase
 deficiency
Mitochondrial myopathy
Dystrophinopathy
Sodium channel myotonia
Malignant hyperthermia

Others
Fibromyalgia
Polymyalgia rheumatica
Postviral myalgia/fatigue

Muscle overuse syndromes
Myopathy with tubular
 aggregates

tion also raises the possibility of an inflammatory myopathy but in many such patients when fatigue and reduced exercise tolerance are the major symptoms, a diagnosis of postviral chronic fatigue syndrome will usually be reached.

In certain instances it may be possible to reach a definitive diagnosis on the basis of the pattern of muscle involvement found on clinical examination or the finding of other distinctive features such as myotonia, fatiguability, muscle contractures, or other systemic features. Although the distribution of muscle involvement in most of the acquired myopathies is relatively non-selective, in the genetic myopathies certain patterns of muscle weakness are distinctive and may be diagnostically helpful although it is being increasingly recognised that the phenotypic manifestations of specific genetic defects may be very variable (for example, the dystrophinopathies). Involvement of the extraocular and eyelid muscles is seen characteristically in oculopharyngeal muscular dystrophy, usually associated with dysphagia and often with limb muscle involvement. They are also involved in the syndrome of chronic progressive external ophthalmoplegia, which is usually due to a mitochondrial myopathy and may occur in isolation, or with a limb myopathy, or other systemic features such as pigmentary retinopathy, heart block, cerebellar ataxia, and sensorineural hearing loss as in the *Kearns-Sayre syndrome*. Involvement of the facial muscles is usually a prominent feature in facioscapulohumeral muscular dystrophy but may also occur in myasthenia gravis, when it is usually associated with involvement of the extraocular muscles, and often of the bulbar and limb muscles; fatiguability is a prominent feature. In myotonic dystrophy there is often also involvement of the facial muscles and, characteristically, there is atrophy and weakness of the sternomastoids and of the distal limb muscles in the later stages of the disease. Other systemic features which point to the diagnosis include cataracts and, in men, frontal baldness and testicular atrophy. Severe weakness of the neck extensor muscles leading to the "dropped head syndrome"[6] may occasionally be the presenting feature in patients with inflammatory myopathy and may also occur in motor neuron disease and longstanding myasthenia gravis. Weakness confined to or most severe in the distal limb muscles also occurs in the distal myopathies and scapuloperoneal syndrome.

The limb-girdle syndrome, in which there is involvement of the girdle and proximal limb muscles, is relatively non-specific and may be seen in several genetic and acquired myopathies. Although in

345

most cases of polymyositis and dermatomyositis there is a predominantly proximal pattern of muscle involvement, in inclusion body myositis the distribution of muscle weakness is characteristically selective, at least in the earlier stages of the condition, with involvement especially of the quadriceps femoris muscles in the lower limbs and the forearm flexors, particularly the flexor digitorum profundus, in the upper limbs.[7] When present, the characteristic skin rash of dermatomyositis over the face and the extensor aspects of the metacarpophalangeal and interphalangeal joints is diagnostic of that condition.

Muscle hypertrophy, when confined to the calves, is seen most typically in Duchenne and Becker dystrophy, but occasionally also in other types of muscular dystrophy, whereas more generalised hypertrophy is common in myotonia congenita. A hypertrophic myopathy may occasionally occur in patients with amyloidosis, sarcoidosis, or cysticercosis. Muscle contractures occur, especially in Emery-Dreifuss muscular dystrophy, and are also a feature of the fibrosing myositis associated with scleromyxoedema.[8] It is always worth looking for muscle tenderness, which, when confined to certain muscles such as those of the calves, may indicate a focal inflammatory or vasculitic process, whereas the characteristic pattern of myofascial tenderness in patients with fibromyalgia is virtually diagnostic of that condition.

Depressed deep tendon reflexes or sensory abnormalities in a patient with a myopathy suggest the presence of an associated peripheral neuropathy. This combination can occur in patients with drug induced neuromyopathy, connective tissue disease, inclusion body myositis, a paraneoplastic syndrome, or mitochondrial myopathy.

Biochemical studies

Creatine kinase

The serum concentration of creatine kinase is the most reliable biochemical indicator of muscle disease. The highest concentrations occur in patients with acute rhabdomyolysis, inflammatory or drug induced myopathies, and Duchenne muscular dystrophy in the early stages when the patient is still ambulant. High concentrations may also occur in some metabolic myopathies such as hypokalaemic or hypothyroid myopathy.[9] Moderately raised concentrations may also be found in patients with chronic neuropathic conditions such as spinal muscular atrophy or motor neuron disease, although it is rare for the creatine kinase concentration to exceed 10 times the normal maximum concentration in these conditions.[10] Raised creatine kinase concentrations may also be found in some people, without clinical evidence of neuromuscular disease[11] and may be useful in detecting those with a genetic risk of malignant hyperthermia, presymptomatic muscular dystrophy, carriers of Duchenne and Becker muscular dystrophy, and early inflammatory myopathy (box 12.3). Serum creatine kinase concentrations are normal in most congenital myopathies, myotonic syndromes, and corticosteroid and thyrotoxic myopathy.

Slight increases in serum creatine kinase (up to about three times the normal maximum level) are not necessarily due to muscle disease and may occur transiently as a result of strenuous exercise, minor muscle trauma including intramuscular injections, and insertion of EMG needle electrodes or viral illnesses.[10] In a situation in which the creatine kinase concentration is unexpectedly raised it is usual to repeat the test after an interval of a week during which the patient is advised not to engage in strenuous physical exercise, and to consider embarking on further investigations only if the concentration remains high or is rising.

Box 12.3   Causes of sustained increased serum creatine kinase concentrations in subjects without clinical signs of muscle disease

- Physical exercise
- Muscle trauma—pressure, falls, injections
- Acute psychosis/delirium
- Dyskinesiae
- Drugs: alcohol, others*
- Hypothyroidism
- Hypokalaemia
- Presymptomatic: malignant hyperthermia, muscular dystrophies, inflammatory myopathies, McArdle's disease
- Carrier state: Duchenne, Becker dystrophy
- Herditary hyperCKaemia

*See box 12.1.

Serum concentrations of other enzymes such as aspartate and alanine aminotransferase, aldolase, and lactate dehydrogenase are of less value than the creatine kinase concentration but may provide a clue to the presence of muscle disease if they are found to be raised as part of an initial biochemical screen in a patient with no other indication of liver disease.

Myoglobin

Myoglobinaemia and myoglobinuria may be due to various causes[12] and result in urinary pigmentation and a positive benzidine dip stick test on the urine as does haemoglobinuria and haematuria. Confirmation of myoglobinuria requires a specific myoglobin radioimmunoassay. Serum myoglobin concentrations are raised in patients with inflammatory[13] and other necrotising myopathies but are not of any additional value to the creatine kinase concentration in diagnosis or in monitoring the response to treatment.

Lactate concentrations

Venous lactate concentrations may be raised at rest and after low levels of exercise in patients with mitochondrial myopathy and defects of the respiratory enzyme chain. Conversely, lactate production is absent or diminished in metabolic myopathies due to defects in glycogenolysis (for example, myophosphorylase or phosphorylase b kinase deficiency) or of the glycolytic pathway (for example, phosphofructokinase, phosphoglycerate mutase, phosphoglycerate kinase, or lactate dehydrogenase deficiency) and is the basis for the forearm exercise test. This was previously performed under ischaemic conditions but, because of the occurrence of severe rhabdomyolysis in some patients with glycogen metabolic defects, this is no longer recommended.[10] Venous blood samples for estimation of lactate and ammonia concentrations are taken at rest and at 1, 2, 4, 6, and 10 minute intervals after a one minute period of repetitive maximum isometric contractions of the forearm flexor muscles. Whereas there is normally a twofold to threefold rise in the lactate concentration within the first two minutes after exercise, this response is absent or diminished in patients with myophosphorylase deficiency or a glycolytic defect. The rise in venous ammonia concentrations that normally occurs after exercise is absent or reduced in patients with myoadenylate deaminase deficiency in which ammonia production during exercise is impaired.[14]

Nuclear magnetic resonance spectroscopy

With nuclear magnetic resonance (NMR) spectroscopy it is possible to monitor changes in muscle metabolite concentrations during exercise non-invasively (for example, inorganic phosphate, phosphocreatine, ATP, lactate concentrations, and intracellular pH). This may be useful in the evaluation of patients with disorders of glycolytic or mitochondrial metabolism.[15] The technique is also useful in the evaluation of patients with fatigue and reduced exercise tolerance to determine whether there is evidence of an underlying defect of muscle energy metabolism.[16]

Other studies

Other biochemical studies which may be relevant in the investigation of some patients with muscle symptoms include serum potassium, calcium, phosphate, thyroxine, and cortisol concentrations, as well as urea and creatinine concentrations and urinary creatine and 3-methyl histidine excretion as indices of skeletal muscle mass and breakdown.[17]

Pharmacological testing

Although in some families with malignant hyperthermia mutations have been found in the ryanodine receptor gene and at risk subjects can therefore be detected using molecular genetic techniques, in many other families as well as in those without a known family history who are suspected of being at risk, it is still necessary to perform in vitro muscle contracture testing. This involves the exposure of muscle tissue obtained at biopsy to caffeine and halothane which, in at risk subjects, induce an exaggerated contractile response.[18] Abnormal responses to caffeine and calcium ions have also been described using the skinned muscle fibre technique.[19] Contracture testing should also be performed in those with unexplained episodes of muscle stiffness or rhabdomyolysis during or after anaesthesia, with infections, or after exercise or heat exposure, and in patients with central core or multicore disease who are also at risk.

349

Electrodiagnostic studies

Electromyography

Conventional EMG is an important investigative procedure in patients with suspected muscle disease.[20] Firstly, it will often provide confirmation of a primary myopathic basis for the patient's condition and allow differentiation from a neurogenic disorder. Characteristically, the duration of motor unit action potentials (MUAPs) is diminished as is MUAP amplitude although this is often less pronounced and more variable, and there is an increased number of polyphasic motor unit potentials. With voluntary contraction there is early recruitment of increased numbers of short duration MUAPs and an unduly full interference pattern which is often reduced in amplitude. Reduced motor unit recruitment and electrical excitability of the muscle are found during attacks of weakness in patients with periodic paralysis. Spontaneous fibrillation potentials, positive sharp waves, and complex repetitive discharges may be found in some myopathic disorders and are particularly prominent in active inflammatory myopathies and certain metabolic and toxic myopathies (for example, hypothyroid and chloroquine myopathy),[21] in some cases of Duchenne muscular dystrophy and distal myopathy, and in myotonic disorders in which they are associated with a pronounced increase in insertional activity and the diagnostic waxing and waning ("dive bomber") myotonic discharges resulting from electrical instability of the muscle cell membrane.[20] The occurrence of spontaneous potentials in the non-myotonic myopathies has been attributed to functional denervation of muscle fibres which have been disconnected from their motor innervation as a result of segmental necrosis. Regenerating muscle fibres which have yet to be innervated may also be a source of spontaneous potentials.

The distribution of EMG changes within individual muscles and in representative proximal and distal limb and axial muscles provides an indication of the extent of the myopathic process and pattern of muscle involvement. This may be useful in selecting a muscle for biopsy, and may also indicate whether the disease process is one which is affecting the muscles in a patchy manner (often the case in the inflammatory myopathies) or more diffusely (as in the muscular dystrophies or metabolic myopathies). The coexistence in the same muscle of typical myopathic MUAPs and longer duration polyphasic potentials is a potentially confusing combination sometimes encountered in patients with very long-standing denervating conditions such as spinal muscular atrophy,[18] and in inclusion body myositis in which there may also be prominent fibrillation potentials as well as increased fibre density and jitter.[20]

Although in many patients with well established myopathies the EMG changes are florid and unmistakable, in some patients with milder forms of myopathy the motor unit changes are less conspicuous. It is in the evaluation of such patients that quantitative techniques employing automated measurement of MUAP variables and motor unit recruitment for given levels of effort are useful.[20]

Neuromuscular transmission studies

Repetitive nerve stimulation studies should be performed if muscle fatigue is prominent or if there are other features suggestive of myasthenia gravis or of the Lambert-Eaton myasthenic syndrome or other neuromuscular junction disorder (box 12.4). In myasthenia gravis the characteristic decrement in the compound muscle action potential (CMAP) occurs with low frequency (2–3 Hz) stimulation and may be associated with postcontraction facilitation and subsequent postactivation exhaustion. The yield with repetitive nerve stimulation studies increases if several muscles

---

Box 12.4   Conditions associated with prominent muscle fatigue

Neuromuscular junction disorders:
- Myasthenia gravis
- Lambert-Eaton syndrome
- Congenital myasthenic syndromes
- Drug induced

Myopathies:
- Mitochondrial myopathies
- Glycolytic disorders

CNS disorders:
- Multiple sclerosis

Chronic fatigue syndrome

---

are studied (for instance, abductor digiti minimi, biceps, deltoid, trapezius, and orbicularis oculi) and the detection rate increases even futher if low frequency stimulation is repeated after a brief period of limb ischaemia as in the double step ischaemic test described by Desmedt and Borenstein.[22] However, these studies are negative in 20% to 30% of patients, particularly those with purely ocular muscle involvement. Decremental responses may also occur in the congenital myasthenic syndromes. In the syndrome associated with motor end plate ACh-esterase deficiency there is characteristically a double or repetitive CMAP after the application of single nerve stimuli.[23]

In the Lambert-Eaton myasthenic syndrome the amplitude of the CMAP is reduced at rest and with low frequency stimulation, which may lead to a further fall in amplitude, whereas stimulation at higher frequencies (for example, 20 and 50 Hz) results in a rapid increase in the amplitude of the CMAP to normal or near normal levels.[20] In many patients a comparable or greater potentiation of the CMAP amplitude occurs after a brief voluntary contraction.[24]

Single fibre electromyography (SFEMG), which can be performed either with voluntary muscle activation or with nerve stimulation, characteristically shows increased jitter (variability in the interval between consecutive firings of muscle fibre pairs belonging to the same motor unit) and intermittent blocking indicating failure of transmission at single motor end plates, and is more sensitive than repetitive nerve stimulation studies in the diagnosis of neuromuscular transmission disorders. In myasthenia gravis SFEMG shows an abnormality in up to 95% of patients with limb muscle involvement and a normal SFEMG study in a patient with clearcut limb weakness and fatigue is strongly against the diagnosis of myasthenia.[20] However, similar abnormalities may be found in several myopathies and other neuromuscular disorders and it is therefore essential that the findings are interpreted in the context of the particular clinical situation.

In vitro microelectrode studies of miniature end plate potentials, quantal content of ACh, and neurally induced end plate potentials and currents may be performed on nerve-muscle preparations obtained from an intercostal muscle biopsy. Such studies, in combination with quantitative studies of motor end plate morphology, ACh receptor numbers, and ACh-esterase content are necessary to define precisely the presynaptic or postsynaptic nature of the transmission defect in patients with unusual myasthenic syndromes.[23]

352

Nerve conduction studies

Motor and sensory nerve conduction studies as well as F wave and H reflex studies may be appropriate to exclude the possibility that the patient's symptoms are due to a peripheral neuropathy. Moreover, a peripheral neuropathy may coexist in some patients with myotonic dystrophy, mitochondrial myopathy, drug induced myopathy, inclusion body myositis, or inflammatory myopathy associated with connective tissue diseases or malignancy.

Muscle imaging

The techniques of computed tomography (CT) or magnetic resonance imaging (MRI) can provide information on the cross sectional area of limb or axial muscles and may therefore be useful in detecting muscle atrophy or hypertrophy and defining selective patterns of muscle involvement in certain conditions such as the muscular dystrophies and inclusion body myositis.[25 26] These techniques may also show differences in muscle properties between conditions such as the muscular dystrophies in which there is extensive fatty infiltration of muscle, and the inflammatory myopathies, but the changes are not sufficiently specific to be of diagnostic value.[27] The techniques are, however, of use in detecting and defining the extent of suppurative lesions of muscle (pyomyositis). Radioisotopic techniques with muscle scanning after administration of technietium pyrophosphate can also be used to detect such lesions as well as areas of active inflammatory myopathy in patients with polymyositis or dermatomyositis, and areas of muscle infarction or pressure necrosis (crush syndrome). Isotopic scanning may also be used to show the extent of subcutaneous calcinosis in patients with dermatomyositis and to monitor changes with treatment.

Muscle biopsy

A biopsy is still required to provide a definitive diagnosis in the case of many muscle diseases. This is especially so in the case of the inflammatory myopathies, in sporadic cases of muscular dystrophy, suspected metabolic myopathies, and in patients in whom there is still uncertainty as to whether the condition is primarily neuropathic or myopathic after clinical and EMG evaluation. In neuropathic disorders a biopsy from an affected muscle will show the characteristic changes of denervation including angulated fibres, grouped fibre atrophy, and, if the condition is protracted, fibre type grouping, but will not necessarily differentiate between anterior horn cell and peripheral nerve disorders. In the more chronic neurogenic disorders—such as the spinal muscular atrophies—histological changes resembling those found in chronic myopathic disorders may also be present (secondary myopathic change).

The effectiveness of muscle biopsy in establishing the diagnosis of myopathy is determined by the correct choice of muscle, the correct biopsy technique, and the application of the appropriate staining and other procedures to the biopsy.[28] In selecting a suitable biopsy site the ideal muscle is one which is only moderately affected (for example, MRC grade 4 muscle power), and which has not been the site of previous intramuscular injections or needle EMG studies. Muscles which are too severely weakened or atrophic should be avoided as the histological changes in such muscles are often non-specific and difficult to interpret. Selection of a needle or open biopsy is determined by personal choice, experience, and availability. Whereas needle biopsy requires only a minor incision and the procedure can be repeated at multiple sites and on more than one occasion, the size of the tissue sample obtained is limited and histological interpretation may be difficult, particularly in diseases in which the muscle involvement is patchy. In many instances, therefore, and especially in the case of suspected inflammatory myopathy or vasculitis, an open biopsy is preferable, having the advantage of providing a larger tissue sample and thereby reducing sampling error.

To maximise the information derived from the muscle biopsy a battery of histological and histochemical stains should be applied routinely to cryostat sections of frozen tissue (box 12.5). In addition, in some cases it will be necessary to apply other selected histochemical or immunohistochemical techniques using monoclonal antibodies for the diagnosis of specific enzyme deficiencies, storage disorders, or other hereditary defects such as the dystrophinopathies and sarcoglycanopathies (figure 12.1). Electron microscopic examination of muscle tissue is also necessary especially in cases of suspected mitochondrial myopathy, inclusion body myositis, and in some congenital myopathies. Tissue should therefore be taken routinely for this purpose at the time of the biopsy and fixed in glutaraldehyde.[28] In metabolic and other inherited myopathies it is also prudent to obtain an additional tissue sample for quantitative biochemical analyses or molecular studies should these be required.

In the hereditary myopathies, immunohistochemistry of muscle biopsies should be used whenever possible to identify the patient or family muscle disease. For example, the autosomal recessive Duchenne-like muscular dystrophies and the limb-girdle dystro-

---

Box 12.5 Staining and labelling procedures applicable to muscle biopsies

Routine histology
- Haematoxylin and eosin (general histology)
- Modified Gomori trichrome (ragged red fibres, nemaline rods)

Routine histochemistry
- Myofibrillar ATPase (fibre types) (pH 9.4, 4.6, 4.3)
- NADH-tetrazolium reductase (mitochondrial myopathy, tubular aggregates)
- Succinic dehydrogenase (mitochondrial myopathy)
- Phosphorylase (McArdle's disease)
- Acid phosphatase (autophagic vacuoles, macrophages)
- Periodic acid-Schiff (PAS) (glycogen storage)
- Oil red O (neutral lipid storage)

Other special stains
- Cytochrome oxidase (COX) (mitochondrial myopathy)
- Phosphofructokinase (PFK deficiency)
- Congo red (amyloid, IBM)
- Microbial stains (bacteria, fungi)

Immunohistochemistry
- Extracellular matrix (collagen, laminin)
- Cytoskeletal proteins (dystrophin, spectrin, desmin, adhalin, vimentin, merosin)
- Myofibrillar proteins (fibre typing)
- Mononuclear cells (T and B cells, macrophages)
- Immune complexes
- Complement (MAC)
- MHC class I and II antigens (inflammatory myopathies)
- Intercellular adhesion molecules (I-CAM)
- Ubiquitin (IBM)

In situ hybridisation
- DNA probes (viruses, mtDNA deletions)

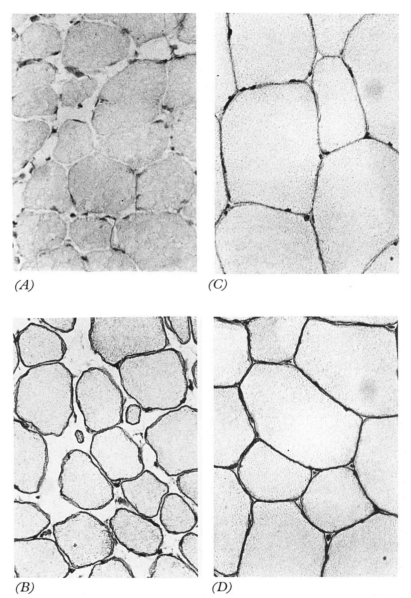

(A) *(C)*

(B) *(D)*

Figure 12.1   *Adhalin deficiency in an eight year old girl with an unclassified muscular dystrophy: (A) antiadhalin; (B) antispectrin; (C) normal muscle antiadhalin; (D) normal muscle antispectrin. Immunoperoxidase*

356

phies can be very difficult to distinguish from Duchenne and Becker dystrophy clinically, whereas antibodies can make the distinction very easily. Up until recently these cases were among the residual of patients all muscle clinics have who are difficult to categorise. For example, Bonnemann et al[29] in their recent characterisation of mutations in β-sarcoglycan screened 62 patients with possible β-sarcoglycan involvement out of a bank of 2500 muscle biopsies to identify their one β-sarcoglycan patient. In our own clinic, screening of nine families which had been undiagnosed for years, with antibodies to α-sarcoglycan (adhalin), showed that three of the families were adhalin negative (RD Johnson and BA Kakulas, unpublished observations) and thus are at risk from a sarcoglycanopathy. Immunohistochemistry or immunoblotting can also predict the severity of disease—for example, in both the dystrophinopathies[30-32] and the sarcoglycanopathies.[29 33] On the other hand, molecular analysis cannot always predict severity of disease, as people with apparently the same mutation can have different severities of disease[34] perhaps due to alternate splicing around the mutation.[35 36]

Molecular diagnosis

Molecular biology, particularly positional cloning, has led to the recent major increase in understanding of the causes of inherited diseases, through identifying the genes mutated in these diseases and thus the faulty proteins.[37] In the clinic, similar molecular techniques can be used for four major purposes:
● Identifying the precise disease affecting an individual patient and family.
● Accurate, simple prenatal diagnosis
● Identifying asymptomatic members of families who are at risk from having more severely affected offspring
● Presymptomatic diagnosis.
All of these lead to more accurate and appropriate genetic counselling.

Identifying the precise disease affecting an individual patient and family

Molecular diagnosis is especially useful for conditions which are difficult to distinguish clinically or by other laboratory techniques. The sarcoglycanopathies,[38] in which mutations in adhalin, β-

357

sarcoglycan, and γ-sarcoglycan all look similar by immunohisto-chemistry, are a good example of diseases only distinguishable by molecular analysis.[39]

Accurate, simple prenatal diagnosis

Identifying the precise mutation or mutations causing the disease in a family also provides the only really practical route to prenatal diagnosis where that is appropriate. The only current alternative for inherited muscle diseases would be fetal muscle biopsy.[40]

Identifying asymptomatic members of families who are at risk from having more severely affected offspring

Molecular diagnosis allows the identification of minimally affected or asymptomatic persons. This is important for identifying carriers of X linked diseases such as Duchenne and Becker muscular dystrophy, Emery-Dreifuss dystrophy, and X linked centronuclear myopathy who are at risk of having affected male offspring. It is also important for tracing at risk subjects—for example, in myotonic dystrophy pedigrees—through cascade screening.

Presymptomatic diagnosis

Presymptomatic diagnosis using molecular techniques has been applied, for example to diagnose the cause of the raised creatine kinase and screen other family members after neonatal or infant screening for Duchenne muscular dystrophy.[41 42] Presymptomatic diagnosis is also possible by molecular techniques in any of the disease with later onset, such as hypokalaemic periodic paralysis.[43]

The polymerase chain reaction (PCR),[44] which amplifies specific regions of DNA, has played a major part in the molecular revolution and is being manipulated for ever more purposes—such as reverse transcriptase PCR (RT-PCR) which allows the PCR to amplify specific cDNA messages[45] or the creation of restriction enzyme sites to discriminate between normal and mutant alleles.[46]

Degrees of ease of molecular diagnosis

There are perhaps three degrees of difficulty for molecular diagnosis: easy, difficult, and average. Easy diseases to diagnose are those in which most cases are caused by a single mutation, or a few mutations, or mutations which are simple to detect. Difficult diseases to diagnose are: (*a*) those in which most cases are caused by many different missense mutations which alter only a single amino acid and thus do not truncate the protein; (*b*) diseases in which linkage to a particular locus has been identified but the disease gene has not been identified; or (*c*) diseases with significant genetic heterogeneity—that is, where the same clinical phenotype may be caused by mutations in a number of different genes. Average diseases to diagnose are those caused in most cases by nonsense mutations which produce a premature stop codon and therefore truncated proteins.

Easy diseases to diagnose by molecular analysis

Diseases which currently fall into this category are:

(1) Myotonic dystrophy, in which the triplet repeat expansion can be detected and sized by a PCR reaction, and/or Southern blotting using EcoRI, BglI, or BamHI digestion.[47]

(2) Duchenne and Becker muscular dystrophy (for most patients) as most disease causing mutations are large deletions of the dystrophin gene. These deletions can be detected by multiplex PCR analysis of DNA from affected boys to identify the deleted exons.[30 48-50]

(3) Spinal muscular atrophy (autosomal recessive), in which the common deletion can be detected by two single strand conformation polymorphism (SSCP) analyses, one for exon 7 of the survival motor neuron gene and one for exon 8.[51 52]

(4) Hypokalaemic periodic paralysis, in which mutations to two residues in the dihydropyridine receptor calcium channel (CACNL1A3) account for all cases so far described.[53]

(5) Mitochondrial myopathies, in which the common point mutations can be tested for using PCR followed by enzyme digestion[46 54] or SSCP analysis.[55]

Difficult diseases to diagnose by molecular analysis

Diseases in which most cases are caused by many different missense mutations—Finding the mutations causing disease in such conditions is the most difficult task for molecular analysis. This is because the entire gene sequence has to be screened, and the difficulty is therefore increased if the gene message is large, which is the case for many of the structural proteins of muscle. The difficulty of identifying missense mutations was reinforced again in a recent summary of current methods of screening genes for unknown mutations,[56] which states that, "Detection of mutations, particularly at the 100% level is time consuming and expensive" and "The 'one best method' still remains elusive". Indeed, the plethora of techniques currently on the market for identifying unknown mutations in genes indicates that none is ideal. A previous review[57] summarised the techniques then current such as the simple single strand conformation analysis (SSCA), denaturing gradient gel electrophoresis (DGGE), heteroduplex analysis (HA), RNAase A cleavage, chemical mismatch cleavage (CMC), and direct sequencing. Techniques which should perhaps be added to the list include restriction endonuclease fingerprinting (REF),[58] dideoxyfingerprinting,[59] and enzymatic mismatch cleavage (EMC).[60 61]

The heroic way to look for mutations is to search genomic DNA. This will often involve synthesising PCR primers for regions flanking each of the exons of the gene followed by, for example, SSCP analysis of each exon. This would necessitate synthesising 80 primers for a gene such as the cardiac β-myosin heavy chain gene (MYH7) involved in familial hypertrophic cardiomyopathy—as MYH7 has 40 exons—and then performing 40 separate SSCPs. The short cut alternative is to examine the cDNA for mutations.[57] This reduces the number of base pairs that have to be screened compared with examining the genomic sequence of the gene. Analysis of cDNA will also instantly disclose any deletions or duplications of the message and splice site mutations which also significantly alter the size of the transcript, leading to rapid identification of one type of single base mutation.[62 63] To examine the cDNA however, a source of RNA is required from the patient in whom the candidate gene is expressed. This should be relatively simple, as nearly all patients with a muscle disease should have had a muscle biopsy, and RNA can easily be extracted from frozen muscle tissue and cDNA synthesised for examination. Analysis of cDNA made from illegitimate transcription messages[64] should always be considered as a possible means of obtaining cDNA for muscle disease genes. However, in some cases it may be more appropriate to analyse cDNA from muscle, as alternate splicing may mask the mutations and the mutations in skeletal muscle may be different and more relevant than those in circulating lymphocytes.[65]

Suggesting that a missense mutation in any message is responsible for disease—especially in a giant message such as the dystrophin message[66]—is fraught with difficulties.[67] The criteria normally used to decide that an identified alteration in a DNA sequence is a mutation that causes disease include a major change of an amino acid, change of an amino acid conserved in many species, the change not being seen in a large number of controls, and the change being in a candidate gene. However, even when all these criteria are fulfilled, the change may still not be disease causing.[67] A missense mutation found only in a single patient, or a small family, probably requires a functional assay (not necessarily a transgenic mouse) or at least characterisation in an expression system to be certain that the missense mutation causes the disease.[68] Unless there is this degree of certainty about the status of the identified alteration in DNA, it should not be used for prenatal diagnosis.

Diseases in which there is only linkage but the precise disease gene has not been identified—Distal myopathy,[69 70] dominant limb girdle muscular dystrophy,[71 72] X linked centronuclear (myotubular) myopathy,[73] oculopharyngeal muscular dystrophy,[74] and recessive nemaline myopathy[75] are all diseases in which there is at present linkage but no identified disease gene. When there is only linkage for a disease, the use of linkage for diagnosis should perhaps be restricted to individual families in which the significant LOD score of 3 has been obtained, especially if there is evidence of genetic heterogeneity for the disease.

Diseases with significant genetic heterogeneity—Perhaps the best example of this at present is malignant hyperthermia, in which although many families show linkage to the ryanodine receptor gene on chromosome 19[76] many others apparently do not[77 78] and virtually only single families have shown linkage to other regions of the genome.[79] The limb-girdle muscular dystrophies may also be included in this category. Some of the different types can now be identified as sarcoglycanopathies or dystrophinopathies by immunohistochemistry, but it is still a large task to precisely identify the gene involved by molecular diagnosis.

Average diseases to diagnose by molecular analysis

Average diseases are those in which most mutations causing disease are nonsense mutations, as these can be detected using the protein truncation test (PTT).[80 81] This test uses an in vitro translation system to synthesise protein from cDNA. If there is a mutation in the protein coding region leading to a premature stop codon, the

361

protein synthesised in vitro will be shorter than normal and can be identified by electrophoresis. The PTT was first applied widely to the identification of nonsense, premature stop codon producing mutations in familial adenomatous polyposis coli[80] and Duchenne muscular dystrophy,[81] (figure 12.2), but it has also been applied to neurofibromatosis.[82 83] The PTT should perhaps be used for all recessive disorders, especially severe ones, as these are often caused by nonsense mutations. For example, the PTT would have detected many of the mutations so far described in the sarcoglycanopathies, especially the severe cases,[24 32 38 84] in which prenatal diagnosis would be most appropriate and there would be most likelihood of pressure to find the family mutation rapidly.

Obviously some diseases fit into both the easy and difficult categories or both the easy and average categories. Duchenne muscular dystrophy is both easy for most mutations and average for the minority. Mitochondrial myopathies are easy for most cases and difficult for the others. The common mtDNA point mutations can be tested easily, but all the other possible mutations are difficult to screen for and to separate from polymorphisms not causing disease.[85] This is also true for other diseases. However, testing only for the common known mutations becomes a self fulfilling prophecy and unless the rest of the transcript is screened for mutations, many mutations causing disease may be missed.

As emphasised by Forrest et al[56] it is essential that comprehensive databases of gene mutations and perhaps, even more importantly, databases of normal polymorphisms should be created and widely disseminated, so that individual diagnostic laboratories can cross check whether a base change identified in a patient is a known mutation causing disease, a known polymorphism, or entirely new.

Muscular dystrophies

The classification of the muscular dystrophies has undergone considerable change with the recognition of the disease genes and molecular basis for some of these conditions, in particular, the X linked and the limb-girdle dystrophies (box 12.6). The availability of genetic or molecular markers for many of these conditions has meant that the diagnosis can now be established with greater precision and that diseases manifesting with similar phenotypes can be readily distinguished. For example, in some patients with

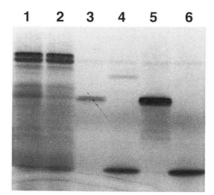

Figure 12.2 *Protein truncation for the deletion prone part of the dystrophine gene carried out on mRNA from muscle biopsies. Lanes 1 and 2 control muscle biopsies; lanes 3, 4, 5, and 6 showing variously truncated proteins in four patients with Duchenne muscular dystrophy.*

Becker dystrophy who have a dystrophin mutation the clinical phenotype may closely resemble that of limb-girdle muscular dystrophy, which is now known to have at least seven different genetic varieties (box 12.6). Other examples include the differentiation of merosin deficiency from a dystrophinopathy in infants with congenital muscular dystrophy and the differentiation of adhalin deficiency from dystrophinopathy in the severe childhood autosomal recessive form of muscular dystrophy (now classified as LGMD2C). The molecular definition of these conditions has also had important implications for the identification of heterozygote carriers and for prenatal diagnosis, especially in the X linked dystrophies. It has also led to the recognition that there is a wide range of phenotypic expression and clinical severity, particularly in the dystrophinopathies and sarcoglycanopathies.[84-86]

Diagnostic approach

The diagnostic approach to the patient with a suspected muscular dystrophy initially involves a detailed clinical assessment of the affected patient and family history which, when positive, may point to an X linked disorder or to one of the distinctive forms of dominantly inherited myopathy such as facioscapulohumeral dystrophy or distal myopathy. Electromyography is helpful in confirming the myopathic nature of the condition and excluding myotonic or

Box 12.6   Muscular dystrophies

X linked	Locus	Gene
Dystrophinopathies	Xp21·2	Dystrophin
Duchenne		
Becker		
Quadriceps myopathy		
Myalgia and cramps		
HyperCKaemia		
Emery-Dreifuss	Xq28	Emerin
Myotubular myopathy	Xq28	?
Autosomal dominant		
Facioscapulohumeral		
FSHD	4q35	?
FSHD2	?	?
Limb-girdle★		
LGMD1A	5q22–q34	?
LGMD1B	?	?
Distal★		
MPD1	14q	?
Oculopharyngeal★		
OPMD	14q11·2–q13	?
Autosomal recessive		
Limb-girdle		
LGMD2A	15q15·1–q21·1	Calpain
LGMD2B	2p16–p13	?
LGMD2C (SCARMD)	13q12	γ-Sarcoglycan
LGMD2D	17q12–q21·33	Adhalin (α-sarcoglycan)
LGMD2E	4q12	β-Sarcoglycan
Congenital		
LAMA2	6q2	Merosin
Fukuyama	9q31–q33	?
Distal (Myoshi)★	2p	?
Oculopharyngeal★	?	?

★Autosomal dominant or recessive.

chronic neurogenic conditions. A raised serum creatine kinase concentration, although not specific, may also be a diagnostic pointer particularly if the concentration is very high as is usually the case in the early stages of Duchenne or Becker muscular dystrophy when concentrations of up to 300 times normal may occur. However, in the other dystrophies less pronounced increases or normal concentrations may be found. The high serum creatine kinase in affected boys with Duchenne dystrophy at birth has been the basis for the development of neonatal screening programmes for newborn males in some countries.[87] The detection of isolated cases by neonatal screening makes it possible to prevent the birth of secondary cases in families and it has been estimated that it is possible to prevent 15 to 20% of new cases of Duchenne dystrophy with this type of screening.

In most instances definitive diagnosis of a muscular dystrophy and recognition of the particular type still require a muscle biopsy for routine histology and immunohistochemical staining for dystrophin and for the other proteins of the dystrophin-glycoprotein complex such as the sarcoglycans (figure 12.1). The immunohistochemical demonstration of complete or partial dystrophin deficiency is the gold standard for establishing the diagnosis of Duchenne and Becker muscular dystrophy. Complete or virtually complete absence of dystrophin is characteristic of Duchenne dystrophy whereas in Becker dystrophy there is usually patchy preservation of the protein on the sarcolemma of muscle fibres. Dystrophin immunohistochemistry may therefore be of prognostic as well as diagnostic value in differentiating Duchenne and Becker dystrophy in young boys. The importance of using a panel of antibodies to different regions of the dystrophin molecule from the N to the C terminus has been emphasised.[88]

Immunoblotting for dystrophin in muscle tissue is a more sensitive technique, which may show more subtle changes in the molecular size or amount of dystrophin. Hoffman et al[31] showed that patients with Duchenne muscular dystrophy had less than 3% of the normal quantity of dystrophin, intermediate patients had up to 60% of normal levels of dystrophin, whereas patients with Becker dystrophy most often had abnormal sized dystrophin rather than abnormal quantities.

Molecular diagnosis

Dystrophinopathies

The main applications of molecular diagnosis are accurate diagnosis if other methods have failed or are inappropriate, accurate diagnosis of asymptomatic subjects (in the case of these X linked diseases this largely means carriers), and prenatal diagnosis.

The dystrophin gene was the first major disease gene to be identified by positional cloning. The dystrophin message and the distribution of deletion mutations which cause about 70% of cases of Duchenne and Becker muscular dystrophy were first described in 1987.[89] However, pulsed field gel electrophoresis had already indicated that most mutations causing Duchenne dystrophy were large deletions.[90] The identification of the dystrophin gene immediately allowed much more accurate differential diagnosis of Duchenne and Becker muscular dystrophy using the available cDNA probes.[91-93] Molecular diagnosis of boys affected with dystrophinopathies is now carried out by multiplex PCR of genomic DNA (figure 12.3), which gives a diagnosis in hours rather than the previous days or weeks.[30 48-50] Prenatal diagnosis is also achieved with multiplex PCR when a family deletion has been identified, and by linkage using microsatellites[94] for the dystrophin gene in the

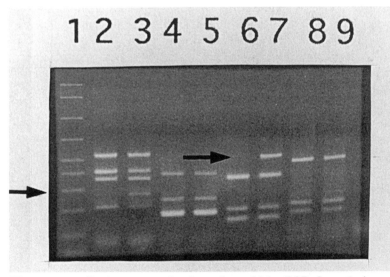

Figure 12.3   *Duchenne muscular dystrophy multiplex PCR: Lane 1: size standard; lanes 2, 4, 6, 8: patient with Duchenne muscular dystrophy; lanes 3, 5, 7, 9: control; lanes 2 and 3 (from top down): promoter, exons 3, 8, 50, 53; lanes 4 and 5: exons 13, 16, 74; lanes 6 and 7: exons 48, 43, 47, 60; lanes 8 and 9: exons 19, 42, 4. The patient is deleted for at least exons 48 and 50 (arrows)*

large minority of families in which deletions have not been identified. Splice site mutations in the gene can be identified by RT-PCR.[62 63]

Identification of carriers of dystrophinopathies has been achieved with dosage Southern blotting,[95-97] presence of junction fragments,[90] and non-inheritance of alleles.[98] However, as with all aspects of molecular diagnosis, carrier detection has moved to PCR; PCR dosage has been used with great accuracy to identify carriers[99 100] as has RT-PCR from illegitimate transcription of the dystrophin message in circulating lymphocytes.[45]

The increasing diversity of dystrophinopathy phenotypes has been reviewed by Beggs *et al*[101] and includes quadriceps myopathy,[102] cramps, and myalgia,[103 104] hyperCKaemia,[105] and X linked cardiomyopathy.[106 107]

Limb-girdle muscular dystrophies

The first recessive limb-girdle muscular dystrophy gene to be localised (LGMD2A) was on chromosome 15[108 109] through linkage in families from the island of Reunion. Mutations in the calcium activated protease gene calpain were subsequently identified both in the families from Reunion and in the Amish families which showed linkage to the chromosome 15 region.[110] (Two different autosomal recessive limb-girdle muscular dystrophies segregate in the Amish community—the other is LGMD2E.[39]) The identification of calpain as the mutant gene in LGMD2A was the first implication of a non-structural protein in a muscular dystrophy.[110] No abnormalities in the dystrophin associated glycoproteins were detected in patients with LGMD2A.[110-112] There are four other localised or identified recessive limb-girdle muscular dystrophy genes: LGMD2C, LGMD2D, and LGMD2E are the sarcoglycanopathies whereas LGMD2B, localised to the short arm of 2p,[113] is an as yet unidentified gene.

There are at least two genes for autosomal dominant limb-girdle muscular dystrophy, one (LGMD1A) localised on chromosome 5.[71 72] The other (LGMD1B) is not yet localised.[109]

Sarcoglycanopathies

Adhalinopathy (α-sarcoglycanopathy) was the first sarcoglycanopathy to be identified, initially by deficiency in immunohistochemical staining[115] and later by mutations in the adhalin gene.[33 116 117] Adhalinopathy is also known as recessive limb-girdle

367

muscular dystrophy type D (LGMD2D). Mutations in the other two sarcoglycans have now been demonstrated. Mutations in the β-sarcoglycan gene on chromosome 4 are associated with LGMD2E, the second limb-girdle muscular dystrophy found among the Amish[39] and also other communities.[28] Mutations in the γ-sarcoglycan gene on chromosome 13 are associated with severe congenital autosomal recessive muscular dystrophy (SCARMD, LGMD2C).[38] In each of these diseases there is a reduction of immunohistochemical staining for all three sarcoglycans. Thus reduction of immunostaining for any of the sarcoglycans in the absence of reduction in dystrophin staining indicates mutation in one of, at present, three genes. As Lim et al[39] state in the discussion of their paper, only molecular investigation of all the candidate genes can provide a definitive diagnosis.

Congenital muscular dystrophy

Congenital muscular dystrophies are characterised by severe dystrophic changes of muscle from birth.[118] Tomé et al[112] were the first to show merosin (LAMA2) deficiency in cases of congenital muscular dystrophy of the occidental type. However, not all of the clinically indistinguishable cases showed merosin deficiency, and this heterogeneity is yet to be explained on a molecular basis. It is estimated that 40% of occidental congenital muscular dystrophy cases show LAMA2 deficiency.[118] Subsequently mutations of the LAMA2 gene were identified in patients with congenital muscular dystrophy.[119]

The LAMA2 gene maps to the long arm of chromosome 6, the Japanese form of congenital muscular dystrophy, Fukuyama muscular dystrophy to the long arm of chromosome 9,[120] and thus a different, as yet unidentified gene must be involved. Fukuyama muscular dystrophy and Walker-Wallberg syndrome may be genetically identical.[121]

Facioscapulohumeral muscular dystrophy

A gene for facioscapulohumeral muscular dystrophy (FSHD) was first mapped in 1990 to chromosome 4q35 near the telomere.[122] Subsequently, altered sized fragments involving a repeated sequence with homeodomain homology were identified in familial and sporadic cases of facioscapulohumeral muscular dystrophy.[123 124] The precise gene or genes affected by the chromosomal rearrangements have not, however, been identified and thus the mechanism of pathogenesis remains a mystery. In addition, recombination with the altered sized fragments has been documented[125] and not all facioscapulohumeral muscular dystrophy families show linkage to 4q35.[126] Facioscapulohumeral muscular dystrophy is thus still a problematic disease for molecular diagnosis.

Oculopharyngeal muscular dystrophy

A gene for oculopharyngeal muscular dystrophy among French Canadians has been linked to the proximal long arm of chromosome 14 close to the genes for cardiac α-myosin and β-myosin[74] and in the same region as a gene for dominant distal myopathy.[70]

Emery-Dreifuss muscular dystrophy

The Emery-Dreifuss muscular dystrophy gene has been identified and its protein product named emerin.[127] Emerin seems to be a transmembrane protein but its function is uncertain.

Distal myopathy

Two genes for distal muscular dystrophy have been localised. One (MPD1) with a phenotype similar to that originally described by Gowers[70] and the other for the recessive Miyoshi myopathy.[69] It is interesting that the MPD1 gene maps to a similar region of chromosome 14 as a gene for oculopharyngeal muscular dystrophy[74] and that the Miyoshi myopathy gene is in a similar region of chromosome 2 to a gene for autosomal recessive limb-girdle muscular dystrophy (LGMD2B)[113] raising the possibility that in both cases the two conditions may be caused by mutations in the same gene.[128]

Myotonic syndromes

Box 12.7 gives a classification of these conditions, based on the underlying molecular defects. Differentiation of the various types is usually possible on the basis of clinical features such as the age of onset, pattern of inheritance, provocative factors for the myotonia, and the presence or absence of dystrophic muscle weakness or other systemic features.

Myotonic dystrophy

This is the most common of the genetic forms of myotonia and is transmitted as an autosomal dominant trait with considerable variability in the degree of phenotypic expression and age of onset

369

Box 12.7   Classification of hereditary myotonias

Myotonias	Gene
Chloride channel myotonias:	
Autosomal dominant (Thomsen)	CLCN1
Autosomal recessive (Becker)	CLCN1
Sodium channel myotonias:	
Paramyotonia congenita	SCN4A
Myotonia fluctuans	SCN4A
Myotonia permanens	SCN4A
Dystrophic myotonias:	
Myotonic dystrophy	Myotonin protein kinase (?)
Proximal myotonic myopathy	?

---

of symptoms. The congenital form, in which there is generalised hypotonia and weakness, often with facial diplegia and a distinctive tent shaped mouth, may occur in the offspring of either affected males or females but the more severe cases are usually the offspring of female heterozygotes who may themselves be only very mildly affected.[129] [130] Mental retardation and delay in motor and speech development are common in early onset cases. Myotonia is not present in affected infants but is usually readily demonstrable in the tongue, hand, and forearm muscles in patients presenting during adolescence or early adult life, and tends to become progressively less severe with the passage of time. Weakness and atrophy of the forearm, calf, and sternomastoid muscles occur as the condition progresses and in some cases weakness of the facial, bulbar, and respiratory muscles also develops and may be associated with irregular breathing patterns, sleep apnoea, and respiratory failure.[131] Ventilatory function studies as well as monitoring of breathing and arterial blood gases during sleep should be performed if these problems are suspected.

Other distinctive features in the adult include frontal baldness and testicular atrophy in the male and distinctive subcapsular cataracts, which are best seen with slit lamp examination.[130] Cardiac involvement also occurs and electrocardiographic abnormalities which include atrioventricular and intraventricular conduction defects and atrial or ventricular arrhythmias, are common and may cause Stokes-Adams attacks or even sudden death.[130-132] The incidence of mitral valve prolapse is also increased in some families.[133] Investigation of cardiac function, including ECG and echocardiography, should therefore be performed routinely and, when indicated, ECG monitoring and radionuclide angiocardiography may also be indicated. Other systemic manifestations which may require investigation in their own right include diabetes mellitus, disorders of the thyroid or immune function, and gastrointestinal and genitourinary abnormalities.[130]

Myotonic dystrophy is one of the easy muscle diseases to diagnose by molecular techniques, as virtually all cases have variations of the same mutation: the expansion of the CTG triplet repeat in the myotonin protein kinase gene on chromosome 19.[134-136] The large triplet repeat expansions causing severe disease can be identified by Southern blotting after digestion of genomic DNA with EcoRI, and smaller expansions can be identified by digestion with BglI or BamHI.[47] The PCR can identify normal subjects by the presence of two alleles within the normal size range and the very small expansions in minimally affected or asymptomatic subjects (figure 12.4).[136 137] Often, this identifies where the disease came from in a family with someone other than the person the family has always suspected. Thus by cascade screening it is possible to detect and warn those family members at risk from possible cardiac complications and sudden death.

A dominantly inherited myotonic myopathy with proximal muscle weakness and cataracts without the characteristic trinucleotide repeat expansion has recently been described[138 139] and has been shown not to be allelic with the genes for myotonic dystrophy or for the chloride or sodium channel myotonias.[138]

Chloride channel myotonia

It is now known that both the autosomal dominant (Thomsen) and recessive (Becker) forms of myotonia congenita are caused by mutations in the muscle chloride channel (CLCN1) gene on chromosome 7.[53] Symptoms may be present from birth in the dominant form but often do not develop until early childhood or adolescence. The myotonia is widespread, usually painless, and more severe in the recessive form, being accentuated by rest, cold, and emotion and improving with repeated muscle contraction. It is commonly associated with diffuse muscular hypertrophy, par-

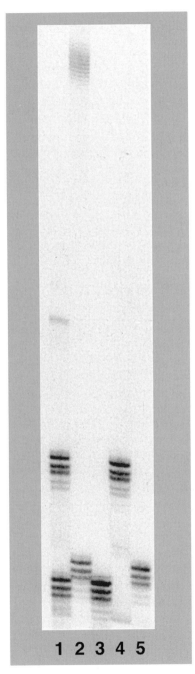

Figure 12.4 *Myotonic dystrophy: Analysis of the myotonic dystrophy triplet expansion by PCR. Lane 1: grandmother showing two normal sized alleles; lane 2: asymptomatic grandfather showing one normal sized allele and a small expansion; lane 3: uncle of proband (son) of lanes 1 and 2 showing non-inheritance of grandfather's allele (expansion too big to PCR), lane 4: mother of proband (daughter) of lanes 1 and 2 showing non-inheritance of grandfather's allele (expansion too big to PCR); lane 5; proband (daughter of lane 4) showing non-inheritance of mother's allele, expansion too large to PCR*

ticularly in affected males. Muscle weakness may develop after exercise, particularly in cases of the recessive form of the condition, and is associated with a reduction in the amplitude of the evoked CMAP and twitch tension.[140] In addition, some degree of fixed weakness and atrophy with EMG evidence of myopathy develops, particularly in the forearm and sternomastoid muscles, in about two thirds of patients with the recessive condition.[141]

To date, 19 separate mutations in the CLCN1 gene have been identified, six being associated with dominant disease and 13 with the recessive disease.[53] Most (four out of five) of the truncating mutations cause recessive disease. The mutations are spread throughout the coding region of the gene and many have been found in single families, indicating that other mutations are highly likely to be found in other families. Myotonia congenita is therefore one of the difficult diseases to diagnose, with molecular techniques requiring screening of the entire coding region of the gene.

Sodium channel myotonia

These varieties of myotonia have all been localised to the same locus and have been associated with different mutations in the α subunit of the sodium muscle channel gene (SCN4A) on chromosome 17.[53 142] In paramyotonia congenita myotonia is characteristically induced by cold exposure, particularly in the facial and hand muscles, and may be associated with attacks of weakness (cold paresis) which improve with warming. In most cases the myotonia is increased by repeated muscle contraction (paradoxical myotonia) rather than improving as in most other myotonic disorders. In potassium sensitive paramyotonia (paralysis periodica paramyotonica) paradoxical myotonia and episodes of weakness are precipitated by potassium administration. Such cases account for the overlap between paramyotonia and hyperkalaemic periodic paralysis in some families.

A third variety of sodium channel myotonia has been designated *myotonia fluctuans*. In this condition, which is dominantly inherited, myotonia is of variable severity at different times, may be associated with painful muscle spasms, with a tendency to increase in severity after exercise, ingestion of potassium, and administration of depolarizing agents, and is responsive to treatment with acetazolamide[142] or, in some families, mexilitine.[143] A fourth variety of sodium channel myotonia with continuous severe myotonia, muscle stiffness, and hypertrophy has also been described and designated myotonia permanens.[53]

The mutations in these conditions are spread through a large part of the coding region of the SCN4A gene making molecular diagnosis difficult, although two mutations, Thr1313Met and Gly1306Val, predominate in paramyotonia congenita and should be initially screened for.

Periodic paralysis

Some conditions may cause episodic weakness or paralysis of the limb muscles (box 12.8). It is difficult to evaluate the importance of a complaint of episodic weakness unless the patient is watched during an attack. Most patients who complain of episodes of weakness are in fact referring to fatigue. In those patients who do have episodes of documented weakness it is first necessary to exclude disorders of neuromuscular transmission such as myasthenia gravis, demyelinating disorders of the peripheral or central nervous system, transient ischaemic episodes, or attacks of hysterical weakness. If these conditions can be excluded, the possibility of one of the primary periodic paralyses arises, particularly if there are other affected family members (box 12.8).

Box 12.8   Classification of hereditary periodic paralyses

Hereditary:
Hypokalaemic (DHP receptor; 1q31–32)
Potassium sensitive (SCN4A; 17q23–25)
   Hyperkalaemic
   Paramyotonia congenita
   Paralysis periodica paramyotonica
   Andersen's syndrome

Acquired:
Hypokalaemic
Hyperkalaemic
Thyrotoxic

Differentiation between the main varieties of primary periodic paralysis is usually possible on the basis of the duration of the attacks of weakness, provocative factors, and serum potassium concentrations during attacks. In hypokalaemic periodic paralysis the attacks are often precipitated by carbohydrate ingestion and tend to be less frequent and of longer duration (up to 24 hours) than in the potassium sensitive periodic paralyses (for example, hyperkalaemic periodic paralysis) in which the attacks are often precipitated by fasting or by resting after exercise.[14] Although the serum potassium concentration during an attack of weakness may help to distinguish the hypokalaemic from the hyperkalaemic form, potassium concentrations are often normal in the second and may occasionally also be normal in the hypokalaemic form.[10] The serum creatine kinase concentration is often raised in severe attacks of both forms and may be somewhat raised even between attacks. Myotonia, when present clinically or evident on EMG, is more suggestive of hyperkalaemic periodic paralysis or paramyotonia but may occasionally occur in the eyelid muscles in hypokalaemic periodic paralysis.[9]

When carried out during an attack of weakness EMG shows a progressive reduction in motor unit recruitment and in the amplitude of the compound muscle action potential evoked by motor nerve stimulation, whereas repetitive nerve stimulation shows a transient potentiation of the compound muscle action potential.[144] A myopathic EMG pattern may be found even during the attack free interval particularly in patients who develop fixed muscle weakness, as often occurs in those who have had the condition for several years.[145] Changes in the evoked compound muscle action potential also occur with exercise and are the basis for the hand exercise test described by McManis et al.[146] Serial measurements of compound muscle action potential amplitudes show a greater than normal increase during exercise and decrease in the post-exercise period in patients with periodic paralysis. The test was found to be abnormal in 70% of cases of periodic paralysis but did not distinguish between the different forms.

Another form of exercise testing, which is useful in detecting some cases of hypokalaemic periodic paralysis, including asymptomatic cases, is that described by Kantola and Tarssinen,[147] which involves a 30 minute period of bicycle ergometry. Affected persons do not show the normal rise in plasma potassium concentrations after the exercise period. Muscle biopsy shows a characteristic vacuolar change in muscle fibres, and sometimes necrotic muscle fibres, particularly during an attack of weakness, but sometimes even during attack free intervals, in both major forms of periodic paralysis. Vacuolar change may be found even in some family members without definite attacks of weakness.[147] Although the biopsy changes are distinctive, a biopsy is seldom necessary as the results of provocative tests and molecular genetic analysis are usually diagnostic.

As the plasma potassium concentrations during an attack of weakness are sometimes misleading, provocative tests remain important in evaluating people with a negative family history or those from families in which the mutation is not known.[10 14] In hypokalaemic periodic paralysis, attacks of weakness may be induced by giving an oral glucose load (1·5 gm/kg over three minutes; maximum 100 g). Muscle strength in selected groups, serum electrolytes, and ECG should be monitored every 30 minutes for three to five hours. If weakness does not develop, an intravenous glucose load (3 g/kg in water) is given over a period of one hour. If weakness does not develop after 30 minutes, intravenous insulin (0·1 U/kg) is given and repeated at 60 minutes if weakness fails to develop. Regular measurements of muscle strength and of plasma electrolyte and glucose concentrations, and ECG should be performed throughout the test and the period of induced weakness.[10 14]

In the potassium sensitive forms of periodic paralysis attacks of weakness may be induced by oral potassium loading.[10 14] A widely used protocol involves giving 0·05 g/kg of potassium chloride in a glucose free solution over a period of three minutes. Muscle strength, serum electrolytes, and ECG are monitored every 15 minutes in the first two hours and every 30 minutes in the next two hours and weakness usually develops after 90 to 180 minutes. If the initial test is negative, higher potassium loads of 0·1 to 0·15 g/kg may be used. The test is contraindicated in patients with insulin dependent diabetes mellitus or renal insufficiency. Cold testing, involving immersion of the arm in water at 10°C for 30 minutes, may be useful in confirming the diagnosis of paramyotonia in patients with a history of episodes of cold induced weakness or myotonia.[10]

The molecular basis for both the hypokalaemic and hyperkalaemic forms of periodic paralysis have now been defined. Hypokalaemic periodic paralysis has been shown to be caused by three mutations in the dihydropyridine receptor calcium channel gene (CACNLIA3) on chromosome 1q31–32 affecting two amino acid residues.[43 53 148 149] The mutations can be detected by PCR followed by enzyme digestion as they either create or destroy restriction enzyme sites[148] or by SSCP.[43] Mutations in the gene encoding the α subunit of the skeletal muscle sodium channel (SCN4A) causing hyperkalaemic periodic paralysis were first described in 1991.[150 151] A recent review by Lehmann-Horn and Rüdel[53] catalogues the five mutations of SCN4A now known to be associated with hyperkalaemic periodic paralysis. Two of the mutations, Thr704Met and Met1592Val, predominate and can be screened for first. There is perhaps a degree of genetic heterogeneity in hyperkalaemic periodic paralysis as one family with a convincing clinical diagnosis of the disease did not map to the SCN4A gene.[67] Mutations in the same gene have also been found in some families with paramyotonia congenita[53] and in some cases of hyperkalaemic periodic paralysis associated with cardiac arrhythmias (Andersen's syndrome).[152 153]

Congenital myopathies

The congenital myopathies are a heterogeneous group of disorders which may result in hypotonia in infancy or may present later in childhood with weakness and delayed motor milestones (box 12.9).[10 154 155] Some, such as central core disease, are benign and relatively non-progressive whereas others such as X linked centronuclear myopathy are usually fatal in infancy. Skeletal abnormalities such as talipes, scoliosis, and hip dislocation as well as dysmorphic features are not uncommon. Ptosis and ophthalmoplegia are often a feature in centronuclear myopathy and may also occur in minicore disease. Respiratory insufficiency may occur, particularly in nemaline myopathy, myotubular myopathy, and cytoplasmic body myopathy. The congenital myopathies should be considered in the differential diagnosis of the floppy infant and need to be distinguished from other neuromuscular and CNS disorders which may produce infantile hypotonia.[10]

In all of these conditions a definitive diagnosis relies on a muscle biopsy with full histochemical and electron microscopic examination of muscle tissue. These will identify specific morphological changes such as central cores, nemaline rods, central nucleation, and abnormalities of myofibre differentiation and fibre type pro-

377

Box 12.9   Congenital myopathies

Central core disease*
Nemaline myopathy
Centronuclear myopathy
Minicore disease*
Congenital fibre type disproportion
Myopathies with cytoplasmic inclusions
● Fingerprint body myopathy
● Reducing body myopathy
● Cytoplasmic body myopathy
● Hyaline body myopathy
● Myopathy with tubular aggregates
● Zebra body myopathy
● Sarcotubular myopathy

*Predisposition to malignant hyperthermia

---

portions[156] or distinctive inclusion bodies (for example, cytoplasmic bodies, fingerprint bodies, spheroid bodies, hyaline bodies, reducing bodies, zebra bodies, and tubular aggregates). This will also exclude other conditions such as congenital muscular dystrophy, metabolic myopathies, and neurogenic disorders such as spinal muscular atrophy and congenital peripheral neuropathies.[10 154] The genetic basis for some of the congenital myopathies such as nemaline myopathy and central core disease have now been defined. To date, one gene for autosomal dominant nemaline myopathy has been linked to chromosome 1[156] and a mutation in the α-tropomyosin gene TPM3 has been shown to segregate with the disease.[157] A gene for recessive nemaline myopathy has been localised to chromosome 2.[75] Neither of the loci map to the known locations for the α-actinin genes.[158] This and the mutation in tropomyosin may indicate that nemaline myopathy is a disease of the thin filament rather than of the Z disc.[128] Central core disease was first linked to the same region of chromosome 19 as malignant hyperthermia[159 160] and then mutations associated with central core disease were identified in the RYR1 gene.[162–164] Thus both malignant hyperthermia and central core disease are caused by mutations in the RYR1 gene and whether central cores manifest or not may depend on the degree of calcium loading of the individual muscle fibres.[162]

Mitochondrial myopathies

Since the discovery of the first mitochondrial DNA mutations in 1988[164 165] it has become apparent that the clinical spectrum of mitochondrial diseases is extremely diverse, ranging from relatively mild and slowly progressive myopathies confined to the extraocular muscles (chronic progressive external ophthalmoplegia) to severe fatal infantile myopathies (for example, cytochrome c oxidase deficiency) and multisystem encephalomyopathies (such as the Kearns-Sayre, MELAS, and MERFF syndromes[10 166–170]) (box 12.10). In addition, deficiencies of mitochondrial enzymes encoded by nuclear DNA have been identified (for example, succinate dehydrogenase deficiency).

Box 12.10   Mitochondrial myopathies and encephalomyopathies

Progressive external ophthalmoplegia
  Sporadic
  Familial

Kearns-Sayre syndrome
  Ophthalmoplegia
  Pigmentary retinopathy
  Cardiac conduction defects
  Cerebellar ataxia
  Sensorineural deafness

Limb-girdle myopathy

Infantile myopathy
  Benign reversible
  Severe fatal

MERFF syndrome
  Myoclonus
  Epilepsy
  Myopathy

MELAS syndrome
  Myopathy
  Lactic acidosis
  Stroke-like episodes

Clinical phenotypes and genotypes

Box 12.11 shows that mitochondrial defects may be associated not only with myopathic disorders but with a wide variety of other neurological and non-neurological manifestations. Although some classic syndromes have been defined (box 12.10), there is a certain amount of overlap between these and new phenotypic combinations are still being identified. Moreover, there is considerable variability in the age of onset, rate of progression, and extent of phenotypic expression in different tissues even within the major syndromes and in patients with the same mutation.[170] This heterogeneity is characteristic of this group of disorders[171] and is attributable to the random distribution of mitochondria containing the mutated DNA within different tissues and to the admixture of normal and abnormal populations of mitochondria within the cells of these tissues (heteroplasmy) as a result of which different tissues in the same patient and different members of the same family may be involved to different degrees.[169]

The classic syndromes have been associated with different types of genomic defect. For example, patients with the pure form of

---

Box 12.11   Clinical manifestations of mitochondrial disease

Neurological	*Non-neurological*
External ophthalmoplegia	Short stature
Limb myopathy	Cardiac conduction defects
Fatiguability and poor exercise tolerance	Cardiomyopathy
	Pigmentary retinopathy
Cerebellar ataxia	Cataracts
Epilepsy	Lactic acidosis
Myoclonus	Diabetes mellitus
Sensorineural deafness	Hypoparathyroidism
Peripheral neuropathy	Renal tubular defects
Dementia	Episodic nausea and vomiting
Stroke	Pancytopenia
Vascular headache	Intestinal pseudo-obstruction
Dystonia	Multiple lipomas
Basal ganglion calcification	

chronic progressive external ophthalmoplegia (CPEO) usually have single major deletions[166 167] but point mutations have been found in some patients.[2] Similarly, those patients with the Kearns-Sayre syndrome have single large mtDNA deletions which occur sporadically.[164 172] In patients with familial CPEO two distinct syndromes have been identified. In the first, which is maternally inherited, deletions are not found, whereas in the second, which is dominantly inherited, large scale multiple mtDNA deletions are usually present and are thought to be secondary to a mutation in a nuclear gene encoding a factor which controls mtDNA replication.[10 173] Such a gene has recently been linked to chromosome 10q23·3–24·3 in a Finnish family with autosomal dominant CPEO.[174] Cases presenting purely with a proximal myopathy may also be dominantly inherited[175] but are uncommon and the genotypic basis for these cases has not been defined. In the encephalomyopathy syndromes different point mutations have been found in tRNA-lys (nucleotides 8344 or 8356) in the MERRF syndrome[176] and tRNA-leu (nucleotides 3243, 3251, 3252, 3271 or 3291) in the MELAS syndrome.[2 167]

Diagnostic approach

In patients with CPEO, Kearns-Sayre syndrome, or one of the other classic syndromes, the clinical features are often sufficiently distinctive to strongly suggest the diagnosis of a mitochondrial disorder, and in familial cases, a maternal pattern of transmission would also raise the possibility of such a diagnosis. A raised fasting venous lactate concentration is an additional diagnostic pointer. Lactate concentrations are usually normal in cases of CPEO, but venous and CSF concentrations are often raised in the MELAS syndrome and may also be increased in Kearns-Sayre syndrome and in patients with a proximal myopathy or encephalomyopathy.[166] A muscle biopsy is the most important diagnostic investigation, the characteristic findings being of ragged red fibres with the modified Gomori trichrome stain, with abnormally prominent subsarcolemmal mitochondrial aggregates with the oxidative enzyme stains (NADH dehydrogenase, succinate dehydrogenase) and abnormal mitochondrial morphology with mitochondrial inclusions on electron microscopy. In addition, histochemical staining for cytochrome oxidase activity shows a characteristic mosaic pattern of fibres lacking enzyme activity in most cases.[177] Immunohistochemical techniques may be applied to

381

determine whether nuclear or mtDNA encoded subunits of cytochrome oxidase are absent. In situ hybridisation with probes to different parts of the mtDNA molecule may also be used to study the distribution of mutant mitochondria in muscle fibres.[178]

The identified common mutations in the mitochondrial genome associated with MERRF or MELAS can be tested using PCR followed by enzyme digestion[43 54] or SSCP analysis.[55] The major deletions of the mtDNA associated with Kearns-Sayre syndrome or CPEO may be identified either using Southern blotting[85] or PCR[179] including long range PCR, which can amplify the entire 16 569 base pairs of the mtDNA in one reaction.[180] The severity of the disease relates to the percentage of mutant mitochondria,[65] which can be estimated either after Southern blotting, or enzyme digestion after PCR, or from SSCP.[176]

Whether all the base changes shown to be associated with mitochondrial related disease actually cause disease may be debatable; some may merely be linked to other disease causing mutations.[181] On the other hand, the polymorphisms of mtDNA may contribute to disease.[182] The mitochondrial genome is thus problematic for molecular diagnosis, the relevance of some "mutations" to disease being unclear.

Acute rhabdomyolysis and myoglobinuria

Various hereditary and acquired disorders may lead to episodes of severe widespread muscle fibre destruction and myoglobinuria.[12] Clinically, there is widespread muscle weakness which may be profound and in severe cases there is often severe muscle pain, tenderness, and depression of the deep tendon reflexes. When myoglobinuria is severe it may lead to the development of acute renal failure. In patients with malignant hyperthermia muscle rigidity, hyperpyrexia, and rhabdomyolysis usually develop during anaesthesia when susceptible subjects are exposed to halothane and some other inhalational anaesthetic agents, but episodes of rhabdomyolysis may also be precipitated by stress, strenuous physical activity, or systemic infective illnesses.

Patients presenting in this way for the first time should undergo a detailed clinical assessment for a drug induced, toxic, or infective cause and hypokalaemia, hypothyroidism, and other metabolic disorders should be excluded. Patients in whom no obvious cause can be identified—especially those in whom there is a history of previous episodes—should have a muscle biopsy and appropriate biochemical investigations for an underlying genetic disorder such as malignant hyperpyrexia or a disorder of glycolysis or fatty acid metabolism.[12 183]

Susceptibility to malignant hyperthermia in humans was first linked to the region containing the ryanodine receptor calcium release channel on chromosome 19[76 184] after the mutation for swine malignant hyperthermia was linked to the glucose phosphate isomerase gene which maps in humans to chromosome 19. A few mutations have now been identified in the relatively large (15 kb) RYR1 gene message[185] in a minority of malignant hyperthermia families.[79] The aim of molecular diagnosis in this condition must be to reduce the reliance on the extremely invasive current gold standard of the muscle contracture test, with which the molecular diagnosis is not always in agreement.[79] However, until a clearer and more comprehensive list of mutations in the RYR1 gene causing malignant hyperthermia is available, including resolution of the apparent genetic heterogeneity, and the discrepancies between molecular diagnosis and the contracture test are resolved, molecular diagnosis for susceptibility to malignant hyperthermia will remain problematical.

Painful muscle conditions

Muscle pain may be a feature in some myopathies and other conditions (box 12.2). The pain may be focal or diffuse and may occur at rest, during, or after exercise. When myalgia develops after an infective illness, an alcoholic binge, exposure to a myotoxic drug, or after an episode of envenomation, the cause is usually apparent. A wide variety of drugs may cause myalgia and muscle cramps without significant muscular weakness and the symptoms usually resolve promptly after withdrawal of the offending agent (box 12.1). The finding of significant muscular weakness, tenderness, and increase in the serum creatine kinase suggests a necrotising myopathy and a muscle biopsy is usually warranted to confirm the diagnosis. A biopsy is also indicated when an inflammatory myopathy is suspected and should include the overlying fascia, if there is a possibility of fasciitis. Muscle pain and stiffness are common symptoms in hypothyroidism and in patients with metabolic bone disease. The diagnosis in such patients can usually be confirmed by appropriate biochemical and other studies without resorting to muscle biopsy.

Muscle pain and cramping which develop during exercise suggest a disorder of muscle energy metabolism, such as deficiency of myophosphorylase, phosphofructokinase, or other glycolytic enzyme defect, or of carnitine palmityl transferase, especially if there is a history of discolouration of the urine after exercise, suggesting myoglobinuria. Such patients warrant further investigation including the forearm exercise test (see above) and assays of carnitine and carnitine palmityl transferase activity as well as a muscle biopsy for histochemical and biochemical studies to confirm the diagnosis of these metabolic disorders. With molecular studies mutations causing disease have been identified in some of these conditions but such studies are not usually necessary for the diagnosis. A muscle biopsy is also necessary for the diagnosis of mitochondrial myopathy, malignant hyperthermia, dystrophin deficiency, and tubular aggregates, all of which may sometimes present with unexplained myalgia, cramps, or exercise intolerance.

The vast majority of patients with complaints of muscle pain, stiffness, or cramping do not have any significant muscular weakness or other evidence of muscle disease. It is important in such patients to look for evidence of muscular and myofascial tenderness. The finding of point tenderness in the typical sites is diagnostic of the condition of fibromyalgia and invasive investigations such as EMG and muscle biopsy can usually be avoided. Similarly, a pattern of proximal or axial muscle pain and stiffness with malaise in elderly patients with preserved muscle strength and a raised erythrocyte sedimentation rate is diagnostic of polymyalgia rheumatica and warrants a therapeutic trial of prednisone without muscle biopsy, although the possibility of an underlying connective tissue or metabolic disorder or malignancy should always be considered and investigated appropriately. In a third group of patients, with the postviral myalgia/fatigue syndrome, there are no diagnostic clinical or laboratory abnormalities. Electromyography and muscle biopsy may, however, be indicated in such patients to exclude an inflammatory or metabolic myopathy, particularly when symptoms are disabling and if the serum creatine kinase concentration is raised.

Inflammatory myopathies

The diagnosis of an inflammatory myopathy may be readily made on clinical grounds in patients with the characteristic skin changes of dermatomyositis or with the typical pattern of muscle weakness seen in inclusion body myositis and may also be suspected in patients with a connective tissue disorder such as systemic lupus erythematosus, progressive systemic sclerosis, mixed connective tissue disease, Sjögren's syndrome, or other autoimmune disease who develop a proximal myopathy and would be supported by the finding of raised serum creatine kinase and an abnormal EMG (see above). However, it is important that the diagnosis should be firmly established on histological grounds and a muscle biopsy should always be performed before commencing treatment. An open biopsy, usually from the deltoid or vastus lateralis muscle, is preferable for the diagnosis of inflammatory myopathy. In addition to routine histological preparations, mononuclear cell populations, immune complex deposition, MHC, and intercellular adhesion molecule expression can be assessed with immunohistochemical techniques.[186 187]

Other investigations are directed towards identifying any underlying immune or infective disorder or malignancy. These should include an autoantibody screen for antinuclear factor, rheumatoid factor, anti-RNP and, when appropriate, other autoantibodies such as PM-Scl and Ku, which are frequently associated with the polymyositis/scleroderma overlap syndrome, and antibodies to the aminoacyl-tRNA synthetases such as Jo-1 which are found in patients with myositis and associated interstitial lung disease and other overlap features.[188] As patients with HIV and HTLV-1 infection may develop an inflammatory myopathy similar to polymyositis,[189] serological testing for HIV and HTLV-1 infection as well as studies of lymphocyte subsets are also indicated, especially in areas where infection with these agents is prevalent. The possibility of an underlying malignancy should be considered, particularly in adults presenting with dermatomyositis but it is rare in patients with juvenile dermatomyositis, connective tissue disease, or inclusion body myositis.[190] The search for a malignancy should include a detailed clinical evaluation, including pelvic and rectal examination, routine haematological and biochemical studies, chest radiography, and mammography in females. In addition, in patients with dysphagia a barium swallow or upper gastrointestinal endoscopy should be performed to exclude carcinoma of the oesophagus or gastro-oesophageal junction before attributing the dysphagia to the myositis.

Cardiac involvement, resulting in arrhythmias, heart block, or congestive cardiac failure may sometimes occur even in patients with isolated polymyositis or dermatomyositis.[183] Electrocardiography, and when appropriate other investigations of cardiac function, should therefore be performed during the active phase of the disease. In addition, assessment of respiratory function should be performed, especially in patients with severe muscle disease or suspected interstitial lung disease.[190 191]

Quantitative assessment of muscle strength in representative upper and lower limb muscle groups using a myometer or isokinetic dynamometer is important in assessing the patient's response to treatment and makes it possible to recognise an upward or downward trend in muscle performance even before there is a change in the patient's functional state or MRC grading.[191] Serial measurements of the serum creatine kinase concentration are also of value in assessing the response to treatment and a rising creatine kinase concentration, even within the normal range, may be the first indication of reactivation of the myositis in a patient who has previously been in remission.[191] Measurements of serum concentrations of myoglobin and of soluble interleukin 2 receptor concentrations in the blood have been reported to be sensitive indicators of disease activity[13 192] but are not widely used.

Muscle fatigue

Chronic or intermittent fatigue and reduced physical endurance in the absence of any abnormality on neurological examination is rarely a symptom of neuromuscular disease and is more often encountered in a setting of depressive illness or the chronic fatigue syndrome which may follow an acute viral illness or develop spontaneously (see box 12.4). However, before reaching such a diagnosis it is important to carry out a detailed clinical evaluation and appropriate laboratory investigations to exclude systemic conditions such as haematological, thyroid, hepatic, or renal disorders as well as neuromuscular or other neurological disorders. In the last two conditions, a detailed examination will usually show some evidence of muscular weakness or pathological fatiguability of the limb or other muscle groups such as the ocular or bulbar muscles in myasthenia gravis or potentiation of muscle strength and of the deep tendon reflexes with repetitive muscle contraction in the Lambert-Eaton myasthenic syndrome.

Confirmation of the diagnosis of a disorder of neuromuscular transmission may be provided by the use of repetitive nerve stimulation studies and single fibre EMG (see above). A positive response to intravenous edrophonium is virtually diagnostic of myasthenia gravis although false positive responses may occasionally occur. Raised titres of ACh receptor antibodies are found in 80 to 90% of patients with generalised myasthenia gravis but only about 50% of patients with ocular disease and are diagnostically helpful when there is a significant increase but normal titres do not exclude the diagnosis.[23] Antibodies to the presynaptic voltage gated calcium channel are found in many cases of the Lambert-Eaton syndrome[193] and react mainly with the P/Q-type of calcium channel.[194]

Patients with myasthenia gravis should be investigated for the presence of a thymoma, which is present in about 15% of cases[195], and those with the Lambert-Eaton syndrome for an underlying bronchogenic or other malignancy, which is present in about two thirds of cases.[196] Both myasthenia gravis and the Lambert-Eaton syndrome may be associated with other autoimmune disorders and patients with both conditions should therefore have a complete autoantibody screen as well as thyroid function tests and haematological studies.[195 197]

Spinal muscular atrophy

Autosomal recessive spinal muscular atrophy was shown in 1990 to link to the proximal long arm of chromosome 5[198 199] with severe type 1 (Werdnig-Hoffman disease), type II, and type III (Kugelberg-Welander syndrome) all mapping to the same region.[200] Homozygous deletions of the survival motor neuron (SMN) gene region were demonstrated in 1995 in the vast majority of cases (98%) (figure 12.5).[51] The deletions can be used for accurate prenatal diagnosis of the condition,[201] more accurately than the previous linkage technique,[202] as new mutations seem to arise at a reasonable high frequency.[52] Such a new mutation rate might be expected in this often lethal recessive condition, unless there has been an as yet unidentified heterozygotous advantage.[203] The fact that the factors controlling severity of disease (which may involve contiguous deletion of neighbouring genes)[204] and that some clinically unaffected parents and siblings of patients with spinal muscular atrophy also show homozygous deletion[205] means that the mechanism of causation of disease has yet to be fully understood. The homozygous deletion of unaffected persons may

387

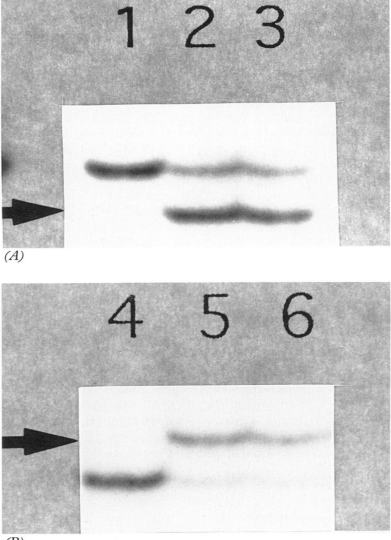

Figure 12.5   *Spinal muscular atrophy SSCP: (A) lanes 1, 2, and 3: SSCP for exon 7 of the survival motor neuron (SMN) gene on chromosome 5: lane 1: proband showing deletion (arrow) of the telomeric gene copy of exon 7; lanes 2 and 3 mother and father not deleted. (B) Lanes 4, 5, and 6: SSCP for exon 8 of the survival motor neuron (SMN) gene on chromosome 5, lane 4: proband showing deletion (arrow) of the telomeric gene copy of exon 8: lanes 5 and 6: mother and father not deleted*

indicate that autosomal recessive spinal muscular atrophy shows incomplete penetrance.

We are grateful to Professor B A Kakulas and Mr R Johnson for providing photomicrographs in figure 12.1, Ms L Kelloway for figure 12.2, Mr M Davis, Ms J Dench, and Ms N Harber for figures 12.3–12.5, and Mrs S Moncrieff for secretarial assistance.

1 Neuromuscular disorders: gene location. *Neuromuscul Disord* 1995;6:I-III.
2 Mitochondrial encephalomyopathies: gene mutation. *Neuromuscul Disord* 1995;6:V-VI.
3 Argov Z, Mastaglia FL. Drug-induced neuromuscular disorders in man. In: Walton JN, Karpati G, Hilton-Jones D, eds. *Disorders of voluntary muscle.* 6th ed. Edinburgh: Churchill Livingstone, 1994:898–1029.
4 Lane RJM, Mastaglia FL. Drug-induced myopathies in man. *Lancet* 1978;ii:562–5.
5 Mastaglia FL. Toxic myopathies. In: Rowland LP, DiMauro S, eds. *Handbook of clinical neurology.* Amsterdam: Elsevier, 1992:595–622.
6 Suarez GA, Kelly JJ. The dropped head syndrome. *Neurology* 1992;42:1625–7.
7 Garlepp MJ, Mastaglia FL. Inclusion body myositis. *J Neurol Neurosurg Psychiatry* 1996;60:251–5.
8 Harvey JM, Mastaglia FL, Zilko PJ, Ojeda VJ, Cheah PS. Scleromyxedema and inflammatory myopathy: a clinicopathological study of three patients. *Aust NZ J Med* 1986;16:329–35.
9 Mastaglia FL, Ojeda VJ, Sarnat HB, Kakulas BA. Myopathies associated with hypothyroidism. A review based upon 13 cases. *Aust NZ J Med* 1988;18:799–806.
10 Griggs RC, Mendell JR, Miller RG. Evaluation and treatment of myopathies. *Contemporary neurology series.* Philadelphia: FA Davis, 1995.
11 Sunohara N, Takagi A, Nonaka I, Sugita H, Satoyoshi E. Idiopathic hyperCKemia. *Neurology* 1984;34:544–7.
12 Tien I, DiMauro S, Rowland LP. Myoglobinuria. In: Rowland LP, DiMauro S, eds. *Handbook of clinical neurology.* Amsterdam: Elsevier, 1992:553–93.
13 Kagen LJ. Myoglobinaemia in inflammatory myopathies. *JAMA* 1977;237:1448–52.
14 Moxley RT. Metabolic and endocrine myopathies. In: Walton JN, Karpati G, Hilton-Jones D, eds. *Disorders of voluntary muscle.* 6th ed. Edinburgh: Churchill Livingstone, 1994:647–716.
15 Argov Z, Bank WJ. Phosphorus magnetic resonance spectroscopy (^{31}pMRS) in neuromuscular disorders. *Ann Neurol* 1991;30:90–7.
16 Moussavi RS, Carson PJ, Boska MD, Weiner MW, Miller RG. Nonmetabolic fatigue in exercising human muscle. *Neurology* 1989;39:1222–6.
17 McKeran RO, Hallidan D, Purkiss P, Royston P. 3-methylhistidine excretion as an index of myofibrillar protein catabolism in neuromuscular disease. *J Neurol Neurosurg Psychiatry* 1979;42:536–41.
18 Nelson TE, Flewellen EH. The malignant hyperthermia syndrome. *New Engl J Med* 1983;309:416–8.
19 Ohkoshi N, Yoshizawa T, Mizusawa H, et al. Malignant hyperthermia in a patient with Becker muscular dystrophy: dystrophin analysis and caffeine contracture study. *Neuromuscul Disord* 1995;5:53–8.
20 Fawcett PRW, Barwick DD. The clinical neurophysiology of neuromuscular disease. In: Walton JN, Karpati G, Hilton-Jones D, eds. *Disorders of voluntary muscle.* 6th ed. Edinburgh: Churchill Livingstone, 1994:1033–104.
21 Mastaglia FL, Papadimitriou JM, Dawkins RL, Beveridge B, Vacuolar myopathy associated with chloroquine, lupus erythematosus and thymoma. *J Neurol Sci* 1977;34:315–28.
22 Desmedt JE, Borenstein S. Double-step nerve stimulation test for myasthenic block: sensitisation of post-activation exhustion by ischaemia. *Ann Neurol* 1977;1:55–60.
23 Engel AG. Myasthenia gravis and myasthenic syndromes. *Ann Neurol* 1984;16:519–34.
24 Tim RW, Sanders DB. Repetitive nerve stimulation studies in the Lambert-Eaton myasthenic syndrome. *Muscle Nerve* 1994;17:995–1001.
25 Grindrod S, Tofts P, Edwards R. Investigation of human skeletal muscle structure and composition by X-ray computerised tomography. *Eur J Clin Invest* 1983;13:465–8.

26 Kiers L. Diabetic muscle infarction: magnetic resonance imaging (MRI) avoids the need for biopsy. *Muscle Nerve* 1995;**18**:129–30.

27 De Visser M, Verbeeten B. Computed tomography of the skeletal musculature in Becker-type muscular dystrophy and benign infantile spinal muscular atrophy. *Muscle Nerve* 1985;**8**:435–44.

28 Pamphlett R. Muscle biopsy. In: Mastaglia FL, Walton JN, eds. *Skeletal muscle pathology.* 2nd ed. Edinburgh: Churchill Livingstone, 1992:95–121.

29 Bönnemann CG, Modi R, Noguchi S, *et al.* β-sarcoglycan (A3b) mutations cause autosomal recessive muscular dystrophy with loss of sarcoglycan complex. *Nature Genet* 1995;**11**:266–73.

30 Beggs AH, Kunkel LM. Improved diagnosis of Duchenne/Becker muscular dystrophy. *J Clin Invest* 1990;**85**:613–9.

31 Hoffman EP, Fischbeck KH, Brown RH, *et al.* Characterization of dystropin in muscle-biopsy specimens from patients with Duchenne's or Becker's muscular dystrophy. *N Engl J Med* 1988;**318**:1363–8.

32 Hoffman EP, Kunkel LM, Angelini C, Clarke A, Johnson M, Harris JB. Improved diagnosis of Becker muscular dystrophy by dystrophin testing. *Neurology* 1989;**39**:1011–7.

33 Piccolo F, Roberds SL, Jeanpierre M, *et al.* Primary adhalinopathy: a common cause of autosomal recessive muscular dystrophy of variable severity. *Nature Genet* 1995;**10**: 243–5.

34 Malhotra SB, Hart KA, Klamut HJ, *et al.* Frame-shift deletions in patients with Duchenne and Becker muscular dystrophy. *Science* 1988;**242**:755–9.

35 Chelly J, Gilgenkrantz H, Lambert M, *et al.* Effect of dystrophin gene deletions on mRNA levels and processing in Duchenne and Becker muscular dystrophies. *Cell* 1990;**63**: 1239–48.

36 Morisaki H, Morisaki T, Newby LK, Holmes EW. Alternative splicing: a mechanism for phenotypic rescue of a common inherited defect. *J Clin Invest* 1993;**91**:2275–80.

37 Collins FS. Positional cloning moves from perditional to traditional. *Nature Genet* 1995;**9**:347–50.

38 Noguchi S, McNally EM, Othmane KB, *et al.* Mutations in the dystrophin-associated protein γ-sarcoglycan in chromosome 13 muscular dystrophy. *Science* 1995;**270**:819–22.

39 Lim LE, Duclos F, Broux O, *et al.* β-sarcoglycan: characterization and role in limb-girdle muscular dystrophy linked to 4q12. *Nature Genet* 1995;**11**:257–65.

40 Evans MI, Greb A, Kunkel LM, *et al.* In utero fetal muscle biopsy for the diagnosis of Duchenne muscular dystrophy. *Am J Obstet Gynecol* 1991;**165**:728–32.

41 Bradley DM, Parsons EP, Clarke AJ. Experience with screening newborns for Duchenne muscular dystrophy in Wales. *BMJ* 1993;**306**:357–60.

42 Greenberg CR, Jacobs HK, Halliday W, Wrogmann K. Three years experience with neonatal screening for Duchenne/Becker muscular dystrophy: gene analysis, gene expression and phenotype prediction. *Am J Med Genet* 1991;**39**:68–75.

43 Ptacek LJ, Tawil R, Griggs RC, *et al.* Dihydropyridine receptor mutations cause hypokalaemic periodic paralysis. *Cell* 1994;**77**:863–8.

44 Mullis KB, Faloona FA. Specific synthesis of DNA in vitro via a polymerase-catalysed chain reaction. *Meth Enzymol* 1987;**155**:335–50.

45 Roberts RG, Bentley DR, Barby TFM, *et al.* Direct diagnosis of carriers of Duchenne and Becker muscular dystrophy by amplification of lymphocyte RNA. *Lancet* 1990; **336**:1523–6.

46 Zeviani M, Amati P, Bresolin N, *et al.* Rapid detection of the A–G mutation of mtDNA in Italian families with myoclonus epilepsy and ragged red fibers: *Am J Hum Genet* 1991;**48**:203–11.

47 Shelbourne P, Winquist R, Kunert E, *et al.* Unstable DNA may be responsible for the incomplete penetrance of the myotonic dystrophy phenotype. *Human Molecular Genetics* 1992;**1**:467–73.

48 Abbs S, Yau SC, Clark S, Mathew CG, Bobrow M. A convenient multiplex PCR system for the detection of dystrophin gene deletions: a comparative analysis with cDNA hybridisation shows mistypings by both methods. *J Med Genet* 1991;**28**:304–11.

49 Chamberlain JS, Gibbs RA, Ranier JE, Nguyen PN, Caskey CT. Deletion screening of the Duchenne muscular dystrophy locus via multiplex DNA amplification. *Nucleic Acids Res* 1988;**16**:11141–56.

50 Chamberlain JS, Gibbs RA, Ranier JE, Caskey CT. Multiplex PCR for the diagnosis of Duchenne muscular dystrophy. In: Innis M, Gelfland D, Sninsky J, White T, eds. *PCR*

protocols: a guide to methods and applications. San Diego: Academic Press, 1990:272–81.

51 Lefebvre S, Burglen L, Reboullet S, *et al.* Identification and characterization of a spinal muscular atrophy-determining gene. *Cell* 1995;**80**:155–65.

52 Rodrigues NR, Owen N, Talbot K, Ignatius J, Dubowitz V, Davies KE. Deletions in the survival motor neuron gene on 5q13 in autosomal recessive spinal muscular atrophy. *Human Molecular Genetics* 1995;**4**:631–4.

53 Lehmann-Horn F, Rüdel R. Hereditary nondystrophic myotonias and periodic paralyses. *Curr Opin Neurol Neurosurg* 1995;**8**:402–10.

54 Wallace DC: Mitochondrial DNA mutations and neuromuscular disease. *TIGS* 1989;**5**:9–13.

55 Suomalainen A, *et al.* Single strand conformation polymorphism analysis of point mutations in human mitochondrial DNA. *J Neurol Sci* 1992;**111**:222–6.

56 Forrest S, Cotton R, Landegren U, Southern E. How to find all those mutations. *Nature Genet* 1995;**10**:375–6.

57 Grompe M. The rapid detection of unknown mutations in nucleic acids. *Nature Genet* 1993;**5**:111–7.

58 Liu Q, Sommer SS. Restriction endonuclease fingerprinting (REF): a sensitive method for screening for mutations in long, contiguous segments of DNA. *Biotechniques* 1995;**18**:470–7.

59 Sarkar G, Yoon H-S, Sommer SS. Dideoxy fingerprinting (ddf): a rapid and efficient screen for the presence of mutations. *Genomics* 1992;**13**:441–3.

60 Mashal RD, Koontz J, Sklar J. Detection of mutations by cleavage of DNA heteroduplexes with bacteriophage resolvases. *Nature Genet* 1995;**9**:177–83.

61 Youil R, Kemper BW, Cotton RGH. Screening for mutations by enzyme mismatch cleavage with T4 endonuclease VII. *Proc Natl Acad Sci USA* 1995;**92**:87–91.

62 Wilton SD, Johnsen RD, Pedretti JR, Laing NG. Two distinct mutations in a single dystrophin gene: identification of an altered splice-site as the primary Becker muscular dystrophy mutation. *Am J Med Genet* 1993;**46**:563–9.

63 Wilton SD, Chandler DC, Kakulas BA, Laing NG. Identification of a point mutation and germinal mosaicism in a Duchenne muscular dystrophy family. *Human Mutation* 1994;**3**:133–40.

64 Chelly J, Gilgenkrantz H, Hugnot JP, *et al.* Illegitimate transcription: application to the analysis of truncated transcripts of the dystrophin gene in nonmuscle cultured cells from Duchenne and Becker patients. *J Clin Invest* 1991;**88**:1161–6.

65 Wallace DC. Mitochondrial diseases: genotype versus phenotype. *TIGS* 1993;**9**:128–33.

66 Prior TW, Papp AC, Snyder PJ, *et al.* A missense mutation in the dystrophin gene in a Duchenne muscular dystrophy patient. *Nature Genet* 1993;**4**:357–60.

67 Wang J, Zhou J, Todorovic SM, *et al.* Molecular genetic and genetic correlations in sodium channelopathies: lack of founder effect and evidence for a second gene. *Am J Hum Genet* 1993;**52**:1074–84.

68 Ohno K, Hutchinson DO, Milone M, *et al.* Congenital myasthenic syndrome caused by prolonged acetylcholine receptor channel openings due to a mutation in the M2 domain of the ε subunit. *Proc Natl Acad Sci USA* 1995;**92**:758–62.

69 Bejaoui K, Hirabayashi K, Hentati F, *et al.* Linkage of Miyoshi myopathy (distal autosomal recessive muscular dystrophy) locus to chromosome 2p12–14. *Neurology* 1995;**45**:768–72.

70 Laing NG, Laing BA, Meredith C, *et al.* Autosomal dominant distal myopathy: linkage to chromosome 14. *Am J Hum Genet* 1995;**56**:422–7.

71 Speer MC, Yamaoka LH, Gilchrist JH, *et al.* Confirmation of genetic heterogeneity in limb-girdle muscular dystrophy: linkage of an autosomal dominant form to chromosome 5q. *Am J Hum Genet* 1992;**50**:1211–7.

72 Yamaoka LH, Westbrook CA, Speer MC, *et al.* Development of a microsatellite genetic map spanning 5q31–33 and subsequent placement of the LGMD1A locus between D5S178 and IL9. *Neuromuscul Disord* 1994;**4**:471–5.

73 Janssen EAM, Hensels GW, van Oost BA, *et al.* The gene for X-linked myotubular myopathy is located in an 8 Mb region at the border of Xq27·3 and Xq28. *Neuromuscul Disord* 1994;**4**:455–61.

74 Brais B, Xie Y-G, Sanson M, Morgan K, *et al.* The oculopharyngeal muscular dystrophy locus maps to the region of the cardiac α and β myosin heavy chain genes on chromosome 14q11·2–q13. *Human Molecular Genetics* 1995;**4**:429–34.

75 Wallgren-Pettersson C, Avela K, Marchand S, *et al.* A gene for autosomal recessive nema-

line myopathy assigned to chromosome 2q by linkage analysis. *Neuromuscul Disord* 1995;5:441–3.

76 McCarthy TV, Healy JMS, Heffron JJA, *et al.* Localization of malignant hyperthermia susceptibility locus to human chromosome 19q12–13·2. *Nature* 1990;343:562–4.

77 Deufel T, Golla A, Iles D, *et al.* Evidence for genetic heterogeneity of malignant hyperthermia susceptibility. *Am J Hum Genet* 1992;50:1151–61.

78 Levitt RC, Nouri N, Jedlicka AE, *et al.* Evidence for genetic heterogeneity in malignant hyperthermia susceptibility. *Genomics* 1991;11:543–7.

79 MacLennan DH. Discordance between phenotype and genotype in malignant hyperthermia. *Curr Opin Neurol Neurosurg* 1995;8:397–401.

80 Powell SM, Petersen GM, Krush AJ, *et al.* Molecular diagnosis of familial adenomatous polyposis. *N Engl J Med* 1993;2:1982–7.

81 Roest PAM, Roberts RG, Sugino S, van Ommen G-JB, den Dunnen JT. Protein truncation test (PTT) for rapid detection of translation-terminating mutations. *Human Molecular Genetics* 1993;2:1719–21.

82 Heim RA, Silverman LM, Kam-Morgan LNW, Luce MC. Screening for truncated NF1 proteins. *Nature Genet* 1994;8:318–9.

83 Heim RA, Kam-Morgan LNW, Binnie CG, *et al.* Distribution of 13 truncating mutations in the neurofibromatosis 1 gene. *Human Molecular Genetics* 1995;4:975–81.

84 Campbell KP. Adhalin gene mutations and autosomal recessive limb-girdle muscular dystrophy. *Ann Neurol* 1995;38:353–4.

85 Byrne E. Mitochondrial DNA abnormalities in human disease. *Med J Aust* 1991;154:646–7.

86 Kakulas BA. The spectrum of dystrophinopathies. In: Lane RJM, ed. *Handbook of muscle disease.* New York: Marcell Dekker 1996 (in press).

87 Van Ommen GJB, Scheuerbrandt G. Neonatal screening for muscular dystrophy. Consensus recommendation of the 14th workshop sponsored by the European Neuromuscular Center (ENMC). *Neuromuscul Disord* 1993;3:231–9.

88 Muntoni F, Mateddu A, Cianchetti C, *et al.* Dystrophin analysis using a panel of antidystrophin antibodies in Duchenne and Becker muscular dystrophy. *J Neurol Neurosurg Psychiatry* 1993;56:26–31.

89 Koenig M, Hoffman EP, Bertelson CJ, Monaco AP, Feener C, Kunkel LM. Complete cloning of the Duchenne muscular dystrophy (DMD) cDNA and preliminary genomic organization of the DMD gene in normal and affected individuals. *Cell* 1987;50:509–17.

90 den Dunnen J, Bakker E, Klein-Breteler E, Pearson P, van Ommen G. Direct detection of more than 50% of the Duchenne muscular dystrophy mutations by field inversion gels. *Nature* 1987;329:640–2.

91 Laing NG, Mears ME, Thomas HE, *et al.* Differentiation of Becker muscular dystrophy from limb-girdle muscular dystrophy and Kugelberg-Welander disease using a cDNA probe. *Med J Aust* 1990;152:270–1.

92 Lunt PW, Cumming WJK, Kingston H, *et al.* DNA probes in differential diagnosis of Becker muscular dystrophy and spinal muscular atrophy. *Lancet* 1989;i:46–7.

93 Norman A, Thomas N, Coakley J, Harper P. Distinction of Becker from limb-girdle muscular dystrophy by means of dystrophin cDNA probes. *Lancet* 1989;i:466–8.

94 Weber JL, May PE. Abundant class of human DNA polymorphisms which can be typed by the polymerase chain reaction. *Am J Hum Genet* 1989;44:388–96.

95 Hejtmancik J, Harris S, Tsao C, Ward P, Caskey C. Carrier diagnosis of Duchenne muscular dystrophy using restriction fragment length polymorphisms. *Neurology* 1986;36:1553–62.

96 Laing NG, Siddique T, Bartlett RJ, *et al.* Duchenne muscular dystrophy: detection of deletion carriers by spectrophotometric densitometry. *Clin Genet* 1989;35:393–8.

97 Mao Y, Cremer M. Detection of Duchenne muscular dystrophy carriers by dosage analysis using the DMD cDNA clone 8. *Hum Genet* 1989;81:193–5.

98 Bartlett RJ, Pericak-Vance MA, Lanman JT, *et al.* Prenatal detection of an inherited Duchenne muscular dystrophy deletion allele. *Neurology* 1987;37:355–6.

99 Abbs S, Bobrow M. Analysis of quantitative PCR for the diagnosis of deletion and duplication carriers in the dystrophin gene. *J Med Genet* 1992;29:191–6.

100 Ioannou P, Christopoulos G, Panayides K, Kleanthous M, Middleton L. Detection of Duchenne and Becker muscular dystrophy carriers by quantitative multiplex polymerase chain reaction analysis. *Neurology* 1992;42:1783–90.

101 Beggs AH, Hoffman EP, Snyder JR, *et al.* Exploring the molecular basis for variability

INVESTIGATION OF MUSCLE DISEASE

among patients with Becker muscular dystrophy: dystrophin gene and protein studies.
Am J Hum Genet 1991;49:54–7.
102 Sunohara N, Arahata K, Hoffman EP, *et al*. Quadriceps myopathy: forme fruste of Becker muscular dystrophy. *Ann Neurol* 1990;28:634–9.
103 Gospe SM, Lazaro RP, Lava NS, Grootscholten BS, Scott MO, Fischbeck KH. Familial X-linked myalgia and cramps: a non-progressive myopathy associated with a deletion in the dystrophin gene. *Neurology* 1989;39:1277–80.
104 Malapert D, Recan D, Leturcq F, Degos JD, Gherardi RK. Sporadic lower limb hypertrophy and exercise induced myalgia in a woman with dystrophin gene deletion. *J Neurol Neurosurg Psychiatry* 1995;59:552–4.
105 Servidei S, Manfredi G, Mirabella M, *et al*. Familial hyperCKemia can be a variant of Becker muscular dystrophy. *Neurology* 1993;43:A293.
106 Piccolo G, Azan G, Tonin P, *et al*. Dilated cardiomyopathy requiring cardiac transplantation as initial manifestation of Xp21 Becker type muscular dystrophy. *Neuromuscul Disord* 1994;4:143–6.
107 Yoshida K, Ikeda S-I, Nakamura A, *et al*. Molecular analysis of the Duchenne muscular dystrophy gene in patients with Becker muscular dystrophy presenting with dilated cardiomyopathy. *Muscle Nerve* 1993;16:1161–6.
108 Beckmann JS, Richard I, Hillaire D, *et al*. A gene for limb-girdle muscular dystrophy maps to chromosome 15 by linkage. *C R Acad Sci (Paris)* 1991;312:141–8.
109 Fougerousse F, Broux O, Richard I, *et al*. Mapping of a chromosome 15 region involved in limb girdle muscular dystrophy. *Human Molecular Genetics* 1994;3:285–93.
110 Richard I, Broux O, Allamand V, *et al*. Mutations in the proteolytic enzyme calpain 3 cause limb-girdle muscular dystrophy type 2A. *Cell* 1995;81:27–40.
111 Matsumura K, Nonaka I, Campbell KP. Abnormal expression of dystrophin-associated proteins in Fukuyama-type congenital muscular dystrophy. *Lancet* 1993;341:521–2.
112 Tome FMS, Evangelista T, Leclerc A, *et al*. Congenital muscular dystrophy with merosin deficiency. *C R Acad Sci (Paris)* 1994;317:351–7.
113 Bashir R, Strachan T, Keers S, *et al*. A gene for autosomal recessive limb-girdle muscular dystrophy, maps to chromosome 2p. *Human Molecular Genetics* 1994;3:455–7.
114 Speer MC, Yamaoka LH, Gilchrist JM, *et al*. Evidence for genetic heterogeneity in the dominant form of limb-girdle muscular dystrophy. *Am J Hum Genet* 1993;53:A1082.
115 Matsumura K, Tome FMS, Collin H, *et al*. Deficiency of the 50K dystrophin-associated glycoprotein in severe childhood autosomal recessive muscular dystrophy. *Nature* 1992;359:320–2.
116 Ljunggren A, Duggan D, McNally E, *et al*. Primary adhalin deficiency as a cause of muscular dystrophy in patients with normal dystrophin. *Ann Neurol* 1995;38:367–72.
117 Roberds SL, Leturq F, Allamand V, *et al*. Missense mutations in the adhalin gene linked to autosomal recessive muscular dystrophy. *Cell* 1994;78:625–33.
118 Arahata K, Ishii H, Hayashi YK. Congenital muscular dystrophies. *Curr Opin Neurol Neurosurg* 1995;8:385–90.
119 Helbling-Leclerc A, Zhang X, Topaloglu H, *et al*. Mutations in the laminin a2-chain gene (LAMA2) cause merosin-deficient congenital muscular dystrophy. *Nature Genet* 1995;11:216–8.
120 Toda T, Segawa M, Nomura Y, *et al*. Localization of a gene for Fukuyama type congenital muscular dystrophy to chromosome 9q31–33. *Nature Genet* 1993;5:283–6.
121 Toda T, Yoshioka M, Nakahori Y, *et al*. Genetic identity of Fukuyama-type congenital muscular dystrophy and Walker-Warburg syndrome. *Ann Neurol* 1995;37:99–101.
122 Wijmenga C, Frants RR, Brouwer OF, Moerer P, Weber JL, Padberg GW. Localisation of facioscapulohumeral muscular dystrophy gene on chromosome 4. *Lancet* 1990;336:651–3.
123 Wijmenga C, Brouwer OF, Padberg GW, Frants RR. Transmission of de novo mutation associated with facioscapulohumeral muscular dystrophy. *Lancet* 1992;340:985–6.
124 Wijmenga C, Hewitt JE, Sandkuijl LA, *et al*. Chromosome 4q DNA rearrangements associated with facioscapulohumeral muscular dystrophy. *Nature Genet* 1992;2:26–30.
125 Weiffenbach B, Dubois J, Storvick D, *et al*. Mapping the facioscapulohumeral muscular dystrophy gene is complicated by chromosome 4q35 recombination events. *Nature Genet* 1993;4:165–9.
126 Gilbert JR, Stajich JM, Wall S, *et al*. Evidence for heterogeneity in facioscapulohumeral muscular dystrophy (FSHD). *Am J Hum Genet* 1993;53:401–8.
127 Bione S, Maestrini E, Rivella S, *et al*. Identification of a novel X-linked gene responsible

393

for Emery-Dreifuss muscular dystrophy. *Nature Genet* 1994;8:323–7.

128 Laing NG. Inherited disorders of contractile proteins in skeletal and cardiac muscle. *Curr Opin Neurol Neurosurg* 1995;8:391–6.

129 Hageman ATM, Gabreëls, Liem KD, Renkawek K, Boon JM. Congenital myotonic dystrophy; a report on thirteen cases and a review of the literature. *J Neurol Sci* 1993;115:95–101.

130 Harper PS. *Myotonic dystrophy. Major problems in neurology.* Vol 9. Philadelphia: WB Saunders, 1979.

131 Serisier DE, Mastaglia FL, Gibson GJ. Respiratory muscle function and ventilatory control I in patients with motor neurone disease, II in patients with myotonic dystrophy. *Q J Med* 1982;202:205–26.

132 Viitasalo MT, Kala R, Karli P, Eisalo A. Ambulatory electro-cardiographic recording in mild or moderate myotonic dystrophy and myotonia congenita (Thomsen's disease). *J Neurol Sci* 1983;62:181–90.

1338 Winters SJ, Schreiner B, Griggs RC, Rowley P, Nanda NC. Familial mitral valve prolapse and myotonic dystrophy. *Ann Intern Med* 1976;85:19–22.

134 Buxton J, Shelbourne P, Davies J, *et al.* Detection of an unstable fragment of DNA specific to individuals with myotonic dystrophy. *Nature* 1992;355:547–8.

135 Fu Y-H, Pizzuti A, Fenwick Jr RG, *et al.* An unstable triplet repeat in a gene related to myotonic muscular dystrophy. *Science* 1992;255:1256–8.

136 Mahadevan M, Tsilfidis C, Sabourin L, *et al.* Myotonic dystrophy mutation: an unstable CTG repeat in the 3' untranslated region of the gene. *Science* 1992;255:1253–5.

137 Reardon W, Harley HG, Brook JD, *et al.* Minimal expression of myotonic dystrophy: a clinical and molecular analysis. *J Med Genet* 1992;29:770–3.

138 Ricker K, Koch MC, Lehmann-Horn F, *et al.* Proximal myotonic myopathy. *Neurology* 1994;44:1448–52.

139 Thornton CA, Griggs RC, Moxley RT. Myotonic dystrophy with no trinucleotide repeat expansion. *Ann Neurol* 1994;35:269–72.

140 Sun SF, Streib EW. Autosomal recessive generalised myotonia. *Muscle Nerve* 1983;6:143–7.

141 Becker PE. Syndromes associated with myotonia: clinical-genetic classification. In: Rowland LP, ed. *Pathogenesis of human muscular dystrophies.* Amsterdam: Excerpta Medica 1977:699–705.

142 Hudson AJ, Ebers GC, Bulman DE. The skeletal muscle sodium and chloride channel diseases. *Brain* 1995;118:547–63.

143 Ricker K, Moxley RT, Heine R, Lehmann-Horn F. Myotonia fluctuans. A third type of muscle sodium channel disease. *Arch Neurol* 1994;51:1095–102.

144 Campa JA, Sanders DB. Familial hypokalaemic periodic paralysis. *Arch Neurol* 1974;31:110–5.

145 Links TP, Smit AJ, Molenaar WM, Zwarts MJ, Oosterhyis HJGH. Familial hypokalaemic period paralysis. Clinical, diagnostic and therapeutic aspects. *J Neurol Sci* 1994;122:33–44.

146 McManis PG, Lambert EH, Daube JR. The exercise test in periodic paralysis. *Muscle Nerve* 1986;9:704–10.

147 Kantola IM, Tarssanen LT. Diagnosis of familial hypokalemic periodic paralysis: role of the potassium exercise test. *Neurology* 1992;42:2158–61.

148 Elbaz A, Vale-Santos J, Jurkat-Rott K, *et al.* Hypokalaemic periodic paralysis and the dihydropyridine receptor (CACNL1A3): genotype/phenotype correlations for two predominant mutations and evidence for the absence of a founder effect in 16 Caucasian families. *Am J Hum Genet* 1995;56:374–80.

149 Jurkat-Rott K, Lehmann-Horn F, Elbaz A, *et al.* A calcium channel mutation causing hypokalaemic periodic paralysis. *Human Molecular Genetics* 1994;3:1415–9.

150 Ptacek LJ, Trimmer JS, Agnew WS, *et al.* Paramyotonia congenita and hyperkalaemic periodic paralysis map to the same sodium channel gene locus. *Am J Hum Genet* 1991;49:851–4.

151 Rojas CV, Wang J, Schwarts LS, Hoffman EP, Powell BR, Brown RHJ. A MET to VAL mutation in the skeletal muscle Na$^+$ channel α- subunit in hyperkalaemic periodic paralysis. *Nature* 1991;354:387–9.

152 Baquero JL, Ayala RA, Wang J, *et al.* Hyperkalemic periodic paralysis with cardiac dysrhythmia: a novel sodium channel mutation? *Ann Neurol* 1995;37:408–11.

153 Tawil R, Ptacek LJ, Pavlakis SG, *et al.* Andersen's syndrome: potassium-sensitive peri-

odic paralysis, ventricular ectopy, and dysmorphic features. *Ann Neurol* 1994;**35**:326–30.

154 Fardeau M. Congenital myopathies. In: Mastaglia FL, Walton JN, eds. *Skeletal muscle pathology*. 2nd ed. Edinburgh: Churchill Livingstone, 1992:237–81.

155 Sarnat HB. New insights into the pathogenesis of congenital myopathies. *J Child Neurol* 1994;**9**:193–201.

156 Laing NG, Majda BT, Akkari PA, *et al.* Assignment of a gene (NEM1) for autosomal dominant nemaline myopathy to chromosome 1. *Am J Hum Genet* 1992;**50**:576–83.

157 Laing NG, Wilton SD, Akkari PA, *et al.* A mutation in the α-tropomyosin gene TPM3 associated with autosomal dominant nemaline myopathy. *Nature Genet* 1995;**9**:75–9.

158 Beggs AH, Byers TJ, Knoll JHM, Boyce FM, Bruns GAP, Kunkel L. Cloning and characterization of two human skeletal muscle alpha-actinin genes on chromosome one and eleven. *J Biol Chem* 1992;**267**:9281–8.

159 Haan EA, Freemantle CJ, McCure JA, Friend KL, Mulley JC. Assignment of the gene for central core disease to chromosome 19. *Hum Genet* 1990;**86**:187–90.

160 Kausch K, Lehmann-Horn F, Janka M, Wieringa B, Grimm T, Muller CR. Evidence for linkage of the central core disease locus to the proximal long arm of human chromosome 19. *Genomics* 1991;**10**:765–9.

161 Quane KA, Healy JMS, Keating KE, *et al.* Mutations in the ryanodine receptor gene in central core disease and malignant hyperthermia. *Nature Genet* 1983;**5**:51–5.

162 Quane KA, Keating KE, Healy JMS, *et al.* Mutation screening of the RYR1 gene in malignant hyperthermia: detection of a novel tyr-ser mutation in a pedigree with associated central cores. *Genomics* 1994;**23**:236–9.

163 Zhang Y, Chen HS, Khanna VK, *et al.* A mutation in the human ryanodine receptor gene associated with central core disease. *Nature Genet* 1993;**5**:46–50.

164 Holt IJ, Harding AE, Morgan-Hughes JA. Deletions of muscle mitochondrial DNA in patients with mitochondrial myopathies. *Nature* 1988;**331**:717–9.

165 Wallace DC, Singh G, Lott MT, *et al.* Mitochondrial DNA mutations associated with Leber's hereditary optic neuropathy. *Science* 1988;**242**:1427–30.

166 Jackson MJ, Schaefer JA, Johnson MA, Morris AAM, Turnbull DM, Bindoff LA. Presentation and clinical investigation of mitochondrial respiratory chain disease. *Brain* 1995;**118**:339–57.

167 Johns DR. Mitochondrial DNA and disease. *New Engl J Med* 1995;**333**:638–44.

168 Morgan-Hughes JA. Mitochondrial diseases. In: Mastaglia FL, Walton JN, eds. *Skeletal muscle pathology*. 2nd ed. Edinburgh: Churchill Livingstone, 1992:367–424.

169 DiMauro S, Moraes CT. Mitochondrial encephalomyopathies. *Arch Neurol* 1993; **50**:1197–208.

170 Hammans SR, Sweeney MG, Hanna MG, Brackington M, Morgan-Hughes JA, Harding AE. The mitochondrial DNA transfer RNA$^{Leu(UUR)}$ A→G$^{(3243)}$ mutation. A clinical and genetic study. *Brain* 1995;**118**:721–34.

171 Mechler F, Johnson MA, Mastaglia FL, *et al.* Mitochondrial myopathies. A clinico-pathological study of cases with and without extra-ocular muscle involvement. *Aust NZ J Med* 1986;**16**:185–92.

172 Zeviani M, Moraes CT, DiMauro S, *et al.* Deletions of mitochondrial DNA in Kearns-Sayre syndrome. *Neurology* 1988;**38**:1339–46.

173 Zeviani M, Servidei S, Gellera C, Bertini E, DiMauro S, DiDonato S. An autosomal dominant disorder with multiple deletions of mitochondrial DNA starting at the D-loop region. *Nature* 1989;**339**:309–11.

174 Suomalainen A, Kaukonen J, Amati P, *et al.* An autosomal locus predisposing to deletions of mitochondrial DNA. *Nature Genet* 1995;**5**:146–51.

175 Mechler F, Fawcett PRW, Mastaglia FL, Hudson P. Mitochondrial myopathy: a study of clinically affected and asymptomatic members of a six-generation family. *J Neurol Sci* 1981;**50**:191–200.

176 Ozawa M, Goto Y-I, Sakuta R, Tanno Y, Tsuji S, Nonaka I. The 8,344 mutation in mitochondrial DNA: a comparison between the proportion of mutant DNA and clinico-pathological findings. *Neuromuscul Disord* 1995;**5**:483–8.

177 Johnson MA, Bindoff LA, Turnbull DM. Cytochrome c oxidase activity in single muscle fibres: assay techniques and diagnostic applications. *Ann Neurol* 1993;**33**:28–35.

178 Hammans SR, Sweeney MG, Wicks DAG, Morgan-Hughes JA, Harding AE. A molecular genetic study of focal histochemical defects in mitochondrial encephalomyopathies. *Brain* 1992;**115**:343–65.

179 Kawai H, Akaike M, Yokoi K, *et al.* Mitochondrial encephalomyopathy with autosomal

dominant inheritance: a clinical and genetic entity of mitochondrial diseases. *Muscle Nerve* 1995;**18**:753–60.

180 Cheng S, Higuchi R, Stoneking M. Complete mitochondrial genome amplification. *Nature Genet* 1994;**7**:350–1.

181 Howell N, Kubacka I, Halvorson S, *et al*. Phylogenetic analysis of the mitochondrial genomes from Leber hereditary optic neuropathy pedigrees. *Genetics* 1995;**140**:285–302.

182 Lertrit P, Kapsa RMI, Jean-Francois MJB, *et al*. Mitochondrial DNA polymorphism in disease: a possible contributor to respiratory dysfunction. *Human Molecular Genetics* 1994;**3**:1973–81.

183 DiMauro S, Tonin P, Servidei S. Metabolic myopathies. In: Rowland LP, DiMauro S, eds. *Handbook of clinical neurology*. Amsterdam: Elsevier, 1992:479–526.

184 MacLennan DH, Duff C, Zorzato F, *et al*. Ryanodine receptor gene is a candidate for predisposition to malignant hyperthermia. *Nature* 1990;**343**:559–61.

185 Zorzato F, Fujii J, Otsu K, *et al*. Molecular cloning of cDNA encoding human and rabbit forms of the Ca^{2+} release channel (ryanodine receptor) of skeletal muscle. *J Biol Chem* 1990;**265**:2244–56.

186 Arahata K, Engel AG. Monoclonal antibody analysis of mononuclear cells in myopathies. I. Quantitation of subsets according to diagnosis and sites of accumulation and demonstration and counts of muscle fibers invaded by T cells. *Ann Neurol* 1984;**16**:193–208.

187 Karpati G, Carpenter S. Pathology of the inflammatory myopathies. In: Mastaglia FL, ed. *Inflammatory myopathies. Bailliere's Clinical Neurology* 1993;**2/3**:527–56.

188 Bernstein RM. Autoantibodies in myositis. In: Mastaglia FL, ed. *Inflammatory myopathies. Bailliere's Clinical Neurology* 1993;**2/3**:599–615.

189 Dalakas MC, Pezeshpour GH. Neuromuscular diseases associated with human immunodeficiency virus infection. *Ann Neurol* 1988;**23**(suppl):S38–S48.

190 Mastaglia FL, Ojeda VJ. Inflammatory myopathies: Part I. *Ann Neurol* 1985;**17**:215–27.

191 Mastaglia FL, Laing BA, Zilko P. Treatment of inflammatory myopathies. In: Mastaglia FL, ed. *Inflammatory myopathies. Bailliere's Clinical Neurology* 1993;**2/3**:717–40.

192 Woolf RE, Baethge BA. Interleukin-1α, interleukin-2 and soluble interleukin-2 receptors in polymyositis. *Arth Rheum* 1990;**33**:1007–14.

193 Leys K, Lang B, Johnston I, Newsom-Davis J. Calcium channel autoantibodies in the Lambert-Eaton myasthenic syndrome. *Ann Neurol* 1991;**29**:307–14.

194 Lennon VA, Kryzer TJ, Griesmann GE, *et al*. Calcium-channel antibodies in the Lambert-Eaton syndrome and other paraneoplastic syndromes. *N Engl J Med* 1995;**332**:1467–74.

195 Drachman DB, Kuncl RW. Myasthenia gravis. In: Hohlfeld R, ed. *Immunology of neuromuscular disease*, Dordrecht: Kluwer Academic Publications, 1994:165–207.

196 O'Neill JH, Murray NM, Newsom-Davis J. The Lambert-Eaton syndrome. A review of 50 cases. *Brain* 1988;**111**:577–96.

197 Vincent A, Newsom-Davis J. Immunology of the motor nerve terminal. In: Hohlfeld R, ed. *Immunology of neuromuscular disease*. Dordrecht: Kluwer Academic Publications, 1994:147–63.

198 Brzustowicz LM, Lehner T, Castilla LH, *et al*. Genetic mapping of chronic childhood-onset spinal muscular atrophy to chromosome 5q11.2–13.3. *Nature* 1990;;**344**:540–1.

199 Melki J, Sheth P, Abdelhak S, *et al*. Investigators at FSMA. Mapping acute (type I) spinal muscular atrophy to chromosome 5q12–q14. *Lancet* 1990;**336**:271–3.

200 Gilliam TC, Brzustowicz LM, Castilla LH, *et al*. Genetic homogeneity between acute and chronic forms of spinal muscular atrophy. *Nature* 1990;**345**:823–5.

201 Rodrigues NR, Campbell L, Owen N, Rodeck CH, Davies KE. Prenatal diagnosis of spinal muscular atrophy by gene deletion analysis. *Lancet* 1995;**345**:1049.

202 Morrison KE, Daniels RJ, Suthers GK, *et al*. Two novel microsatellite markers for prenatal prediction of spinal muscular atrophy (SMA). *Hum Genet* 1993;**92**:133–8.

203 Gelehrter TD, Collins FS. *Principles of medical genetics*. Baltimore: Williams and Wilkins, 1990.

204 Roy N, Mahadevan MS, McLean M, *et al*. The gene for neuronal apoptosis inhibitory protein (NAIP) is partially deleted in individuals with spinal muscular atrophy. *Cell* 1995;**80**:167–78.

205 Hahnen E, Forkert R, Marke C, *et al*. Molecular analysis of candidate genes on chromosomes 5q13 in autosomal recessive spinal muscular atrophy: evidence of homozygous deletions of the SMN gene in unaffected individuals. *Human Molecular Genetics* 1995;**4**:1927–33.

13 Investigation of the neurogenic bladder

CLARE J FOWLER

Methods of examination which have been used to investigate the neurogenic bladder include tests of bladder function, so-called "urodynamics", and neurophysiological tests of sphincter and pelvic floor innervation. A possible consequence of a neurogenic bladder is damage to the upper urinary tract but the investigation of such complications is essentially urological and is only briefly mentioned in this review.

History of the development of investigations

Urodynamics

The term "urodynamics" encompasses any investigation of urinary tract function although it is often used colloquially as a synonym for cystometry. Cystometry, the measurement of bladder pressure, has been the main tool used to show abnormal behaviour of the neurogenic bladder.

The earliest reference to a study measuring bladder pressure is commonly given as the paper by Mosso and Pellacani published in 1882.[1] With a water manometer they showed that bladder pressure rose at the start of micturition and then gradually declined but that during storage the pressure measured within the organ gave little indication of what volume it contained. However, the paper which described a technique for cystometry producing what is regarded as the precursor of modern day urodynamic recordings was published in *Brain* in 1933 by Denny-Brown and Robertson[2] from the National Hospital for Nervous Diseases, Queen Square.

397

Using an ingenious system of mirror manometers they recorded intravesical and intraurethral pressure with two transurethral catheters (one inside the other), as well as recording rectal, perineal, and abdominal wall pressures in three neurologically normal men. From their findings they defined the physiological sequence of processes which occur with bladder filling, the initiation of micturition, and voiding to completion.

The introduction of cystometry into clinical practice was gradual and by the 1960s it was being used in only a few specialised urological centres.[3] When commercial equipment first became available it consisted of a series of pen recorders which recorded pressure changes as analogue signals but with the advances in electronics and development of microchip technology the machines have become progressively more complex, more "intelligent", and mostly easier to use. Today measured pressures are digitised allowing on line, real time computer analysis of signals.

During the development of urodynamics an important advance came with the introduction of facilities to record pressure measurements superimposed on the fluoroscopic appearances of the bladder, a "videocystometrogram".[4] This combination provides a complete picture of the behaviour of the bladder both during filling and emptying although it has the disadvantages of expense and exposure of the patient to x rays. However, much can be learnt from simple cystometry alone and it is this investigation which is now a standard facility in almost every district general hospital with a urology department.

The hydrodynamic problems of measuring fluid flow are different from measuring pressure within an organ. Introduction of simple and cheap equipment for measuring urinary flow rate[5] has led to this becoming routine; combined with ultrasound measurement of the postmicturition residual volume, it provides a simple noninvasive means by which much valuable information can be obtained about lower urinary tract function.

Neurophysiological investigations

Various types of neurophysiological investigation of the pelvic floor and the sphincters have been developed over the years. A neurophysiological method for recording the bulbocavernosus reflex, regarded as clinically valuable in assessing patients with neurogenic bladder disorders, was first reported in 1967.[6] Neurophysiological recordings of various pelvic floor reflexes were much in vogue in the 1970s but have since lapsed and have been transiently replaced by an enthusiasm for recording the pudendal evoked potential.

Recording from the striated muscle of the urethral sphincter or anal sphincter during cystometry was first recommended as a means of detecting inappropriate sphincter contraction during detrusor contraction, the disorder known as detrusor sphincter dyssynergia.[7] However, for several reasons this type of kinesiological EMG is now little used although sphincter EMG performed as a separate neurophysiological test remains a valuable investigation in some circumstances.

Principle underlying investigations

Cystometry

Cystometry is the recording of the pressure-volume relation of the bladder. The intravesical pressure is measured and by subtracting the intra-abdominal pressure from this figure an estimate of the true pressure produced by the smooth muscle of the detrusor is obtained. This is best seen by looking at the preparatory stages of cystometric recordings when the patient is asked to cough (figure 13.1). Coughing raises the intra-abdominal pressure and thus the measured intravesical pressure but under physiological conditions the detrusor does not then contract so that the derived detrusor pressure (pdet) remains unchanged or becomes slightly negative because the intra-abdominal pressure may rise more than the intravesical pressure. To measure the intravesical and intrabdominal pressures a fine catheter is passed through the urethra into the bladder and another into the rectum. The catheter used to monitor intravesical pressure is passed together with a somewhat wider diameter catheter through which the bladder is filled. Important information is obtained if detrusor pressure is measured both during filling and while the patient attempts to micturate. In the interests of saving time an unphysiologically rapid rate of filling of 50 ml/min is commonly used in cystometric studies.

Recently, methods have become available for recording bladder pressures over periods of many hours and the bladder is left to fill naturally, so-called "ambulatory urodynamics".[8]

In patients with neurogenic incontinence the commonest finding is of an abrupt rise in detrusor pressure which the patient is unable to suppress and which is usually accompanied by reports of

399

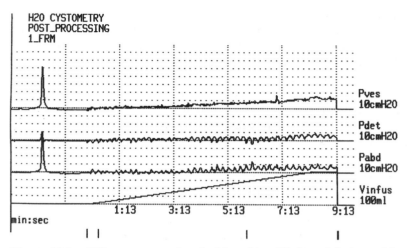

Figure 13.1   *Filling cystometry in a healthy subject. Vinfus = infusion at 50 ml/min; Pabd = intra-abdominal pressure measured by the rectal line; Pves = intravesical pressure; Pdet = Pves-Pabd. Respiratory movements, which were not recorded with the intravesical pressure measurements, were recorded with the rectal pressure line so that these appear as an artefact due to subtraction on Pdet. In the early part of the trace the subject was asked to cough and the subtraction of Pabd from Pves was complete so that no rise in Pdet is recorded*

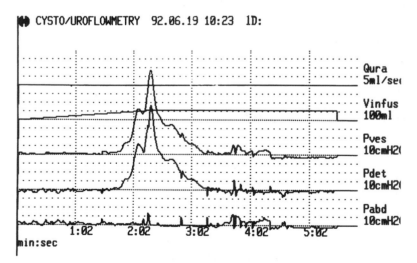

Figure 13.2   *Detrusor hyperreflexia in a woman with multiple sclerosis. After filling to 100 ml (Vinfus) there was a detrusor contraction which resulted in a pressure rise of 90 cm H_2O*

400

urinary urgency (figure 13.2). If the patient is recognised as having a neurological condition, this is called "detrusor hyperreflexia", the condition is otherwise referred to as "detrusor instability"[9]—the cystometric changes in the two conditions being indistinguishable. The cause of detrusor instability is unknown but the weight of opinion is shifting from thinking that it has a psychogenic cause or is due to an occult neurological lesion to the view that it may be due to a disorder of the detrusor muscle itself.[10] Likewise the causes of failure of bladder emptying cannot be identified from cystometry, and urological and neurological disorders can cause indistinguishable cystometric abnormality. Because bladder behaviour cannot always be predicted from the patient's history it has been argued that urodynamic investigations are important in the investigation of urinary complaints but the failure of urodynamics to provide anything more than a description of bladder dysfunction has not been properly acknowledged. This has resulted in a large body of medical literature in which patients are classified according to their urodynamic findings rather than by the underlying pathophysiological cause and diagnosis.

In patients with suspected obstruction of outflow, particularly men with prostatic hypertrophy, measurement of detrusor pressure during voiding is important. This, together with urinary flow rate provides information about the outflow tract[11] and an estimate of the presence of obstruction can be made (figure 13.3).

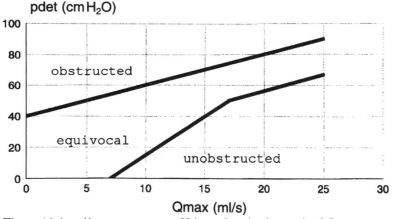

Figure 13.3   *Abrams nomogram. Using values for the maximal flow (Qmax) and the corresponding voiding detrusor pressure (Pdet) a point can be plotted on the nomogram that determines whether the bladder outlet is obstructed, unobstructed, or equivocally abstructed*

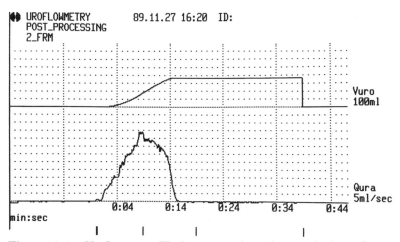

Figure 13.4   *Uroflowmetry. The lower trace shows the rate of urinary flow, which reaches a maximum of 40 ml/s in three seconds and then declines. The upper trace is the result of integrating the flow rate and shows that a total of 275 ml was passed*

Uroflowmetry

Uroflowmetry is the measurement of urinary flow rate. This is a non-invasive investigation. The patient presents with a full bladder and voids into a receptacle in the base of which is a spinning wheel. Urinary flow slows the rate of rotation and from this a graphical output of flow rate can be obtained (figure 13.4).

Abnormalities of flow can be due to local urological problems such as prostatic hypertrophy, or a urethral stricture, or neurogenic disorders of the bladder outlet mechanism. Detrusor sphinc-

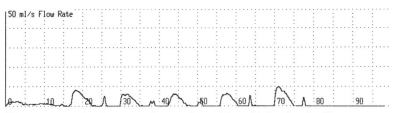

Figure 13.5   *Uroflowmetry in a patient with multiple sclerosis. He was paraparetic and had frequency and urgency but also symptoms of difficulty voiding and was shown to have incomplete bladder emptying. This interrupted flow pattern is the result of contractions of the striated urethral sphincter occurring during the detrusor contraction—that is, "detrusor sphincter dyssynergia"*

ter dyssynergia, which occurs with spinal cord disease, is a common example of this, and results in interrupted flow (figure 13.5). Uroflowmetry combined with ultrasound scanning of the postmicturition residual volume is used as a screening test to exclude serious outflow obstruction and can also provide information for planning bladder management in patients with neurological disease.

Ultrasound scanning of the urinary tract

The residual volume left after voiding is important, and can readily be measured with a small inexpensive ultrasound scanner. Great precision is not needed—it is simply enough to know whether there is more or less than 100 ml—an obvious abnormality on ultrasound scanning which does not need great expertise to recognise. Most scanners have cursors that can be placed on the black outline of the urine in the bladder and from this, assuming a spherical shape to the bladder, bladder volume can be calculated.

Ultrasound scanning has largely overtaken intravenous urography as the method of choice to examine the upper renal tract to detect dilatation, but intravenous urography remains the preferred method to look for ureteric stones. With modern, highly complex three dimensional scanning, details of the structure of the lower urinary tract can be discerned.[12] This has exciting possibilities for both urologists and urogynaecologists.

Neurophysiological investigations of the sphincters and pelvic floor

Clinical neurophysiological techniques for examining the pelvic floor have been used for many years. These studies have greatly enhanced our understanding of the physiological and pathophysiological mechanisms of neural control of the lower urinary tract.

The first neurophysiological measurements made were of sacral reflexes starting with the bulbocavernosus reflex.[6 13] To record this reflex either a surface or a needle electrode was placed over or in the bulbocavernosus muscle and electrical stimuli were applied to the dorsal nerve of the penis. The time taken for the reflex contraction of the muscle to occur after the stimulus was measured. After the introduction of this technique various other pelvic floor reflex contractions were recorded[14] and it was shown that equally useful responses could be obtained by recording from the urethral or anal sphincter or other parts of the striated muscle of the pelvic floor.[15-17] It was argued that abnormalities of the sacral roots, both efferent and afferent, would lead to a delay in this reflex and this did indeed prove to be the case in patients with established cauda equina lesions.[13 18 19] However, it was found that reflex responses could still be elicited in patients with partial cauda equina lesions[20] and more importantly these tests were of little value when applied to patients with uncertain neurological lesions presenting with hypocontractile bladders or impotence. The explanation for this is probably that, as with other reflexes measured using clinical neurophysiological techniques only the responses mediated by large myelinated fibres are recorded. The small myelinated or unmyelinated fibres which either innervate the smooth muscle or constitute the functionally important afferent nerve supply of the region are not tested. Possibly tests of the autonomic innervation of the genital region will prove more useful.[21]

Recording the pudendal evoked potential is similar to recording tibial evoked potentials. The same cortical recording electrodes can be used and it is advisable to record the tibial evoked responses first to familiarise the patient with the technique. The patient is then asked to hold the stimulating electrode on the dorsal nerve of the penis or clitoris and a similar number of stimuli as needed for obtaining the tibial evoked potentials are given. Surprisingly the latency of tibial and pudendal responses is similar despite the difference in conduction distance. This is thought to be due to the slower conduction velocity of the pudendal afferents compared with fast conducting muscle afferents which respond when the tibial nerve at the ankle is stimulated.[22]

The introduction of a method to record the pudendal evoked potential was initially hailed as promising.[23] It was considered that this would provide a means of testing the afferent innervation from the sacral region and certainly the responses were delayed in patients with conditions such as multiple sclerosis.[24-26] Like the lower limb somatosensory evoked potentials, the pudendal evoked potential is delayed if there is spinal cord disease but this is also usually apparent on clinical examination. Recent studies have shown that the pudendal evoked potential is very rarely abnormal unless there are other clinical signs of neurological disease[27-29] and furthermore if the lesion is predominantly unilateral the pudendal evoked potential can be within normal limits.[29] It seems that there is little diagnostic gain in recording the pudendal evoked potential although it is sometimes reassuring to show that it is normal in patients in whom neurological problems are suspected.

A technique for measurement of the terminal motor latency of the pudendal and perineal nerves (PTML) was devised at St Mark's Hospital.[30] It has been used to show pathophysiological changes in these nerves in women with faecal,[30] urinary,[31] or double incontinence.[32] The pudendal nerve is stimulated transrectally near the ischial spine through the wall of the rectum using an electrode mounted on the tip of the examiner's finger. An electrode is mounted at the base of the finger, which records from the anal sphincter, and a ring electrode mounted on a Foley catheter can be used to record from the periurethral striated muscle. The latency of the response has been found to be prolonged in women with urinary stress incontinence after childbirth and women with faecal incontinence due to sphincter weakness. It is thought that stretching of the nerves during parturition and also with straining at defaecation in chronic constipation results in pudendal nerve injury.[33] Although of considerable research value this test is not used in the routine assessment of women with urinary stress incontinence, nor has it proved to be as useful as electromyography of the anal sphincter in the assessment of faecal incontinence.[34]

Electromyography (EMG) of the striated musculature of the pelvic floor is of value in recognising changes of denervation and chronic reinnervation in patients with cauda equina lesions as well those with suspected multiple system atrophy. A single fibre needle may be used to show changes in fibre density[35] or a concentric needle electrode to show changes in configuration of individual motor units which result from reinnervation.[36]

The striated muscles of the sphincters are innervated by anterior horn cells that lie in Onuf's nucleus in the sacral part of the spinal cord. Neurophysiological studies showed loss of cells in Onuf's nucleus in patients dying with Shy-Drager syndrome.[37] These pathological changes may be reflected in abnormalities of sphincter EMG in life. This was first shown by Sakouta et al[38] and then in a systematic study by Kirby et al.[39] Sphincter EMG is now used to distinguish between patients with bladder symptoms and multiple system atrophy and atypical parkinsonism and those with idiopathic Parkinson's disease,[40 41] and a urological disorder as in the first condition changes of reinnervation can be found which

405

are not present in the second. Changes of reinnervation in multiple system atrophy are non-specific and some caution must be exercised in interpreting EMG findings in multiparous women or patients who have had extensive pelvic surgery. However, the changes which occur in the motor units in multiple system atrophy are so extreme as to make the test reliable and robust.

Using a concentric needle electrode 10 different motor units are recorded from either the urethral or anal sphincter, the anal sphincter being more accessible and therefore less uncomfortable for the patient but equally valuable for giving a significant result. The mean duration of the 10 motor units is measured as well as the number of units which exceed 10 ms in duration. In multiple system atrophy, some motor units remain of normal duration, but others become excessively prolonged. By contrast with this—for example, after multiple deliveries—all the units might be mildly prolonged. The values used to define normal are a mean duration of less than 8·5 ms and less than 20% of units having a duration of less than 10 ms.[40] A mean duration of more than 10 ms is highly abnormal and suggestive of multiple system atrophy but there is inevitably an area of uncertainty when the mean value is less than this.

The other condition in which urethral sphincter EMG has proved to be of particular value is in the investigation of young women with urinary retention.[42] These patients have no neurological signs on clinical examination and in particular no evidence of spinal cord disease.[43] It was previously suggested that they were either presenting with urinary retention as the first symptom of multiple sclerosis or that they had a hysterical disorder. The first is now easy to disprove as imaging and neurophysiological investigation in these women show no appropriate abnormality. Sphincter EMG shows a myotonic-like activity called "complex repetitive discharges and decelerating bursts".[44] Detailed EMG analysis of this activity, measuring the jitter of the component potentials, has shown that in common with other complex repetitive discharges, it is due to ephaptic transmission between muscle fibres[44] and it has been suggested that it is this activity which can be recorded as a continuous phenomenon which prevents the muscle from relaxing. The striated muscle of the urethral sphincter is a circularly placed horseshoe-like structure and it is not difficult to see how a failure of it to relax would result in either obstructed voiding or urinary retention. Why the abnormal activity should develop remains unknown but it is not uncommon for women with urinary retention to have clinical features of polycystic ovaries.[45] A speculative hypothesis is that the striated muscle of the urethral sphincter, being hormonally sensitive, undergoes a breakdown in membrane stabilisation secondary to the pervading hormonal abnormality of polycystic ovary syndrome allowing ephaptic transmission between muscle fibres to occur. Unfortunately no specific treatment has yet been effective and the women manage best by performing intermittent self catheterisation.

A similar abnormality has not been found in men and extensive neurophysiological testing has failed to show a defect in the less commonly encountered young men with urinary retention without a urological explanation. The role of primary detrusor abnormality in these men needs to be explored as it does in patients with idiopathic detrusor instability. Unfortunately there is as yet no neurophysiological means of investigating detrusor smooth muscle function.

Planning investigations

Investigations of bladder symptoms are carried out for two very different purposes: in a patient with bladder symptoms and established neurological disease urodynamic investigations may be performed to try and understand the pathophysiological basis for the patient's symptoms and obtain information on which to base recommendations for management of incontinence.

When the question being asked is "is this a neurogenic bladder?" a different approach is required. In this instance investigations are of a neurological or neurophysiological nature.

Urodynamic investigations in patients with established neurological disease

Poor bladder control is a common and troublesome feature of many types of neurological disease, especially of the spinal cord. The commonest complaints are of urgency, frequency, and urge incontinence and in patients with established neurological disease these can be assumed to reflect detrusor hyperreflexia. However, patients with neurogenic bladder disorders often have a disorder of emptying as well; incomplete emptying is probably due to a combination of detrusor sphincter dyssynergia and poorly sustained detrusor contractions. If the bladder does not empty completely the persistent postmicturition residual volume acts as a stimulus for repeated detrusor contractions so that efforts to treat detrusor hyperreflexia are unlikely to succeed until effective emptying is achieved. The most effective treatment for detrusor hyperreflexia is an anticholinergic drug (oxybutynin is currently recommended) but there is no oral medication which improves neurogenic voiding disorders and the best management is intermittent catheterisation, performed by the patient or carer.

In summary the presence of detrusor hyperreflexia may be reliably deduced from clinical history, but incomplete emptying, although contributing appreciably to the problem, can be largely asymptomatic. For this reason the single most important investigation when planning the management of patients with neurogenic incontinence is measurement of the postmicturition residual volume. This can either be done by simple ultrasound (see earlier) or by "in-out" catheterisation. The advantage of using catheterisation is that it familiarises the patient with what is involved in intermittent self catheterisation.

Investigation of the postmicturition residual volume is recommended before starting on an anticholinergic drug, as shown in the summary algorithm (figure 13.6). A further point about treatment with anticholinergic drugs is that although they may be effective in lessening detrusor hyperreflexia they can adversely affect bladder emptying. It is advisable therefore if a patient starts on these drugs and fails to respond to recheck the postmicturition residual volume and make sure that this has not significantly accumulated.

If the patient has recurrent urinary tract infections or fails to respond to the regimen outlined in figure 13.6, it is advisable to refer the patient to a urologist who will carry out investigations to exclude urinary tract stones or some other structural lesion.

Although cystometry is not critical in the routine investigation and management of patients with neurological disability such as multiple sclerosis, there are other neurological conditions in which measurements of bladder pressure are important. This is particularly the case in patients with parkinsonian features and bladder symptoms. There must be a high index of suspicion of multiple system atrophy in such a patient, best investigated by sphincter EMG (see earlier). If, however, sphincter EMG is normal and the disorder seems to be idiopathic Parkinson's disease the question of

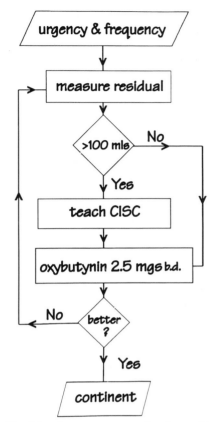

Figure 13.6   *Algorithm for management of patients with neurogenic bladder disorders. By following this both aspects of bladder dysfunction—incomplete emptying and hyperreflexia—are treated*

prostatic obstruction of outflow in men arises and full cystometry with a voiding study is essential.

Cystometry is also of value when investigating patients with an uncertain neurological diagnosis who have among their symptoms complaints of bladder dysfunction. Finding sensory urgency may provide an explanation for bladder symptoms without suggesting a neurogenic basis.

Is this a neurogenic bladder?

The role of urodynamics in trying to decide if a patient has a neurogenic bladder disorder is limited. In most patients sent by urologists to neurologists, filling cystometry has disclosed bladder overactivity. In this instance the neurologist must try to confirm or refute that there is a neurological basis for the problem. Foremost in the patient's assessment is the clinical neurological examination.

The clinical neurological examination

The neural organisation of control of bladder function is widely distributed throughout the neuraxis. The neural programmes which determine whether the bladder is in storage or voiding mode exist in centres in the dorsal tegmentum of the pons.[46] For these programmes to be effected there must be intact connections between the sacral part of the spinal cord, which is the level of efferent and afferent neural connections to the lower urinary tract, and the pons. Spinal cord abnormality is, therefore, a common cause of neurogenic bladder dysfunction. The influence of higher centres and particularly input from the mesial frontal lobes is thought to be important in modulating the activity of the pontine micturition centres and there is probably also input from other suprapontine regions although these have been less clearly defined. Thus any lesion between the frontal lobes and the sacral part of the spinal cord is likely to result in bladder dysfunction.

Because of the relative levels at which the innervation of the lower limbs and the bladder arise, it is unusual to have a lesion between the pons and the sacral part of the cord giving rise to a neurogenic bladder that does not also produce signs of an upper motor neuron lesion in the lower limbs. This is undoubtedly the case in patients with multiple sclerosis[47] but it also seems to hold for most other instances of spinal abnormality unless the lesion is very small and intramedullary. A predictable exception to this rule might be expected from a conus or cauda equina lesion affecting only S2-S4. It seems, however, that even with such extreme caudal lesions there are usually neurological abnormalities in the lower limbs and foot deformities may be present if the problem has been of long duration.

Brain stem or pontine abnormalities giving rise to bladder dysfunction often cause other pronounced neurological deficits but occasionally a lesion can be sufficiently dorsal and discrete to produce predominantly a defect of bladder function.[48] An internuclear ophthalmoplegia is a frequent additional sign, due presumably to the proximity of the median longitudinal fasciculus.

410

The contribution of suprapontine disease to neurogenic bladder dysfunction, with the exception of areas in the frontal lobes, is poorly defined. Patients with incontinence due to lesions of the frontal lobe usually have quite profound neuropsychological impairment including a change of personality but are not indifferent to their incontinence unless there has been extensive frontal lobe damage.[49] Hydrocephalus probably causes bladder dysfunction by pressure effects from the distended lateral ventricles on the frontal regions.[50]

The neurologist may be asked if a patient's peripheral neuropathy is responsible for bladder dysfunction. Many forms of neuropathy are length dependent, the maximum deficit being evident in the longest fibres whereas the nerve fibres to the bladder are comparatively short. For the innervation of the bladder to have been affected as part of a generalised neuropathy there should be clinical evidence of extensive disease with loss of both knee and ankle jerks and sensory impairment in small fibres to a level well above the ankles. Even if the neuropathy is selective for small fibres symptomatic bladder involvement occurs relatively late and only in patients with other profound neuropathic symptoms.

Imaging of the nervous system

From the preceding section, emphasising the value of clinical examination, it is apparent that there are regions of the CNS where a lesion can cause bladder symptoms and yet produce only minor or equivocal physical signs. Imaging is particularly indicated to exclude a suprapontine abnormality or a subsacral cauda equina lesion. Magnetic resonance imaging of the lower cord and cauda equina has replaced myelography as the investigation of choice for imaging this region.[51] It seems that a congenital malformation of the lower spinal cord such as a tethered cord cannot be excluded by a plain radiograph as various forms of dysrraphism can occur without spina bifida.

Pelvic floor neurophysiological investigations

There are two conditions in which neurophysiological investigations can disclose an abnormality that might not otherwise be evident.

If there are any other neurological features such as parkinsonism, cerebellar ataxia, postural hypotension, or symptoms suggesting laryngeal stridor, a diagnosis of multiple system atrophy should be considered.[52] Sphincter EMG has proved a valuable test in detecting this disorder by showing pronounced changes of denervation and reinnervation in the motor units (see earlier).

In young women with bladder disturbance but no other convincing neurological deficit, EMG of the urethral sphincter may show the myotonic-like activity, decelerating bursts, and complex repetitive discharges described earlier.[42] Even if sphincter EMG is not available, in a young woman with urinary retention simply indicating an absence of spinal cord signs on clinical examination makes a diagnosis of multiple sclerosis, a condition otherwise likely to be considered as the cause, highly improbable.

Conclusion

The difficulty that neurologists have had with investigating the neurogenic bladder stems from a combination of factors: the range of presenting symptoms is limited to either incontinence or retention, it is not possible to examine the bladder clinically, and the impression that urodynamics may prove a "diagnosis" has obscured the fact that there are many bladder disorders of unknown cause. Finally there has been the neurologists' reluctance to become involved in the management of incontinence. In patients with established neurological disease bladder dysfunction should be regarded as an essentially neurological symptom and investigated and managed appropriately. Bladder symptoms are among the most treatable of neurological deficits and are an unpleasant and troublesome burden for the patient and their carer.

In patients sent from urologists to neurologists the emphasis should be on excluding spinal cord disease, which can be readily done by clinical examination. A high index of suspicion for multiple system atrophy should be maintained for older patients as this is a neurological disease which can present with bladder dysfunction and the patients do not benefit from urological surgery.

1 Mosso A, Pellacani P. Sur les fonctions de la vessie. *Archives Italiennes de Biologie* 1882;**1**:98–128.
2 Denny-Brown D, Robertson E. On the physiology of micturition. *Brain* 1933;**56**:149–90.
3 Scott FB, Quesada EM, Cardus C. The use of combined uroflowmetry, cystometry and electromyography in evaluation of neurogenic bladder dysfunction. In: Boyarsky S, ed. *The neurogenic bladder*. Baltimore: Williams and Wilkins, 1967:106–14.
4 Bates CP, Whiteside CG, Turner-Warwick R. Synchronous cine-pressure flow cystourethrography. *Br J Urol* 1970;**42**:714–23.
5 Christmas T, Chapple C, Rickards D, *et al*. Contemporary flow meters: an assessment of their accuracy and reliability. *Br J Urol* 1989;**63**:460–1.

6 Rushworth G. Diagnostic value of the electromyographic study of reflex activity in man. *Electroencephalogr Clin Neurophysiol* 1967;**25**:65–73.

7 Blaivas JG, Sinha HP, Zayed AAH, *et al.* Detrusor-external sphincter dysynergia: a detailed electromyography study. *J Urol* 1981;**125**:545–8.

8 Griffiths C, Assi M, Styles R, *et al.* Ambulatory monitoring of bladder and detrusor pressure during natural filling. *J Urol* 1989;**142**:780–4.

9 International Continence Society. Fourth report on the standardisation of terminology of lower urinary tract. *Br J Urol* 1981;**53**:333–5.

10 Brading AF, Turner WH. The unstable bladder: towards a common mechanism. *Br J Urol* 1994;**73**:3–8.

11 Abrams P, Griffiths D. The assessment of prostatic obstruction from urodynamic measurements and from residual urine. *Br J Urol* 1979;**51**:129–34.

12 Ng K, Gardener J, Rickards D, *et al.* Three-dimensional imaging of the prostatic urethra—an exciting new tool. *Br J Urol* 1994;**74**:604–8.

13 Ertekin C, Reel F. Bulbocavernosus reflex in normal men and in patients with neurogenic bladder and/or impotence. *J Neurol Sci* 1976;**28**:1–15.

14 Bradley WE. Urethral electromyography. *J Urol* 1972;**108**:563–4.

15 Bilkey WJ, Awad EA, Smith AD. Clinical application of sacral reflex latency. *J Urol* 1983;**129**:1187–9.

16 Vodusek EB, Janko M, Lokar J. Direct and reflex responses in perineal muscles on electrical stimulation. *J Neurol Neurosurg Psychiatry* 1983;**46**:67–71.

17 Varma JS, Smith AN, McInnes A. Electrophysiological observations on the human pudendo-anal reflex. *J Neurol Neurosurg Psychiatry* 1986;**49**:1411–6.

18 Bradley WE, Timm GW, Rockswold GL, Scott FB. Detrusor and urethral electromyelography. *J Urol* 1975;**114**:891–4.

19 Krane RJ, Siroky MB. Studies on sacral-evoked potentials. *J Urol* 1980;**124**:872–6.

20 Blaivas JG, Zayed AAH, Labib KB. The bulbocavernosus reflex in urology: a prospective study of 299 patients. *J Urol* 1981;**126**:197–9.

21 Ertekin C, Almis S, Ertekin N. Sympathetic skin potentials and bulbocavernosus reflex in patients with chronic alcoholism and impotence. *Eur Neurol* 1990;**30**:334–7.

22 Guerit JM, Opsomer RJ. Bit-mapped imaging of somatosensory evoked potentials after stimulation of the posterior tibial nerves and dorsal nerve of the penis/clitoris. *Electroencephalogr Clin Neurophysiol* 1991;**8**:228–37.

23 Haldeman S, Bradley WE, Bhatia N, *et al.* Pudendal evoked responses. *Arch Neurol* 1982;**39**:280–3.

24 Haldeman S, Glick M, Bhatia NN, *et al.* Colonometry, cystometry, and evoked potentials in multiple sclerosis. *Arch Neurol* 1982;**39**:698–701.

25 Kirkeby HJ, Poulsen EU, Petersen T, *et al.* Erectile dysfunction in multiple sclerosis. *Neurol* 1988;**38**:1366–71.

26 Eardley I, Nagendran K, Lecky B, *et al.* The neurophysiology of the striated urethral sphincter in multiple sclerosis. *Br J Urol* 1991;**67**:81–8.

27 Kunesch E, Reiners K, Muller-Mattheis V, *et al.* Neurological risk profile in organic erectile impotence. *J Neurol Neurosurg Psychiatry* 1992;**55**:275–81.

28 Pickard RS, Powell PH, Schofield IS. The clinical application of dorsal penile nerve cerebral-evoked response recording in the investigation of impotence. *Br J Urol* 1994;**74**:231–5.

29 Delodovici ML, Fowler CJ. The clinical value of the pudendal somatosensory evoked potential is examined. *Electroencephalogr Clin Neurophysiol* 1995;**96**:509–15.

30 Kiff ES, Swash M. Normal proximal and delayed distal conduction in the pudendal nerves of patients with idiopathic (neurogenic) faecal incontinence. *J Neurol Neurosurg Psychiatry* 1984;**47**:820–3.

31 Snooks SJ, Badenoch DF, Tiptaft RC, *et al.* Perineal nerve damage in genuine stress incontinence. *Br J Urol* 1985;**57**:422–6.

32 Snooks SJ, Swash M, Setchell M, *et al.* Injury to the pelvic floor sphincter musculature in childbirth. *Lancet* 1984;**ii**:546–50.

33 Swash M, Snooks SJ, Henry MM. A unifying concept of pelvic floor disorders and incontinence. *J R Soc Med* 1985;**78**:906–11.

34 Cheong D, Vaccaro C, Salanga V, *et al.* Electrodiagnostic evaluation of fecal incontinence. *Muscle Nerve* 1995;**18**:612–9.

35 Neill ME, Swash M. Increased motor unit fibre density in the external anal sphincter in ano-rectal incontinence: a single fibre EMG study. *J Neurol Neurosurg Psychiatry*

1980;**43**:343–7.

36 Fowler C. Pelvic floor neurophysiology. In: Osselton J, ed. *Clinical neurophysiology*. Oxford: Butterworth Hienemann, 1995;233–52.

37 Sung JH, Mastri AR, Segal E. Pathology of the Shy-Drager syndrome. *J Neuropathol Exp Neurol* 1978;**38**:253–68.

38 Sakuta M, Nakanishi T, Tohokura Y. Anal muscle electromyograms differ in amyotrophic lateral sclerosis and Shy-Drager syndrome. *Neurology* 1978;**28**:1289–93.

39 Kirby RS, Fowler CJ, Gosling J, *et al*. Urethro-vesical dysfunction in progressive autonomic failure with multiple system atrophy. *J Neurol Neurosurg Psychiatry* 1986;**49**: 554–62.

40 Eardley I, Quinn NP, Fowler CJ. The value of urethral sphincter electromyography in the differential diagnosis of parkinsonism. *Br J Urol* 1989;**64**:360–2.

41 Beck RO, Betts CD, Fowler CJ. Genito-urinary dysfunction in multiple system atrophy: clinical features and treatment in 62 cases. *J Urol* 1994;**151**:1336–41.

42 Fowler CJ, Kirby RS. Electromyography of the urethral sphincter in women with urinary retention. *Lancet* 1986;**i**:1455–6.

43 Fowler CJ, Kirby RS. Abnormal electromyographic activity (decelerating bursts and complex repetitive discharges) in the striated muscle of the urethral sphincter in 5 women with persisting urinary retention. *Br J Urol* 1985;**57**:69–70.

44 Fowler CJ, Kirby RS, Harrison MJG. Decelerating bursts and complex repetitive discharges in the striated muscle of the urethral sphincter associated with urinary retention in women. *J Neurol Neurosurg Psychiatry* 1985;**48**:1004–9.

45 Fowler CJ, Christmas TJ, Chapple CR, *et al*. Abnormal electromyographic activity of the urethral sphincter, voiding dysfunction, and polycystic ovaries: a new syndrome? *BMJ* 1988;**297**:1436–8.

46 de Groat WC. Central neural control of the lower urinary tract. In: Bock G, Whelan J, eds. *Neurobiology of incontinence*. Chichester: John Wiley and Sons, 1990:27–56. (Ciba Foundation Symposium 151.)

47 Betts CD, D'Mellow MT, Fowler CJ. Urinary symptoms and the neurological features of bladder dysfunction in multiple sclerosis. *J Neurol Neurosurg Psychiatry* 1993;**56**:245–50.

48 Betts CD, Kapoor R, Fowler CJ. Pontine pathology and micturition dysfunction. *Br J Urol* 1992;**70**:100–2.

49 Andrew J, Nathan PW. Lesions of the anterior frontal lobes and disturbances of micturition and defaecation. *Brain* 1964;**87**:233–62.

50 Ahlberg J, Norlen L, Blomstrand C. Outcome of shunt operating on urinary incontinence in normal pressure hydrocephalus predicted by lumbar puncture. *J Neurol Neurosurg Psychiatry* 1988;**51**:105–8.

51 Mathew P, Todd NV. Intradural conus and cauda equina tumours: a retrospective review of presentation, diagnosis and early outcome. *J Neurol Neurosurg Psychiatry* 1993; **56**:69–74.

52 Wenning G, Shlomo Y, Magalhaes M, *et al*. Clinical features and natural history of multiple system atrophy. *Brain* 1994;**117**:835–45.

14 Diagnosis of inherited metabolic disorders affecting the nervous system

PHILLIP D SWANSON

The number of metabolic disorders that can produce neurological symptoms is daunting. The clinician cannot simply send off to the laboratory a blood sample and ask for a metabolic "screen" that will detect a hypothetical metabolic abnormality. The range of possible conditions must be narrowed to the most likely before deciding which investigative approach should be taken. Most biochemical disorders encountered by neurologists are genetically determined. Thus one of the most important elements of the history is the family history. It is not sufficient to ask "has anyone in your family had a neurological problem?". The clinician must be aware of the different forms of inheritance patterns (autosomal dominant, autosomal recessive, X linked, mitochondrial) and must obtain enough information to construct a meaningful family tree. Directed questions must be asked about siblings as well as parents, grandparents, uncles, aunts, cousins, and children. Box 14.1 lists features that characterise single gene inheritance patterns.[1-3]

Most of the clear cut genetic diseases are due to single gene abnormalities. There are several different mechanisms, however, that produce abnormal genes. A *point mutation* of a single DNA nucleotide can result in a different amino acid being coded for in the resulting polypeptide or protein. There can be *deletion* of a segment of a gene or *insertion* of one or more nucleotides. *Duplication* of a gene has been reported in Charcot-Marie-Tooth disease type 1A. Unstable expansions of portions of a gene (trinucleotide repeats) are being increasingly found in autosomal dominant

---

Box 14.1   Some characteritics of single gene inheritance

Type of inheritance	Characteristics
● Autosomal dominant	Multiple generations affected Father to son transmission (rules out X linked and mitochondrial inheritance patterns) Males and females equally affected
● Autosomal recessive	Only siblings affected Parental consanguinity common Males and females equally affected
● X Linked	Never father to son transmission Transmission through unaffected mothers Only males affected (rare exceptions) 50% risk to sons of carrier women All daughters of affected men are carriers
● Mitochondrial	Maternally inherited Never father to child transmission Both sons and daughters can be affected

Adapted from table 9–1 in Bird and Farrell.[3]

---

neurodegenerative diseases. The pace of new discoveries in medical genetics is incredibly rapid. Many of the new discoveries have led to diagnostic methods that were unanticipated only a few years ago.

Certain terms used by medical geneticists should be familiar to neurological practitioners. *Anticipation* refers to a disease beginning earlier and often being more severe in succeeding generations. In some autosomal dominant disorders, such as myotonic dystrophy and spinocerebellar ataxia 1, this phenomenon seems to be related to the length of an expanded trinucleotide repeat in the abnormal gene.[4] *Penetrance* refers to the proportion of subjects with the abnormal gene who will develop symptoms if they live long enough. The degree of *expression* of a genetic disease refers to the variation of severity of the phenotype that is seen in a patient population. *Mosaicism* refers to variation among different cells and tissues in the chromosome complement. This occurs normally in women due to *lyonisation*, in which one of each cell's two X chromosomes is randomly inactivated. Mitochondrial disorders (see later) are associated with *heteroplasmy*, a term that refers to variation in the proportion of normal or genetically abnormal mitochondria in different tissues.

In *autosomal dominant* disorders, multiple generations are usually affected, although this might not have occurred if the affected patient represents a new mutation. Male to male transmission only occurs with autosomal dominant transmission. Each child of an affected parent will have a 50% chance of having or not having the abnormal gene.

Autosomal recessive disorders occur when expression of the disease requires the abnormal gene to be inherited from both parents, so that the affected person's cells have two abnormal alleles. Many autosomal recessive disorders are associated with defective enzymes. The low level of enzyme activity often leads to accumulation of the enzyme substrate with resultant toxicity to susceptible cells. The carrier parents seldom manifest symptoms because the normal gene codes for normal enzyme that is active enough to prevent substrate accumulation. Consanguineous marriages between cousins are more common in families with autosomal recessive diseases.

X Linked disorders are due to abnormal genes located on the X chromosome. Clinical disease characteristically occurs in males who have inherited the abnormal gene from a carrier mother. Occasionally the mother or daughter with one normal and one abnormal gene will manifest symptoms, which almost always are milder than in the affected son or father, who has only one X chromosome. Male to male transmission cannot occur because a son receives the X chromosome from his mother.

Mitochondrial disorders are due to abnormalities in genes (deletions, point mutations) located in mitochondrial DNA. Both male and female mitochondria are derived from the ovum rather than the sperm. Both males and females can be affected by mitochondrial disorders, but father to child transmission does not occur. Because tissues and cells vary in the proportion of normal and abnormal mitochondria they carry (*heteroplasmy*), the expression

417

of the disorder in different tissues and in different subjects can be extremely variable.

This contribution will not include much discussion of diseases that primarily affect muscle or nerve, as these are the subjects of other chapters in ths book. Some metabolic conditions, however, including metachromatic leukodystrophy and certain mitochondrial disorders that affect both central and peripheral structures, will be included. Non-genetic metabolic conditions such as hypoglycaemia, hepatic encephalopathy, deficiency diseases, and electrolyte disorders will not be discussed. Emphasis will be on conditions that are seen in adults by neurologists but many of these disorders will be variants of diseases that usually have their first manifestations in infancy or childhood. The first section contains brief discussions of categories of metabolic disease likely to be encountered by neurologists. The second section contains a discussion of differential diagnoses of metabolic conditions that might produce particular complexes of neurological symptoms, including mental retardation, dementia, ataxias, motor neuron disease, movement disorders, and stroke.

Categories of metabolic disorders

Aminoacidurias and organic acidaemias

These are the classic disorders of infancy and childhood associated with mental retardation and seizures. The *aminoacidurias* include phenylketonuria, maple syrup urine disease, homocystinuria, and other disorders listed in box 14.2.[5] Screening the urine for amino acids is routinely done in clinical chemistry laboratories. Although it would be very unusual for first symptoms to occur in adult life, patients with treated phenylketonuria eventually will be seen as adults by neurologists.

Organic acidaemias, including methylmalonic acidaemia and propionic acidaemia, usually have their onset in infancy. Symptoms of dehydration are associated with ketoacidosis, hypoglycaemia, and hyperammonaemia. Diagnosis is made by urinalysis for organic acids, and can be confirmed by measuring activity of the abnormal enzyme in cultured fibroblasts.

These disorders are becoming better understood since the advent of modern molecular investigative techniques. For example, it is now known that there are three genes located on three different chromosomes (Nos 1, 6, 19) that code for the structural

Box 14.2 Aminoacidurias and organic acidaemias

Disease	Clinical features	Increased substances	Enzyme defect
• Phenylketonuria	Mental retardation	Phenylalanine Phenylpyruvic acid	Phenylalanine hydroxylase
• Maple syrup urine disease	Ketoacidosis Infantile seizures Characteristic odour Progressive encephalopathy Milder variants	Branched chain aminoacids (leucine, isoleucine, valine) (urine: branched chain ketoacids)	Branched chain ketoacid dehydrogenase complex
• Homocystinuria	Ectopia lentis, stroke	Homocystine	Cystathionine β-synthase
• Non-ketotic hyperglycinaemia	Coma, progressive encephalopathy	Glycine	Glycine clearance system (four proteins)
• Methylmalonic acidaemia	Ketoacidosis Hyperammonaemia	Methylmalonic acid	Methyl-malonyl CoA mutase
• Propionic acidaemia	Ketoacidosis Hyperammonacinia	3-Hydroxypropionic acid	Propionyl CoA carboxylase
• Isovaleric acidaemia	Ketoacidosis Hyperammonaemia	Isovaleric acid	Isovaleryl CoA dehydrogenase
• Glutaric aciduria	Progressive encephalopathy	Glutaric, 3-hydroxyglutaric acids	Glutaric CoA dehydrogenase
Type 1	Spasticity, choreoathetosis		
Type 2	Three groups— Renal cystic dysplasia Hypoglycaemia, acidosis Muscle weakness	Glutaconic acid	Electron transfer flavoprotein (ETF) and ETF ubiquinone oxidoreductase
γ-Hydroxybutyric aciduria	Mental retardation Seizures Developmental delay and motor abnormalities	γ-Hydroxybutyric acid	Succinic semialdelyde dehydrogenase

419

proteins unique to the deficient enzyme (branched chain ketoacid dehydrogenase complex [BCKAD]) in maple syrup urine disease. Mutations in different components of the complex can lead to variable clinical manifestations.[6]

Lysosomal disorders

The term lysosome was proposed by DeDuve *et al* in 1955 for intracellular granules that were rich in hydrolytic enzymes.[7] A lysosomal disease is associated with an abnormal enzyme that results in defective breakdown of the enzyme substrate.[8] The product accumulates and eventually alters cell function. Because hydrolytic enzymes are present in many tissues, the diagnosis of the accumulated product or of the enzyme deficiency usually can be made with readily accessible tissues such as peripheral white blood cells or skin fibroblasts.[9-11] Although most of these disorders produce symptoms at a young age, some mutations, as in adult onset GM_1 gangliosidosis, lead to onset of symptoms later in life.[12]

Lysosomal disorders can be subcategorised according to the type of accumulated storage product. The two principal groups are lipid storage diseases and mucopolysaccharidoses. As these conditions have been more fully characterised, it has become clear that a great deal of heterogeneity exists among them, in many cases due to different point mutations in the gene. Thus these disorders should be considered in the differential diagnosis of atypical degenerative disorders.

Lipid storage diseases

Box 14.3 lists the lipid storage diseases that cause neurological dysfunction. These disorders are diagnosed either by finding high concentrations of substrate in tissues or by showing pronounced reduction in concentrations of the lysosomal enzyme responsible for degrading the accumulated storage substance.

In each disorder, subtypes have been delineated. In Gaucher's disease, associated with accumulation of glucocerebroside, and in Niemann-Pick disease, with sphingomyelin accumulation, hepatosplenomegaly is prominent in all types; however, only types 2 and 3 Gaucher's disease and types A and C Niemann-Pick disease are associated with neurological deterioration. Globoid leukodystrophy (Krabbe's disease), metachromatic leukodystrophy, and Tay-Sachs disease are inherited as autosomal recessive disorders

Box 14.3 Common lipid storage diseases

Disease	Neurological symptom	Major lipid accumulated	Enzyme defect
Gaucher	Hepatosplenomegaly Neurological deterioration in type 2 Dementia, seizures in type 3	Glucocerebroside	Glucocerebroside-β-glucosidase
Niemann-Pick	Hepatosplenomegaly, psychomotor deterioration in types A and C	Sphingomyelin Cholesterol (type C)	Sphingomyelinase (type A)
Globoid leukodystrophy (Krabbe's)	Progressive encephalopathy, seizures, spasticity, blindness	Galactocerebroside	Galactocerebroside β-Galactosidase
Metachromatic leukodystrophy	Progressive encephalopathy, neuropathy, ataxia, spasticity	Sulphatide	Arylsulphatase A
Fabry	Pain, rare strokes, X linked, renal insufficiency, skin lesions	Ceramide trihexoside	Ceramide trihexoside α-Galactosidase
Tay-Sachs	Progressive encephalopathy	GM_2 ganglioside	Hexosaminidase A
Tay-Sachs variant	More rapid progression	Globoside and GM_2	Hexosaminidase A and B
GM_1 gangliosidosis	Dementia, progressive ataxia, choreoathetosis	GM_1 ganglioside	β-Galactosidase 16 point mutations

421

and can be diagnosed by measurement of enzyme concentrations in peripheral white blood cells or cultured skin fibroblasts. Clinical variants are found in each disorder. In metachromatic leukodystrophy some mutations in the arylsulphatase A gene on chromosome 22 have been correlated with different phenotypes.[13] Similarly, in Tay-Sachs disease over 20 mutations including nucleotide insertions, deletions, and substitutions on the α subunit (chromosome 15) and the β subunit (chromosome 5) of the hexosaminidase enzyme have been described.[14] Late onset cases may develop weakness, fasciculations, ataxia, and psychiatric symptoms.[15]

GM_1 gangliosidosis, due to deficiency of the lysosomal enzyme β-galactosidase, can produce symptoms in infancy, childhood, or adult life. At least 16 mutations have been identified in the β-galactosidase gene.[12 16 17] Severity of the diseases can be correlated with the amount of residual enzyme activity, the infantile form having no demonstrable activity and the adult forms having 4–8% of normal activity. Leinekugel et al found that 10–15% of β-hexosaminidase A and arylsulphatase A activities were sufficient to degrade substrate.[18]

The adult form of the disorder is slowly progressive and may produce gait disorders, involuntary choreoathetoid movements, bradykinesia, or dementia. Storage of GM_1 ganglioside can be much more pronounced in the striatum than in other parts of the brain by contrast with younger onset patients, in whom storage is more widespread.[12 19]

Diagnosis is confirmed by finding much reduced lysosomal acid β-galactosidase activity in leucocytes. Single base mutations can be found on the β-galactosidase gene. The [51]isoleucine (ATC) $\rightarrow$ threonine (ACC) mutation in the gene is common in Japanese adult onset GM_1 gangliosidosis.[12]

Mucopolysaccharidoses

These lysosomal disorders are associated with accumulation of complex glycosoaminoglycans (mucopolysaccharides), due to genetic defects resulting in deficiencies of degradative enzymes.[20 21] The stored substances include dermatan sulphate, heparan sulphate, keratan sulphate, and chondroitin 4/6 sulphates, which are detectable in the urine. Of the 12 described disorders all are autosomal recessive except for Hunter syndrome which is X linked recessive. Among these conditions are Hurler's, Scheie's,

Sanfilippo, Morquio's, and Maroteaux-Lamy diseases, and β-glucuronidase deficiency. Clinical signs such as coarse facial features, corneal clouding, hearing difficulties, hepatosplenomegaly, or joint abnormalities are usually detected during the first year of life. Later, developmental delay or mental regression may become apparent.

Peroxisomal disorders

The peroxisome is an organelle that is found in most tissues. It contains over 40 enzymes including oxidases and catalase. Moser *et al* list 11 disorders attributable to defects in peroxisomal enzymes.[22 23] These include disorders of peroxisome biogenesis (Zellweger syndrome, neonatal adrenoleukodystrophy, infantile Refsum's syndrome, and hyperpipecolic acidaemia). The first two of these disorders can be associated with neonatal seizures, hypotonia, and developmental delay.

Of the disorders associated with peroxisomal enzyme abnormalities, X linked adrenoleukodystrophy is the most likely to be seen by neurologists.

Adrenoleukodystrophy and adrenomyeloneuropathy are X linked disorders and are associated with raised blood concentrations of very long chain fatty acids (VLCFAs) due to impaired peroxisomal β oxidation. The genetic defect seems to result from deletions in the peroxisomal membrane protein gene.[24] Some different phenotypes occur.[22-26] Neurologists are most likely to encounter an adult patient with adrenomyeloneuropathy, with slowly progressive paraparesis as the main neurological manifestation and adrenocortical failure as a common occurrence. Adult onset cerebral adrenoleukodystrophy is manifested by dementia, confusional states, and sometimes progressive ataxia or psychiatric disturbances.[27] Symptom progression is usually slower in patients with adult onset.

Assays for VLCFAs (C24:0, C26:0) are carried out in specialised lipid laboratories using gas liquid chromatography or mass spectrometry. Although the vast majority of patients have raised plasma concentrations of these fatty acids, an occasional family will have VLCFA concentrations within the "normal" range.[28] Molecular genetic analysis now makes it possible to detect point mutations within the adrenoleukodystrophy gene.[29]

Mitochondrial encephalopathies

A high index of suspicion is aroused for the presence of a disorder involving an abnormal mitochondrial gene if there are clinical features of Leigh's disease (subacute necrotising encephalomyelopathy), Kearns-Sayre syndrome (progressive external ophthalmoplegia, retinal pigmentary degeneration, and other symptoms), MELAS (mitochondrial encephalomyelopathy with lactic acidosis and stroke-like episodes), MERRF (myoclonic epilepsy with ragged red fibres), Leber's hereditary optic neuroretinopathy, or NARP (neurogenic muscle weakness, ataxia, and retinitis pigmentosa).[30-36] Various other features have been seen including short stature, deafness, diabetes mellitus, peptic ulceration, severe constipation, and migraine.

Mutations in mitochondrial DNA have been discovered in patients with several clinical presentations. Deletions of mitochondrial DNA are common in Kearns-Sayre syndrome.[2] In MELAS, point mutations include an A → G mutation at nt3243 in 80% of cases, as well as T → C mutations at nt3271 and at nt9957, and an A → G mutation at nt11084. An A → G nt8344 mutation has been found in MERRF, and a T → G or T → C mutation at nt8993 in Leigh's syndrome.[37 38]

Diagnostic laboratory tests include: (*a*) serum pyruvate and lactate concentrations; (*b*) muscle biopsy to assess for the presence of ragged red fibres, and as a source of mitochondria for DNA analysis; and (*c*) molecular genetic studies on blood or muscle in a specialised laboratory to assess for known mutations.

Disorders associated with expanded trinucleotide repeats

One of the most exciting developments in neurology has been the discovery of neurogenetic diseases in which the abnormal gene mutation results in expansion of a repeated sequence of trinucleotides. Box 14.4 lists many of the presently known disorders of this type.[39-50] Most are either X linked or autosomal dominant disorders and include the dominant spinocerebellar ataxias SCA1 and Machado-Joseph disease, Huntington's disease, fragile X syndrome, myotonic dystrophy, and spinal bulbar muscular atrophy (Kennedy's syndrome). Friedrich's ataxia is the only autosomal recessive disorder in this group. The expanded GAA repeat is located in the first intron of the gene X25.[50a] In many of these disorders, the length of the expanded trinucleotide repeat is unstable.

Box 14.4 Disorders associated with unstable expanded trinucleotide repeats

Disorder	Chromosome	Expanded trinucleotide	Number of repeats		Translation of repeat
			Normal	Disease	
• Fragile X syndrome (FRXA)	X	CGG	6–~50	Premutation:52–200 Disease: 200 to >1000	No
• Fragile X E (FRXE)	X	GCC	6–25	>200	No
• Myotonic dystrophy	19q	CTG	<30	Premutation: 42–180 Disease: 200–>1000	No
• Bulbar spinomuscular atrophy (Kennedy's syndrome)	Xq11–12	CAG	17–26	40–52	Yes
• Huntington's disease	4p16.3	CAG	11–34	37–121	Yes
• Spinocerebellar ataxia 1	6p22–23	CAG	19–36	42–81	Yes
• Machado-Joseph disease (spinocerebellar ataxia 3)	14q32.1	CAG	13–36	68–79	Yes
• Dentatorubral-pallidoluysian atrophy (DRPLA)	12p12–ter	CAG	7–23	49–75	Yes
• Friedrich's ataxia	9q13–q21.1	GAA	7–22	200–900	No

425

Succeeding generations have expansions of greater length which may be associated with earlier onset and more severe disease manifestations. It is likely that additional neurodegenerative disorders will be added to this list.[43]

Genetics laboratories have the capability of definitively diagnosing the presence or absence of some of these disorders on a single sample of blood, using molecular genetic techniques. Commercial availability is limited at this time.

Disorders of copper metabolism

Two diagnosable genetic disorders are associated with defects in copper metabolism—namely, Menkes' disease and Wilson's disease.

Menkes' "kinky hair" (steely hair) disease is an X linked disorder with manifestations in early infancy.[51 52] Infants feed poorly, become hypothermic, gain weight slowly, develop seizures, and show progressive neurological deterioration. They have colourless, friable hair which has a characteristic microscopic appearance. Danks et al suggested that the disease was due to a disorder of copper metabolism.[53] The gene has been isolated and is a copper transporting ATPase. Until recently, diagnosis if suspected clinically was established by demonstrating low caeruloplasmin and serum copper concentrations and abnormalities in fibroblast copper uptake.[54 55] In the newborn, however, copper and caeruloplasmin are normally low, so reliable detection of abnormally low concentrations cannot be made until the third or fourth week of life. The diagnosis can be made by DNA analysis.[56]

Wilson's disease is an autosomal recessive disorder due to an abnormal gene at q14.3 on chromosome 13. This gene codes for a copper transporting P-type ATPase that is presumably important for hepatic incorporation of copper into caeruloplasmin and for excretion of copper into bile.[57–59] The enzyme is also expressed in the kidney. Twenty five mutations have been identified in the Wilson's disease gene, accounting for the great variability in clinical symptomatology.[60] The pathogenetic role of reduced synthesis or impaired function of the copper transporting protein caeruloplasmin is not clear.[61] In the course of Wilson's disease, increased storage of copper occurs in liver, brain, cornea (Kayser-Fleischer ring in Descemet's membrane), and kidneys. Neurological and psychiatric symptoms can occur secondary to deposition of copper in the brain or as a result of hepatic encephalopathy due to copper induced liver damage. The diagnosis can and should be made before the onset of symptoms in close relatives of affected patients.[62-64] The diagnosis can be made with the assistance of the following laboratory findings[63]: (*a*) increased excretion of copper into the urine (normal <30 μg/24 h; Wilson's disease 100–1000 μg/24 h); (*b*) decreased serum concentration of total copper (normal 85–145 μg/dl); (*c*) decreased serum concentration of caeruloplasmin (normal range 25–45 mg/dl); about 5% of cases will have normal caeruloplasmin concentrations.[65]

Symptomatic approach to the diagnosis of inherited metabolic disorders

Mental retardation or deterioration

Fragile X syndrome

Over 100 X linked mental retardation syndromes are known at the present time.[66] Of these, fragile X syndrome is the leading genetic cause of mental retardation.[67] The syndrome is so named because of the instability of the X chromosome when incubated in folic acid deficient media.[68 69] This was the first neurological disorder to be associated with an unstable trinucleotide repeat sequence.[70 71] Clinically, patients may have prominent ears, large testicles, high arched palates, and behavioural deficits. Definitive diagnosis can be made by the demonstration of an expanded trinucleotide CGG repeat sequence. Abnormality in the FMR gene results in lack of production of the FMR1 protein.

Diagnosis of mental deterioration or progressive encephalopathy in infants may require various metabolic tests if the suspected diagnosis is not already obvious.[72] A metabolic screen of the urine carried out by a hospital laboratory usually includes a nitroprusside-cyanide test, a ferric chloride test, tests for ketoacids and mucopolysaccharides, and two dimensional amino acid chromatography. Serum analyses for amino acids and organic acids will usually be diagnostic for amino acidurias and organic acidaemias. Studies to search for other disorders mentioned (Menkes' disease, lipid storage diseases) will require special testing by genetics laboratories.

Juvenile or adult patients presenting with dementia

Laboratory investigations are of limited usefulness in dementia diagnosis. The most common dementing illnesses such as

Alzheimer's disease are not yet diagnosable biochemically on a routine basis. In a few families with familial Alzheimer's disease, point mutations have been found in the gene on chromosome 21 that codes for the amyloid precursor protein (APP) gene.[73 74] Most families, however, do not have these mutations. In young onset families, linkage analysis has located the gene defect to a locus on chromosome 14.[75] Point mutations on the genes coding for presenilin 1 and presenilin 2 are responsible for early onset (chromosome 14) and Volga German (chromosome 1) familial cases.[75a, 75b] Ultimately it may be possible to diagnose the disorder by molecular genetic techniques. At present, diagnosis of the known mutations can be carried out only by specialised research laboratories studying this disorder.

In some patients with progressive cognitive impairment, a high degree of suspicion based on clinical or radiological clues may justify carrying out further metabolic studies to confirm a suspected diagnosis (box 14.5). Vitamin B12 deficiency rarely produces dementia alone but should be excluded.

Huntington's disease

The diagnosis of Huntington's disease can now be confirmed by commercially available DNA testing. The presence of an extended CAG repeat in the Huntington's disease gene on chromosome 4 establishes the diagnosis. A normal allele has less than 35 CAG repeats. The Huntington's disease gene has more than 38 repeats in 98–99% of cases.[76]

Leukodystrophies

In addition to multiple sclerosis and progressive multifocal leukoencephalopathy, cerebral white matter can be affected by several metabolic disorders, with dementia as a major symptom. These include adult onset metachromatic leukodystrophy, adrenoleukodystrophy, Pelizaeus-Merzbacher disease, Krabbe's disease, and cerebrotendinous xanthomatosis. In each disorder, symptoms are progressive, usually over months to years. Inherited in an autosomal recessive manner, metachromatic leukodystrophy would likely be associated with clinical or EMG/nerve conduction velocity evidence of a peripheral neuropathy. Adrenoleukodystrophy might be associated with adrenal insufficiency and, as it is an X linked disorder, would occur predominantly in

428

Box 14.5   Disorders associated with dementia

Disorder	Diagnostic test
● Alzheimer's disease	In known families, genetics laboratory for DNA point mutation in the gene for APP, presenilin 1 or presenilin 2
● B12 deficiency	Serum B12 level, Schilling test
● Huntington's disease	Genetics laboratory for DNA screen (CAG > 37 repeats)
● Adrenoleukodystrophy	Lipid laboratory for plasma VLCFA
● Pelizaeus-Merzbacher disease	Genetics laboratory for PLP gene
● Canavan's disease	Urine for N-acetylaspartic acid Fibroblasts for aspartoacyclase
● Metachromatic leukodystrophy	Arylsulphatase A
● GM$_1$ gangliosidosis	β-Galactosidase
● Globoid leukodystrophy (Krabbe's)	Galactocerebrosidase
● Cerebrotendinous xanthomatosis	Lipid laboratory for cholestanol
● Ceroid-lipofuscinosis	EM of buffy coat for curvilinear bodies

VLCFA = very long chain fatty acids; PLP = proteolipid protein; APP = amyloid precursor protein; EM = electron microscopy.

males. Patients with cerebrotendinous xanthomatosis usually develop prominent xanthomas in large tendons such as the Achilles tendon.

Adrenoleukodystrophy This disorder is characterised by varying modes of onset at different ages. Most affected people are male, as the disorder is X linked. Some heterozygous women may, however, develop spastic paraparesis.[22] The phenotypes delineated by Moser *et al* are: childhood cerebral (48%), adolescent cerebral (5%), adult cerebral (3%), adrenomyeloneuropathy (25%), addisonian only (10%), asymptomatic (8%).[26] The disorder is suspected in children with learning disorders and dementia. Adreno-myeloneuropathy usually begins with progressive paraparesis.

Pelizaeus-Merzbacher disease This disorder is X linked. Symptoms usually begin in infancy or childhood, but onset in early adulthood has been reported.[77] Symptoms include psychomotor delay and later, dementia, nystagmus, ataxia, spasticity, and involuntary movements. Mutations in the gene coding for proteolipid protein result in defective myelin. Mutations in the proteolipid protein gene can now be determined in genetics laboratories.[78 79] Prenatal diagnosis is also possible.[80]

Canavan's disease Another rare leukodystrophy is Canavan's disease, characterised by infantile and juvenile forms with severe progressive neurological deterioration. Raised urinary N-acetylaspartic acid and deficiency of the enzyme aspartoacyclase in skin fibroblasts confirm the diagnosis.[81]

Lipid storage diseases

Metachromatic leukodystrophy and Krabbe's disease (globoid leukodystrophy), as well as other lipid storage diseases such as GM_1 gangliosidosis and type 3 Gaucher's disease can produce dementia as part of more generalised neurological deterioration. Urinary sulphatides will be abnormally increased in metachromatic leukodystrophy. In the other conditions, confirmation of clinical suspicion will require white blood cell or fibroblast enzyme determinations carried out by a specialised laboratory.

Neuronal ceroid lipofuscinosis (Batten's disease and variants) This is a disorder associated with storage of a complex lipopigment. Patients usually develop retinal degeneration, myoclonus, seizures, and dementia. The genre for the infantile form (CLN1) is on chromosome 1p32.[82] It codes for the enzyme palmitoyl-protein thioesterase (ppt) which removes thioster-linked fatty acyl groups from 5-acylated proteins and is also a palmitoyl-CoA hydrolase. Mutations result in undetectable brain enzyme activity and intracellular accumulation of the polypeptide. Lymphoblast PPT activity in CLN1 patients was about 40% of control activity.[32a] Juvenile onset neuronal ceroid lipofuscinosis (CLN3), due in 81% of cases to a 1 Kb deletion on chromosome 16p 12.1, can be diagnosed prenatally by detecting the intragenic marker D165298 on a sample of chronic villus.[83, 83a] Diagnosis of these disorders is usually made by demonstrating accumulated storage product in buffy coat or in skin biopsies, which show curvilinear bodies or a "fingerprint" pattern on electron microscopy. The early onset forms are autosomal recessive. Both autosomal dominant and autosomal recessive inheritance have been reported in the adult form (Kufs' disease) which is not associated with pigmentary retinal degeneration.[84 85]

Ataxias

Progressive ataxia can result from several conditions that have metabolic causes. The MRI will have assisted in diagnosing multiple sclerosis, cerebellar neoplasms, and the diagnoses of alcoholic cerebellar degeneration and paraneoplastic syndromes will have been considered.

Genetic causes are of special importance in this group of disorders. As yet the diagnosis of Friedreich's ataxia is based on clinical, not biochemical findings. The genetics laboratory can, however, assist in diagnosing several of these disorders, including spinocerebellar ataxia type I (SCA-1) and Machado-Joseph's disease.[44 86]

Ataxia-telangiectasia, an autosomal recessive disorder, is the most common cause of ataxia in children under the age of 10.[72] Usually the diagnosis is evident clinically, with ataxia, nystagmus, choreoathetosis, and characteristic auricular and conjunctival telangiectases being evident. The abnormal gene on chromosome 11q22–23, which is important for DNA repair, has recently been identified.[87] The gene product is likely to be a phosphatidylinositol-3' kinase. Presumably more definitive DNA diagnostic testing will become available. Symptoms of ataxia-telangiectasia can begin in early adult life.[88] Some serum abnormalities are found in patients with this disorder, including raised α-fetoprotein in 95% of cases, alterations in serum immunoglobulins, and raised carcinoembryonic antigen concentrations.[89]

Autosomal dominant cerebellar ataxias are being reclassified as their genetic defects are discovered. Abnormal genes have been found on chromosomes 6, 11, 12, 14, and 16.[42–46 86 90–92] Dubourg *et al* sampled DNA from 88 families with inherited ataxias and from 16 patients with sporadic ataxia to determine the frequency of the SCA1 mutation on chromosome 6.[4] Twelve of the families and none of the sporadic cases carried the SCA1 mutation (unstable expanded CAG repeat).

Clinical characteristics do not readily distinguish the subtypes of cerebellar ataxias.[93] Many patients will have additional signs

431

such as extensor plantar responses, decreased vibration sense, ophthalmoplegias, and increased or decreased tendon reflexes. In SCA1, instability of the mutation is more common with male transmission and the age of onset of symptoms is lower in patients with a higher number of CAG repeats (anticipation).

Dentatorubral-pallidoluysian atrophy (DRPLA) is a rare autosomal dominant neurodegenerative disorder, usually classified under the ataxias. The disorder can be associated with myoclonus, chorea, dementia, and seizures. Juvenile and adult onsets are reported.[94] The disorder may be misdiagnosed as Huntington's disease.[48] The molecular defect is an expanded CAG repeat on the gene located on chromosome 12p and can be diagnosed by molecular analysis.[49 50]

Another disorder that may present with ataxia is *cerebrotendinous xanthomatosis*. This condition is suspected in a patient who has tendon xanthomas, often in the Achilles tendons.[95] The diagnosis is confirmed by showing raised concentrations of cholestanol (dihydrocholesterol) in blood or tissue.[96] This test will involve contacting a specialised lipid laboratory, but it is important to do, as the disease can be treated by giving chenodeoxycholic acid.[97] Several mutations of the gene on chromosome 2 that codes for the enzyme sterol 27-hydroxylase have been found in families with this disorder.[98-100] Presymptomatic cases and heterozygotes can now be detected by molecular diagnostic techniques.[101]

Ataxia with isolated vitamin E deficiency (AVED) Patients have been described with progressive ataxia and other features of Friedreich's disease, in which vitamin E concentrations were reduced in the absence of malabsorption.[102] In the patient described by Stumpf *et al*, serum vitamin E concentrations were below 1·0 (normal 5–20) μg/ml and could be restored to normal with an oral dose of 800 mg/day DL-α-tocopherol.[103] This disorder is autosomal recessive. The gene maps to chromosome 8q13.[104 105] Affected patients have mutations in the α-tocopherol transfer protein resulting in impaired ability to incorporate α-tocopherol into lipoproteins.[106]

A-β-lipoproteinaemia Patients with this disorder usually develop steatorrhea in infancy followed in the second decade by progressive ataxia and peripheral neuropathy.[72] The patients have absence of serum β-lipoproteins and very low concentrations of α-tocopherol. Dietary supplementation with high doses of vitamin E (100 mg/kg/day) may arrest the neurological

432

manifestations.[107] This condition is associated with defective genes coding for the larger subunit of the microsomal triglyceride transfer protein, resulting in abnormal VLDL secretion and impairing delivery of vitamin E and other fat soluble substrates.[108]

The autosomal recessive disorder *Friedreich's ataxia* is associated with defects in the X25 gene on chromosome 9 that codes for a 210 amino acid protein frataxin.[50a] A few cases have point mutation in the gene, but most have homozygous GAA trinucleotide expansions in the first intron. Because of clinical similarities to AVED, it has been suggested that the Friedreich's ataxia gene may also be involved in α-tocopherol metabolism.[109]

Ataxia associated with mitochondrial disorders—Ataxia can be a feature of several of the mitochondrial disorders, especially the MERRF and MELAS syndromes, and the rare syndrome termed NARP.[34] The presence of retinitis pigmentosa should raise the index of suspicion for NARP, which is sometimes due to a point mutation at bp8993 resulting in substitution of arginine for leucine in sub-sequence 6 of the mitochondrial H-ATPase. Patients with this disorder may have seizures, muscle weakness, mental retardation, and long tract signs with symptoms beginning from infancy to late adulthood.

Periodic ataxia, an autosomal dominant disorder in which ataxia-dysarthria attacks lasting seconds to minutes can result from missense point mutations on a potassium channel gene KCNIA located on chromosome 12p.[109a]

Motor neuron disease

Most patients with suspected amyotrophic lateral sclerosis have no known biochemical defect. Kennedy's syndrome (spinal bulbar muscular atrophy) may clinically resemble the bulbar form of amyotrophic lateral sclerosis, although progression is usually slow. A genetics laboratory can confirm this diagnosis by determining the presence of an expanded CAG repeat on the X chromosome (box 14.4).

About 20% of cases of familial amyotrophic lateral sclerosis have been discovered to have one of several mutations of the gene on chromosome 21 that codes for the Cu/Zn binding superoxide dysmutase enzyme (SOD).[110-112]

In patients with mutations in this gene, the concentration and specific activity of Cu/Zn SOD are reduced in erythrocytes by about 50%[113]; however, these changes do not correlate with dis-

Box 14.6 Metabolic disorders associated with involuntary movements

Disease	Type of movement	Associated features	Diagnostic test
• Huntington's disease	Chorea Dystonia (juvenile)	Dementia	Molecular analysis for CAG repeat expansion
• Wilson's disease	Tremor, dystonia chorea	Hepatic insufficiency Kayser-Fleischer ring	Caeruloplasmin, serum and urine copper
• Dentatorubral pallidoluysian atrophy (DRPLA)	Chorea	Ataxia, myoclonus, dementia	Molecular analysis for CAG repeat expansion
• GM$_1$ gangliosidosis	Dystonia, choreoathetosis	Gait disturbance	Leucocyte lysosomal acid β-galactosidase activity
• Dopa responsive dystonia	Dystonia	Dopa responsiveness	Research laboratory for GTP cyclohydrolase mutation
• Ataxia-telangiectasia	Choreoathetosis	Ataxia, auricular, and conjunctival telangiectases	Decreased α-fetoprotein, immunoglobulin abnormalities

ease severity. Detection of the Cu/Zn SOD mutation requires DNA analysis of a blood sample by a genetics laboratory studying this disorder.

Movement disorders (box 14.6)

Wilson's disease

Patients with Wilson's disease can develop symptoms of hepatic or neurological dysfunction. Symptoms that may bring a patient to a neurologist include involuntary movements (tremor, dystonia, chorea, spasms), and behavioural and personality changes. Psychiatric symptoms account for a high proportion of presenting complaints.[64] A Kayser-Fleischer ring may be seen on examination of the cornea.

Wilson's disease is commonly but not invariably associated with reduction in serum caeruloplasmin concentrations (normal range 25-45 mg/dl). Total serum copper concentrations may not be raised. "Free" serum copper can be calculated by subtracting from the total copper ($\mu g/dl$), that amount bound to caeruloplasmin (multiply by 3 the caeruloplasmin concentration (in mg/dl) to obtain the bound copper in $\mu g/dl$). The free copper concentration should be <10–15 $\mu g/dl$. Laboratory standards are variable, however, so it is recommended that a 24 hour urinary copper be obtained. In Wilson's disease copper excretion is >100 $\mu g/24$ h (normal <30 $\mu g/24$ h).

In an asymptomatic patient at risk for Wilson's disease, liver biopsy may be necessary to detect increased copper content in the liver (patients with Wilson's disease have >200 $\mu g/g$ wet weight).

Other metabolic causes of dystonia

Adult onset of dystonia can occur in GM_1 gangliosidosis.[12] The disorder is autosomal recessive and is diagnosed by showing pronounced reduction of activity of the enzyme β-galactosidase, which can be measured in leucocytes. Progressive dopa responsive dystonia has been recently reported to be associated with mutations in a gene on chromosome 14q22.1–22.2 which codes for the enzyme GTP cyclohydrolase 1.[114]

Other movement disorders

Choreic movements are characteristic of Huntington's disease, which is discussed in the section on dementia. Another disorder in which chorea can occur is ataxia-telangiectasia, discussed in the section on ataxias.

Progressive myoclonus epilepsy

The constellation of seizures, myoclonic jerks, and neurological dysfunction including dementia and seizures can occur in several disorders including the mitochondrial disorder MERRF, Lafora body disease and Baltic myoclonus (Unverricht-Lundborg disease). In the last named condition, mutations have been found in the genre on chromosome 21q22.3 that encodes cystatin B, an inhibitor of proteases. Reduced levels of cystatin B mRNA can be detected in lymphoblastoid cells from affected persons.[114a]

Stroke

Metabolic causes of stroke are rare, but must be considered in children and young adults presenting with an acute ischaemic event. Disorders to consider include MELAS syndrome, homocystinuria, sulphite oxidase deficiency, and Fabry's disease. MELAS syndrome can be associated with stroke-like episodes in young adults.[115] Diagnosis may be difficult (see section on mitochondrial disorders) and requires strong suspicion and communication with a genetics laboratory specialising in mitochondrial disorders.

Homocystinuria is much more common than *sulphite oxidase deficiency*. Both disorders may be suspected by the presence of ectopia lentis. Chronic homocysteine infusions in baboons produce sustained endothelial cell loss and result in accelerated atherosclerosis.[116] It has been suggested that moderate homocysteinaemia in otherwise normal subjects may be a risk factor for atherosclerotic stroke.[117] The disorder is due to an inborn error of cystathionine synthase. Urinary amino acid screen will detect raised concentrations of homocystine. *Sulphite oxidase* deficiency can be associated with stroke-like episodes in infancy and childhood.[118] Amino acid screening of the urine must be done carefully and on fresh urine, and should show the presence of S-sulphocysteine.[119] S-sulphocysteine and sulphite are also detectable in plasma.[120] Basal ganglia infarction in children, and adult onset chorea and dementia have been reported in propionic acidaemia.[121 122]

Fabry's disease

This X linked lysosomal storage disease is associated with accumulation of trihexose ceramide due to deficiency in the enzyme ceramide trihexoside α-galactosidase (box 14.3). At an early age, patients develop pinpoint skin lesions, especially on the abdomen. Trihexose ceramide accumulates in blood vessel walls, in the kidney, and in the myocardium. Death is usually due to renal or heart failure. Patients have been reported to develop episodic stroke-like symptoms and headaches. Small infarcts have been found in cerebral hemispheres, associated with proliferative changes in vessel intima and media, presumably due to glycolipid deposition.[123]

Summary

Knowledge of the molecular causes for genetic diseases that affect the nervous system is rapidly expanding. Especially striking has been the finding in several autosomal dominant neurodegenerative disorders that unstable expansions of trinucleotide repeats are responsible for the genetic disorder and that the length of the repeat can be correlated with the age of onset and the severity of symptoms. Phenotypic heterogeneity in many disorders associated with enzyme deficiencies can often be linked to the amount of residual enzyme activity occurring with different gene mutations.

Making a specific diagnosis of a neurological disorder associated with genetically determined metabolic defects requires access to a laboratory that can assist in arranging for appropriate testing to be carried out. In disorders such as the amino acidurias diagnostic metabolic studies can be performed in hospital clinical chemistry laboratories. In others, such as the lysosomal storage diseases, a laboratory that carries out special lipid analyses and white blood cell enzyme assays will be necessary. DNA mutational analyses are becoming commercially available for diagnosing many disorders such as mitochondrial diseases and those conditions associated with expanded trinucleotide repeats. It may be necessary to contact individual research laboratories when confronted with a disorder that has been newly discovered or that is very rare. A computerised directory of specialised laboratories that perform disease specific testing for genetic disorders should be useful in choosing the appropriate diagnostic or research laboratory.

1 Beaudet AL, Scriver CR, Sly WS, *et al.* Genetics and biochemistry of variant human phenotypes. In: Scriver CR, Beaudet AL, Sly WS, Valle D, eds. *The metabolic basis of inherited disease.* 6th ed. New York: McGraw-Hill, 1989:3–53.

2 Harding AE. The DNA laboratory and neurological practice. *J Neurol Neurosurg Psychiatry* 1993;56:229–33.

3 Bird TD, Farrell DF. Genetics and neurology. In: Swanson PD, ed. *Signs and symptoms in neurology,* Philadelphia: JB Lippincott, 1984:345–77.

4 Dubourg O, Durr A, Cancel G, *et al.* Analysis of the SCA1 CAG repeat in a large number of families with dominant ataxia: clinical and molecular correlations. *Ann Neurol* 1995;37:176–80.

5 Nyhan WL, Haas R. Inborn errors of amino acid metabolism and transport. In: Rosenberg RN, Prusiner SB, DiMauro S, *et al,* eds. *The molecular and genetic basis of neurological disease.* Boston: Butterworth-Heinemann, 1993:145–65.

6 Cox RP, Chuang DT. Maple syrup urine disease: clinical and molecular genetic considerations. In: Rosenberg RN, Prusiner SB, DiMauro S, *et al,* eds. *The molecular and genetic basis of neurological disease.* Boston: Butterworth-Heinemann, 1993:189–207.

7 de Duve C, Pressman BC, Gianetto R, *et al.* Tissue fractionation studies. 6. Intracellular distribution patterns of enzymes in rat-liver tissue. *Biochem J* 1955;60:604–17.

8 Hers HG. Inborn lysosomal diseases. *Gastroenterology* 1965;48:625–33.

9 Brady RO. Biochemical genetics in neurology. *Arch Neurol* 1976;33:145–51.

10 Kolodny EH. Current concepts in genetics. Lysosomal storage diseases. *N Engl J Med* 1976;294:1217–20.

11 Suzuki K. Enzymatic diagnosis of sphingolipidoses. *Methods in enzymology* 1987;138:727–62.

12 Yoshida K, Ikeda S, Kawaguchi K, Yanagisawa N. Adult GM$_1$ gangliosidosis: immunohistochemical and ultrastructural findings in an autopsy case. *Neurology* 1994; 44:2376–82.

13 Kolodny EH. Metachromatic leukodystrophy and multiple sulfatase deficiency: sulfatide lipidosis. In: Rosenberg RN, Prusiner SB, DiMauro S, *et al,* eds. *The molecular and genetic basis of neurological disease.* Boston: Butterworth-Heinemann, 1993:497–503.

14 Kolodny EH. The GM2 Gangliosidoses. In: Rosenberg RN, Prusiner SB, DiMauro S, *et al,* eds. *The molecular and genetic basis of neurological disease.* Boston: Butterworth-Heinemann, 1993:531–40.

15 Navon R, Argov Z, Frisch A. Hexosaminidase A deficiency in adults. *Am J Hum Genet* 1986;24:179–96.

16 Yoshida IC, Oshima A, Sakuraba H, *et al.* GM$_1$ gangliosidosis in adults: clinical and molecular analysis of 16 Japanese patients. *Ann Neurol* 1992;31:328–32.

17 Nishimoto J, Nanba E, Inui K, *et al.* GM1-gangliosidosis (genetic β-galactosidase deficiency): identification of four mutations in different clinical phenotypes among Japanese patients. *Am J Hum Genet* 1991;49:566–72.

18 Leinekugel P, Michel S, Conzelmann E, Sandhoff C. Quantitative correlation between the residual activity of β-hexosaminidase A and arylsulfatase A and the severity of the resulting lysosomal storage disease. *Hum Genet* 1992;88:513–23.

19 Goldman JE, Katz D, Rapin I, *et al.* Chronic G$_{M1}$-gangliosidosis presenting as dystonia: I. clinical and pathological features. *Ann Neurol* 1981;9:465–75.

20 Neufeld EF, Lim TW, Shapiro LJ. Inherited disorders of lysosomal metabolism. *Ann Rev Biochem* 1975;44:357–76.

21 Matalon R, Kaul R, Michals K. The mucopolysaccharidoses and the mucolipidoses. In: Rosenberg RN, Prusiner SB, DiMauro S *et al,* eds. *The molecular and genetic basis of neurological disease,* Boston: Butterworth-Heinemann, 1993:401–9.

22 Moser HW, Moser AE, Singh I, O'Neill BP. Adrenoleukodystrophy: survey of 303 cases: biochemistry, diagnosis and therapy. *Ann Neurol* 1984;16:628–41.

23 Moser HW. Peroxisomal disorders. In: Rosenberg RN, Prusiner SB, DiMauro S, *et al,* eds. *The molecular and genetic basis of neurological disease.* Boston: Butterworth-Heinemann, 1993:351–87.

24 Mosser J, Douar AM, Sarde CO, *et al.* Putative X-linked adrenoleukodystrophy gene shows unexpected homology with ABC transporter. *Nature* 1993;361:726–30.

25 van Geel BM, Assies J, Weverling GJ, Barth PG. Predominance of the adrenomyeloneuropathy phenotype of X-linked adrenoleukodystrophy in The Netherlands: a survey of 30 kindreds. *Neurology* 1994;44:2343–6.

26 Moser HW, Moser AB, Smith KD, *et al.* Adrenoleukodystrophy: phenotypic variability

and implications for therapy. *J Inherit Metab Dis* 1992;15:645–64.

27 Farrell DF, Hamilton SR, Knauss TA, *et al*. X-linked adrenoleukodystrophy: adult cerebral variant. *Neurology* 1993;43:1518–22.

28 Kennedy CR, Allen JT, Fensom AH, Steinberg SJ, Wilson R. X-linked adrenoleukodystrophy with non-diagnostic plasma very long chain fatty acids. *J Neurol Neurosurg Psychiatry* 1994;57:759–61.

29 Vorgerd M, Fuchs S, Tegenthoff M, Malin J-P. A missense point mutation (Ser515Phe) in the adrenoleukodystrophy gene in a family with adrenomyeloneuropathy: a clinical, biochemical, and genetic study. *J Neurol Neurosurg Psychiatry* 1995;58:229–31.

30 Crimmins D, Morris JGL, Walker GL, *et al*. Mitochondrial encephalomyopathy: variable clinical expression within a single kindred. *J Neurol Neurosurg Psychiatry* 1993;56:900–5.

31 DeVivo DC. The expanding clinical spectrum of mitochondrial diseases. *Brain Dev* 1993;15:1–22.

32 Fryer A, Appleton R, Sweeney MG, *et al*. Mitochondrial DNA 8993 (NARP) mutation presenting within a heterogeneous phenotype including "cerebral palsy". *Arch Dis Child* 1994;71:419–22.

33 Lestienne P, Bataille N. Mitochondrial DNA alterations and genetic diseases: a review. *Biomed Pharmacother* 1994;48:199–214.

34 Holt IJ, Harding AE, Petty RKH, Morgan-Hughes JA. A new mitochondrial disease associated with mitochondrial DNA heteroplasmy. *Am J Hum Genet* 1990;46:428–33.

35 Lodi R, Montagna P, Iotti S, *et al*. Brain and muscle energy metabolism studied in vivo by ^{31}P magnetic resonance imaging in NARP syndrome. *J Neurol Neurosurg Psychiatry* 1994;57:1492–6.

36 Zeviani M, Taroni F. Mitochondrial diseases. *Bailliere's Clinical Neurology* 1994;3:315–34.

37 Santorelli FM, Shanske S, Jain K, *et al*. A T → C mutation at nt8993 of mitochondrial DNA in a child with Leigh syndrome. *Neurology* 1994;44:972–4.

38 Tatuch Y, Christodonlon J, Feigenbaum A, *et al*. Heteroplasmic mtDNA mutation (T → G) at 8993 can cause Leigh disease when the percentage of abnormal mtDNA is high. *Am J Hum Genet* 1992;50:852–8.

39 La Spada AR, Paulson HL, Fishbeck KH. Trinucleotide repeat expansion in neurological diseases. *Ann Neurol* 1994;36:814–22.

40 La Spad AR, Wilson EM, Lubahn DB, Harding AE, Fischbeck KH. Androgen receptor gene mutations in X-linked spinal and bulbar muscular atrophy. *Nature* 1991;352:77–9.

41 Plassart E, Fontaine B. Genes with triplet repeats: a new class of mutations causing neurological diseases. *Biomed Pharmacother* 1994;48:191–7.

42 Stevanin G, Le Guern E, Ravise N, *et al*. A third locus for autosomal cerebellar ataxia (ADCA) type 1 maps to chromosome 14q26.3qter: evidence for the existence of a fourth locus. *Am J Hum Genet* 1994;521:11–20.

43 Willems PJ. Dynamic mutations hit double figures. *Nature Genetics* 1994;8:213–5.

44 Kawaguchi Y, Okamoto T, Taniwaki M, *et al*. CAG expansions in a novel gene for Machado-Joseph disease at chromosome 14q32.1. *Nature Genetics* 1994;8:221–7.

45 Ranum LPW, Chung M, Banfi S, *et al*. Molecular and clinical correlations in spinocerebellar ataxia 1 (SCA1): evidence for familial effects on the age of onset. *Am J Hum Genet* 1994;55:244–52.

46 Giunti P, Sweeney MG, Spadaro M, *et al*. The trinucleotide repeat expansion on chromosome 6p (SCA 1) in autosomal dominant cerebellar ataxias. *Brain* 1994;227:645–9.

47 Duryao M, Ambrose C, Myers R, *et al*. Trinucleotide repeat length instability and age of onset in Huntington's disease. *Nature Genetics* 1993;4:387–92.

48 Potter NT, Meyer MA, Zimmerman AW. Molecular and clinical findings in a family with dentatorubral-pallidoluysian atrophy. *Ann Neurol* 1995;37:273–7.

49 Nagafuchi S, Yanagisawa H, Sato K, *et al*. Dentatorubral and pallidoluysian atrophy expansion of an unstable CAG trinucleotide on chromosome 12p. *Nature Genetics* 1994;6:14–8.

50 Nagafuchi S, Yanagisawa H, Ohsaki E, *et al*. Structure and expression of the gene responsible for the triplet repeat disorder, dentatorubral and pallidoluysian atrophy (DRPLA). *Nature Genetics* 1994;8:177–82.

50a Campuzano V, Monterimi L, Molto MD, *et al*. Friedrich's ataxia: autosomal recessive disease caused by an intronic GAA triplet repeat expansion. *Science* 1996;271:1423–7.

51 Menkes JH, Alter M, Steigleder GK, *et al*. A sex-linked recessive disorder with growth retardation, peculiar hair, and focal cerebral and cerebellar degeneration. *Pediatrics*

1962;29;764–79.
52 Menkes JH. Kinky hair disease: twenty-five years later. *Brain Dev* 1988;10:77–9.
53 Danks DM, Campbell PE, Stevens BJ, *et al*. Menkes' kinky hair syndrome: an inherited defect in copper absorption with widespread effects. *Pediatrics* 1972;50:188–201.
54 Gunn TR, Macfarlane S, Phillips LI. Difficulties in the neonatal diagnosis of Menkes' kinky hair syndrome-trichopoliodystrophy. *Clinical Pediatr* 1984;23:514-6.
55 Tonnesen T, Horn N. Prenatal and postnatal diagnosis of Menkes disease, an inherited disorder of copper metabolism. *J Inherit Metab Dis* 1989;12 (suppl):207–14.
56 Tumer Z, Tonnesen T, Bohmann J, *et al*. First trimester prenatal diagnosis of Menkes disease by DNA analysis. *J Med Genet* 1994;31:615–7.
57 Bull PC, Cox DW. Wilson disease and Menkes disease: new handles on heavy-metal transport. *Trends Genet* 1994;10:246–52.
58 Tanzi RE, Petrukhin K, Chernov I, *et al*. The Wilson disease gene is a copper transporting ATPase with homology to the Menkes disease gene. *Nature Genetics* 1993;5:344–50.
59 Yamaguchi Y, Heiny ME, Gitlin JD. Isolation and characterization of a human liver cDNA as a candidate gene for Wilson disease. *Biochem Biophys Res Commun* 1993;197:271–7.
60 Thomas GR, Forbes JR, Roberts EA. The Wilson disease gene: spectrum of mutations and their consequences. *Nature Genetics* 1995;9:210–7.
61 Czaja MJ, Weiner FR, Schwarzenberg FJ, *et al*. Molecular studies of ceruloplasmin deficiency in Wilson's disease. *J Clin Invest* 1987;80:1200–4.
62 Walshe JM. Diagnosis and treatment of presymptomatic Wilson's disease. *Lancet* 1988;ii:435–7.
63 Walshe JM. Wilson's disease: yesterday, today, and tomorrow. *Mov Disord* 1988;3:10–29.
64 Walshe JM, Yealland M. Wilson's disease: the problem of delayed diagnosis. *J Neurol Neurosurg Psychiatry* 1992;55:692–6.
65 Gibbs K, Walshe JM. A study of the caeruloplasmin concentrations found in 75 patients with Wilson's disease, their kinships and various control groups. *Quart J Med* 1979;48:447–63.
66 Neri G, Chiurazzi P, Arena JF, Lubs HA. XLMR genes: update 1994. *Am J Med Genet* 1994;51:542–9.
67 Jacobs PA, Glover TW, Mayer M, *et al*. X-linked mental retardation: a study of 7 families. *Am J Med Genet* 1980;7:471–89.
68 Turner G, Brookwell R, Daniel A, *et al*. Heterozygous expression of X-linked mental retardation and X-chromosome marker fra(X) (q27). *N Engl J Med* 1980;303:662–4.
69 Nielson KB. Diagnosis of the fragile X syndrome: clinical findings in 27 males with the fragile site at Xq28. *Journal of Mental Deficiency Research* 1983;27:211–26.
70 Verkerk AJMH, Pieretti M, Sutcliffe JS, *et al*. Identification of a gene (FMR-1) containing CGG repeat coincident with a breakpoint cluster region exhibiting length variation in fragile X syndrome. *Cell* 1991;65:905–14.
71 Fu Y-H, Kuhl DPA, Pizzuti A. Variation of the CGG repeat at the fragile X site results in genetic instability: resolution of the Sherman paradox. *Cell* 1992;67:1047–58.
72 Menkes JH. *Textbook of child neurology*, 5th ed. Baltimore: Williams and Wilkins, 1995.
73 Goate A, Chartier Harlin MC, Mullan M, *et al*. Segregation of missense mutations in amyloid precursor protein gene with familial Alzheimer's disease. *Nature* 1991;349:704–6.
74 Hardy J. Alzheimer's disease. Molecular genetics. *J Fla Med Assoc* 1994;91:759–61.
75 Schellenberg GD, Bird T, Wijsman E, *et al*. Genetic linkage evidence for a familial Alzheimer's disease locus on chromosome 14. *Science* 1992;258:668–71.
75a Levy-Lahad E, Wasco W, Poorkaj P, *et al*. Candidate gene for the Chromosome 1 familial Alzheimer's disease locus. *Science* 1995;269:973–7.
75b Sherrington R, Rogaer EI, Liang Y, *et al*. Cloning of a gene bearing missense mutations in early-onset familial Alzheimer's disease. *Nature* 1995;375:750–60.
76 Kremer B, Goldberg P, Andrew SE, *et al*. A worldwide study of the Huntington's disease mutation. The sensitivity and specificity of measuring CAG repeats. *N Engl J Med* 1994;330:1401–6.
77 Saito Y, Ando T, Doyu M, *et al*. An adult case of classical Pelizaeus-Merzbacher disease-magnetic resonance images and neuropathological findings. *Rinsho Shinkeigaku. Clinical Neurology* 1993;33:187–93.
78 Pham-Dinh D, Boespflug-Tanguy O, Mimault C, *et al*. Pelizaeus-Merzbacher disease: a frameshift deletion/insertion event in the myelin proteolipid gene. *Human Molecular*

DIAGNOSIS OF INHERITED METABOLIC DISORDERS

Genetics 1993;2:465-7.

79 Boespflug-Tanguy O, Mimault C, Melki J, *et al.* Genetic homogeneity of Pelizaeus-Merzbacher disease: tight linkage to the proteolipoprotein locus in 16 affected families. *Am J Hum Genet* 1994;55:461-7.

80 Strautnieks S, Rutland P, Winter RM, *et al.* Pelizaeus-Merzbacher disease: detection of mutations THR[181] → Pro and Leu[223] → Pro in the proteolipid protein gene, and prenatal diagnosis. *Am J Hum Genet* 1992;51:871-8.

81 Matalon R, Michals K, Sebasta D, *et al.* Aspartoacyclase deficiency and N-acetylaspartic aciduria in patients with Canavan disease. *Am J Med Genet* 1988;29:463-71.

82 Gardiner RM. Genetic analysis of Batten disease. *J Inherit Metab Dis* 1993;16:787-90.

82a Vesa J, Hellsten E, Verkruyse LA, *et al.* Mutations in the palmitoyl protein thioesterase gene causing infantile neuronal ceroid lipofuscinosis. *Nature* 1995;376:584-8.

83 Mitchison HM, Taschner PE, O'Rawe AM, *et al.* Genetic mapping of the Batten disease locus (CLN3) to the interval D16S288-D16S383 by analysis of haplotypes and allelic association. *Genomics* 1994;22:465-8.

83a Munroe PB, Rapola J, Mittison HM, *et al.* Prenatal diagnosis of Batten's disease. *Lancet* 1996;347:1014-5.

84 Ferrer I, Arbizu T, Pena J, Serra JP. A Golgi and ultrastructural study of a dominant form of Kufs' disease. *J Neurol* 1980;222:183-90.

85 Martin J-J. Adult type of neuronal ceroid-lipofuscinosis. *J Inherit Metab Dis* 1993;16:237-40.

86 Rosenberg RN. Autosomal dominant cerebellar phenotypes: the genotype has settled the issue. *Neurology* 1995;45:1-5.

87 Savitsky K, Bar-Shira A, Gilad S, *et al.* A single ataxia telangiectasia gene with a product similar to PI-3 kinase. *Science* 1995;268:1749-53.

88 Serizawa M, Sakamoto M, Hirabayashi K, *et al.* Histological and radiobiological study of adult cases with ataxia telangiectasia. *Rinsho Shinkeigaku. Clinical Neurology* 1994;34:38-42.

89 Boder E. Ataxia-telangiectasia. In: Gomez MR, ed. *Neurocutaneous diseases. A practical approach,* Boston: Butterworths, 1987:95-117.

90 Gardner K, Alderson K, Galster B, *et al.* Autosomal dominant spinocerebellar ataxia: clinical description of a distinct hereditary ataxia and genetic localization to chromosome 16 (SCA4) in a Utah kindred. *Neurology* 1994;921S.

91 Benomar A, Le Guern E, Dure A. Autosomal dominant cerebellar ataxia with retinal degeneration (ADCA type II) is genetically different from ADCA type 1. *Ann Neurol* 1994;35:439-44.

92 Ranum LPW, Schut LJ, Lundgren JK, *et al.* Spinocerebellar ataxia type 5 in a family descended from the grandparents of President Lincoln maps to chromosome 11. *Nature Genetics* 1994;8:280-4.

93 Harding AE. The clinical features and classification of the late onset autosomal dominant cerebellar ataxias. *Brain* 1982;105:1-28.

94 Smith JK, Gonda VE, Malamud N. Unusual form of cerebellar ataxia. Combined dentato-rubral and pallido-luysian degeneration. *Neurology* 1958;8:205-9.

95 Schimschock JR, Alvord EC, Swanson PD. Cerebrotendinous xanthomatosis: clinical and pathological studies. *Arch Neurol* 1968;18:688-98.

96 Menkes JH, Schimschock JR, Swanson PD. Cerebrotendinous xanthomatosis: the storage of cholestanol within the nervous system. *Arch Neurol* 1968;19:47-53.

97 Berginer VM, Salen G, Shefer S. Long-term treatment of cerebrotendinous xanthomatosis with chenodeoxycholic acid. *N Engl J Med* 1984;311:1649-52.

98 Leitersdorf E, Reshef A, Meiner V, *et al.* Frameshift and splice-junction mutations in the sterol 27-hydroxylase gene cause cerebrotendinous xanthomatosis in Jews of Moroccan origin. *J Clin Invest* 1993;91:2488-96.

99 Kim K-S, Kubata S, Kuriyama M, *et al.* Identification of new mutations in sterol 27-hydroxylase gene in Japanese patients with cerebrotendinous xanthomatosis (CTX). *J Lipid Research* 1994;35:1031-9.

100 Nakashima N, Sakai Y, Sakai H, *et al.* A point mutation in the bile acid biosynthetic enzyme sterol 27-hydroxylase in a family with cerebrotendinous xanthomatosis. *J Lipid Research* 1994;35:663-8.

101 Meiner V, Meiner Z, Reshef A, *et al.* Cerebrotendinous xanthomatosis: molecular diagnosis enables presymptomatic detection of a treatable disease. *Neurology* 1994;44:288-90.

102 Harding AE, Matthews S, Jones S, *et al.* Spinocerebellar degeneration associated with a

selective defect of vitamin E absorption. *N Engl J Med* 1985;**313**:32–5.

103 Stumpf DA, Sokol R, Bettis D, *et al.* Friedreich's disease: V. Variant form with vitamin E deficiency and normal fat absorption. *Neurology* 1987;**37**:68–74.

104 Ben Hamida M, Belal S, Sirugo G, *et al.* Friedreich's ataxia phenotype not linked to chromosome 9 and associated with selective autosomal recessive vitamin E deficiency in two inbred Tunisian families. *Neurology* 1993;**43**:2179–83.

105 Ben Hamida C, Doerflinger N, Belal S, *et al.* Localization of Friedreich ataxia phenotype with selective vitamin E deficiency to chromosome 8q by homozygosity mapping. *Nature Genetics* 1993;**5**:195–200.

106 Ouahchi K, Arita M, Kayden H, *et al.* Ataxia with isolated vitamin E deficiency is caused by mutations in the α-tocopherol transfer protein. *Nature Genetics* 1995;**9**:141–5.

107 Kayden HJ. The neurologic syndrome of vitamin E deficiency: a significant cause of ataxia. *Neurology* 1993;**43**:2167–9.

108 Sharp D, Blinderman L, Combs KA, *et al.* Cloning and gene defects in microsomal triglyceride transfer protein associated with abetalipoproteinemia. *Nature* 1993;**365**:65–9.

109 DiDonato S. Can we avoid AVED? *Nature Genetics* 1995;**9**:106–7.

109a Browne DL, Gancher ST, Nutt JG, *et al.* Episodic ataxia myokymia syndrome is associated with point mutations in the human potassium channel, KCNA1. *Nature Genetics* 1994;**8**:136–40.

110 Rosen DR, Siddique T, Patterson D, *et al.* Mutations in Cu/Zn superoxide dismutase gene are associated with familial amyotrophic lateral sclerosis. *Nature* 1993;**362**:59–62.

111 Deng H-X, Hentati A, Tainer JA. Amyotrophic lateral sclerosis and structural defects in Cu,Zn superoxide dismutase. *Science* 1993;**261**:1047–51.

112 Aoki M, Ogasawara M, Matsubara Y, *et al.* Familial amyotrophic lateral sclerosis (ALS) in Japan associated with H46R mutation in Cu/Zn superoxide dismutase gene: a possible new subtype of familial ALS. *J Neurol Sci* 1994;**126**:77–83.

113 Bowling AC, Barkowski EE, McKenna YD, *et al.* Superoxide dismutase concentration and activity in familial amyotrophic lateral sclerosis. *J Neurochem* 1995;**64**:2366–9.

114 Ichinose H, Ohye T, Takahashi E, *et al.* Hereditary progressive dystonia with marked diurnal fluctuation caused by mutations in the GTP cyclohydrolase 1 gene. *Nature Genetics* 1994;**8**:236–41.

114a Pennachio LA, Lehesjoki A-E, Stone NE, *et al.* Mutations in the gene-encoding cystatin B in progressive myoclonus epilepsy (EPM1). *Science* 1996;**271**:1731–4.

115 Lertrit P, Noer AS, Jean-Francis MJB, *et al.* A new disease related mutation for mitochondrial encephalomyopathy, lactic acidosis and stroke-like episodes syndrome affecting the ND4 subunit of complex I. *Am J Hum Genet* 1992;**52**:457–68.

116 Harker LA, Ross R, Slichter SJ, Scott CR. Homocystine-induced arteriosclerosis. The role of endothelial cell injury and platelet response in its genesis. *J Clin Invest* 1976;**58**:731–41.

117 Brattstrom LE, Hardebo JE, Hultberg BC. Moderate homocysteinemia—a possible risk factor for arteriosclerotic cerebrovascular disease. *Stroke* 1984;**15**:1012–6.

118 Riela AR, Roach S. Etiology of stroke in children. *J Child Neurol* 1993;**8**:201–20.

119 Mudd SH, Irreverre F, Laster L. Sulfite oxidase deficiency in man: demonstration of the enzymatic defect. *Science* 1967;**156**:1599–602.

120 Shih VE, Abroms IF, Johnson JL, *et al.* Sulfite oxidase deficiency. Biochemical and clinical investigations of a hereditary metabolic disorder in sulfur metabolism. *New Engl J Med* 1977;**297**:1022–8.

121 Haas RH, Marsden DL, Capistrano-Estrada S, Hamilton R *et al.* Acute basal ganglia infarction in propionic acidemia. *J Child Neurol* 1995;**10**:18–22.

122 Sesthi KD, Ray R, Roesel RA. Adult-onset chorea and dementia with propionic acidemia. **39**:1343–5.

123 Christensen Lou HO, Reske-Nielson E. The central nervous system in Fabry's disease. *Arch Neurol* 1971; **25**:351–9.

15 Cerebrospinal fluid

E J THOMPSON

Normal physiology of blood-brain barriers

Despite the existence of several "barriers" between the blood and the brain, cerebrospinal fluid (CSF) can still be considered as an ultrafiltrate of plasma. There are, nevertheless, exceptions to this generality. Perhaps the most obvious relates to CSF cells, of which about two thirds are found to be lymphocytes and one third monocytes, whereas the blood contains mainly granulocytes. Most immunologists could thus be forgiven for assuming that CSF is a type of lymphatic fluid. More recent trends in immunology[1] have spoken of "regional" immunology in which localised variations in immune modulators cause the nature of the response to vary from region to region—that is, the overall lymphatic/cytokine milieu is different in the brain from that in, say, the gut or the lung. Due to the higher brain concentration of TGF-β, the CNS tends to emphasise the cell mediated (Th2) over the humoral (Th1) response, at least in experimental autoimmune encephalomyelitis.[2]

In normal CSF, about 80% of proteins are transudated from plasma and 20% are synthesised by the brain. Under pathological conditions there are striking alterations. The bulk of the normal CSF proteins are derived from the plasma. There are various rules which govern the process of ultrafiltration but, as the word "ultrafiltrate" suggests, the molecular size is of primary importance. The word "barrier" suggests some sort of impervious limit which cannot ever be breached. All known proteins pass from plasma into CSF, however, and mainly do so in inverse relation to their molecular size.[3] It is important to realise that none is excluded by any

443

"barrier". The barrier is only relative and probably best understood as a function based on hydrated molecular size. There are other functions, notably lipophilicity, which mainly applies to substances with molecular weights less than 500 Da. Molecular charge plays a lesser part in determining ease of entry into the CSF from the plasma. Acidic proteins have a slight advantage over proteins with a more basic charge. Because of the difference in CSF composition compared with a parallel blood (plasma or serum) sample, comparisons between the two fluids are always necessary to detect local synthesis of any given analyte, antigen, or antibody. This demonstration of local synthesis is based on the initial statement that CSF is mainly an ultrafiltrate of plasma. Figure 15.1 shows the six main barriers and sources of CSF production:

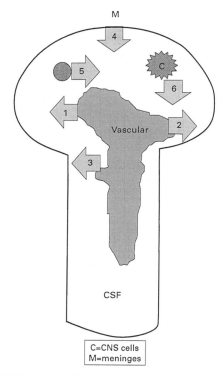

Figure 15.1   *CSF barriers and sources: 1 = blood-CSF barrier; 2 = blood-brain barrier; 3 = blood-dorsal root barrier; 4 = meninges; 5 = wandering cells; 6 = sessile cells (for details see text)*

(1) *The blood-CSF barrier*—The choroid plexus is the main source of CSF, accounting for two thirds of the volume. CSF production is rarely affected by abnormalities of the choroid plexus.

(2) *The blood-brain barrier*—The rest of the brain vasculature accounts for one third of the CSF volume. Many abnormalities affect this route, the most common being brain tumours. Lesions which produce Froin's syndrome give the highest CSF protein concentrations.

(3) *The blood-dorsal root barrier*—The vasculature within the dorsal root ganglia is more permeable than the rest of the brain vasculature. In the Guillain-Barré syndrome there can be dramatic increases in the total protein concentrations surrounding the spinal cord, whereas the total protein in the ventricles is quite low.

(4) *The meninges*—The meninges do not normally produce any CSF. In meningitis there is a dramatic increase in the permeability to cells and serum proteins.

(5) *CSF cells*—The normal CSF contains two thirds lymphocytes and one third monocytes. In various inflammatory diseases, plasma cells are lymphocytes actively secreting antibody whereas polymorphs typically imply bacterial infection;

(6) *The structural cells which constitute the nervous system*—Four marker proteins correspond to the four cell types: neurons—enolase; astrocytes—glial fibrillary acidic protein; oligodendrocytes—myelin basic protein; microglia—ferritin.

Cells enter the CSF using rules other than molecular size. Ignoring red cells, the blood mainly contains granulocytes (polymorphs) but these are essentially absent from normal CSF. As we have noted, lymphocytes are the commonest cells in the CSF and are derived from the blood. Monocytes (macrophages) can either be derived from the blood or from the local microglia (which comprise about one third of brain cells), being a kind of sessile macrophage, which can present antigens to local lymphocytes.

Methods of analysis of CSF and serum

Gram stain and culture using traditional growth media

The growth of bacteria from CSF in acute meningitis using standard molecular techniques is required to define the specific type of bacteria and to test for sensitivities to the appropriate antibiotics. It is essential to prepare a Gram stain to help select the initial antibiotics on the simple basis of whether there are Gram positive cocci or Gram negative rods.

Immunodetection of antigen and antibody

Immunoassays have evolved to detect the various antigens which may be found in the CSF. Initial work was done with counter immunoelectrophoresis which then evolved through latex agglutination, in which the surface of the latex beads was coated with antibody against the antigen in question, and finally the methodology evolved to use enzyme linked immunosorbent assay (ELISA) technology. This is basically a colorimetric technique in small microtitre wells.

In the detection of specific antibodies, the newest move in technology is to examine the oligoclonal antibody response with nitrocellulose immunoblotting, in which the nitrocellulose membrane has been previously impregnated with the relevant antigen. This provides additional information as to the underlying clonal pattern of the antibodies which can be different in the CSF from parallel serum, as will be shown below with the five types of pattern (using total IgG rather than antigen specific IgG).

Cytology: cytospin; immunostaining

The traditional procedure for cell counting is based on the number of cells per μl. The use of the cytospin centrifuge allows 300 μl to be effectively concentrated on to a single slide with the dimension of the cell pellet being only a few millimetres,[4] which can be readily scanned under the microscope. Additional slides can also be prepared for immunostaining with antigen specific reagents.[5]

Malignant cells are occasionally found in the CSF, in cases of primary or secondary CNS tumours. The presence of plasma cells follows the general pattern previously noted that qualitative analysis can be more informative than quantitative analysis—that is, despite unequivocally normal CSF cell counts, there can be atypical, reactive lymphocytes or frank plasma cells. These typically coincide with the presence of oligoclonal IgG indicating local synthesis.[6]

Biochemistry: lactate

Lactate gives more information than the traditional estimation of glucose in distinguishing bacterial (higher lactate) from viral

446

meningitis. The fluoride (or oxalate) bottle, which has usually been dedicated to glucose, can be used to preserve the lactate specimen. In the blood, however, the specimen should be collected into perchloric acid to stop any further metabolism of the lactate present.

Isoelectric focusing

By international consensus five types of banding pattern are recognised when comparing the isoelectric focusing of CSF and parallel serum from the same patient (figure 15.2).

Polymerase chain reaction (PCR)

This technique is now popular for the diagnosis of herpes simplex encephalitis and has largely replaced the use of brain biopsy. Many investigators have found that this is a reliable test for herpes encephalitis, but a slight degree of caution should still be exercised. Although false positives in the PCR technique are notorious, false negative results have also been noted, especially depending on the time of sampling of CSF. Whereas the viral DNA can often be detected in the first seven to 10 days (when the antibody is negative), following this the obverse applies: there will be positive antibody with negative PCR.[7] Therefore CSF should be screened for antibodies against herpes simplex, as well as looking for the herpes DNA.[8] It seems likely that this will be true of other viruses as well. Many other DNA sequences have been looked for using PCR, and also RNA viruses, when reverse transcriptase is used first to convert the RNA into DNA. Recent papers sound a note of caution for some of these techniques.[9] One attempt at quality control produced very sobering results when several different laboratories achieved a wide range of false positives and false negatives for the PCR of DNA from defined specimens containing tubercle bacilli.[10] There is an obvious need to establish international schemes for the quality assurance of PCR for each DNA/RNA sequence being amplified.

According to Baringer and Pisani,[11] postmortem analyses of neurological and non-neurological diseases have shown that some of the neurotropic viruses are found in brain tissue. This may not be surprising, given that a virus such as herpes simplex is essentially endemic in the population and most people over the age of 30 normally have antibodies against herpes in their serum. This reinforces the idea not only of possible false positives, but also the

447

more important question of measurement of the concentrations of DNA in parallel CSF and serum. It would thus be of little consequence to find a positive PCR result from the CSF of a patient who had viraemia when any insult to the blood-brain barriers would simply allow the virus into the CSF.[9] In this case some of the newer techniques for quantitative measurement of herpes antigen would be more relevant.[12] These rely on quantitative chemiluminescence detection of viral antigen using labelled herpes antibody. Attempts to achieve quantitative PCR are unfortunately not simply related to the number of amplifications which are performed in the two parallel fluids (CSF and serum). On balance, PCR for herpes remains reliable, but we recently had a case which was negative on two punctures, yet was positive for antibody and responded well to acyclovir.

Spectroscopic scan: xanthochromia

The analysis of haemoglobin pigments in the CSF requires scanning a broad spectrum from the ultraviolet through visible light to allow expression of the peak height ratios of different wavelengths. Raised total protein concentration usually produces absorption due to tyrosine at 280 nm, whereas the other haemoglobin pigments have distinct wavelengths, which depend on the time the haemoglobin has been in the CSF, as it is further metabolised in vivo into derivative bile products.[13]

ELISA: ferritin (necrosis)

The ELISA technique is likely to replace many radioimmunoassays, and a good example of the technique is the measurement of ferritin. Ferritin concentration in CSF is a particularly good test for intracranial bleeding (causing CNS necrosis) and is more sensitive than the traditional technique of testing for xanthochromia.[14] Because ferritin is normally produced locally by the microglial cells, any increase in activity of these cells due either to phagocytosis (secondary to necrosis) or in response to a strong immunological stimulus such as infection, will result in dramatic increases in ferritin in CSF.

Immunoelectrophoresis: β_2-transferrin (CSF marker)

The β_2-transferrin protein (originally called tau protein) is the best marker to detect spinal fluid in nasal secretions in suspected CSF

448

rhinorrhoea.[15] This is performed using an immunostain of nitro-cellulose blotting with transferrin antibody. The β_2-transferrin protein represents transferrin without the sialic acid residues and is thus an unequivocal marker for an unknown fluid being derived from CSF rather than other analytes (for example, glucose) which are less reliable markers for CSF.

Molecular sizing: small (free light chains); large (polymers)

Free light chains have traditionally been estimated using pre-adsorbed antiserum which can unfortunately still show some cross reactivity with bound light chains. Polyacrylamide gel electrophoresis separates proteins on the basis of their molecular size. Free light chains are by definition not bound to heavy chains and run ahead of the traditional gamma region, where all the intact (bound) immunoglobulins migrate. Two replicate nitrocellulose blots are applied to the polyacrylamide gel, one is immunostained with antikappa and the other with antilambda, to look for a discrepancy in the two light chain patterns, which is then consistent with local synthesis of IgG in the CNS. It also indicates recent antigenic stimulation in the CNS as may be seen in multiple sclerosis relapses.

Haptoglobin polymers (of large molecular size) are the most subtle test for barrier damage. The concentrations are also increased in relation to relapses in multiple sclerosis.[16] The concentrations of haptoglobin polymers increase with normal aging.

CSF flow rates: brain proteins

Cerebrospinal fluid is produced at the rate of some 500 ml per 24 hours, so that the fluid passing over the brain surface is renewed about once every six hours. A single lumbar puncture performed on a patient who has sustained cerebral injury will therefore only reflect the concentration of brain proteins which are found in the CSF at that particular point in time. Additional punctures show whether the concentration of brain specific proteins is increasing or decreasing, and over what interval of time. This kind of "vectorial" analysis gives the most useful information when applied to CSF (and serum) and is clearly set out in the example from Hans et al[17] using the brain form (BB) of creatine kinase. They found that there is an exponential decay of enzyme activity during the first day after injury, with a half life of 4·5 hours.

Serum acute phase monitoring: C reactive protein

The concentrations of CSF C reactive protein (CRP) are highly variable and have less value in clinical practice than the serum concentrations.[18] In response to tissue injury of whatever aetiology, feedback via the cytokine network induces increases in several acute phase proteins, with the most dramatic increases being in the concentrations of CRP. Because of multiple possible causes, CRP cannot be used as a diagnostic test. However, monitoring CRP is helpful in a known disease such as systemic lupus to check for possible intercurrent infection and consequent modulation of the immunosuppressive therapy. It also provides a useful indication of immunological changes in multiple sclerosis as described by Dowling and Cook[19] and confirmed by us.

Urinary substances: neopterin; myelin basic protein

Neopterin, a byproduct of interferon-γ induced macrophage activity, has previously been measured in the CSF and found to be related to recent exacerbations in multiple sclerosis.[20] Increases in neopterin have been found during longitudinal studies of the urine in patients with the progressive form of multiple sclerosis as well as in the traditional relapsing and remitting type.[21] Fragments of myelin basic protein have also been studied in relation to predicting response to therapy as shown below.

Abnormal findings and their clinical relevance

Sensitivity and specificity for a given disease

The correct interpretation of any abnormal result cannot be understood without reference to the incidence of that abnormality in the relevant population, and the prior probability of, say, multiple sclerosis in different geographical areas. The predictive value (PV) for a positive (or a negative) result is largely dependent on this value for the prior probability and this is also reflected in the sensitivity of the test in question—that is, what percentage of patients with a certain disease will show the associated abnormality.[22] As far as the use of various laboratory tests is concerned, the combination of sensitivity and specificity can also be expressed graphically by the receiver and operator curve.[23]

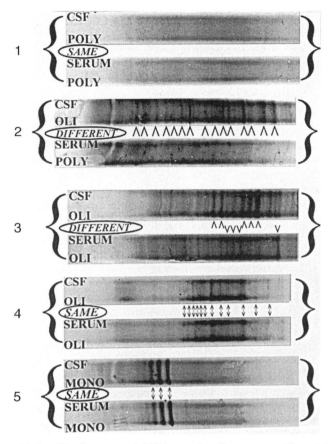

Figure 15.2   *The five types of CSF/serum banding patterns: Type 1 is
normal with a polyclonal response in both CSF and serum; type 2 is a typical
CSF oligoclonal response with the parallel serum showing a normal polyclonal
response; type 3 is the "systemic + superimposed local synthesis" picture in
which there are oligoclonal patterns in both CSF and serum but they differ in
the isoelectric points (pI) of the bands and/or their relative peak height ratios
between the bands in the two fluids. It is also called the "greater than" pattern
since there are a greater number of oligoclonal bands in CSF than in serum;
type 4 has been termed the "mirror" pattern in which the oligoclonal patterns
in CSF and serum are essentially the same. This reflects primarily a systemic
disease or, if there is infection in the brain, such as meningitis, the systemic
response plays the predominant part; type 5 is the monoclonal response which is
typical for paraproteins and shows three to five regularly spaced bands of which
the most prominent is near the cathode. Successively decreasing amounts of
band staining are found towards the anode*

The question of specificity relates essentially to pathological controls—patients with diseases other than that in question—what percentage will show the specified abnormality? The finding of oligoclonal bands in the CSF but not the serum will reflect intrathecal inflammation, which is more common in chronic than acute diseases, as it takes about seven to 10 days for the plasma cells to begin to secrete IgG molecules.

The combined sensitivity and specificity of CSF oligoclonal bands gives considerable weight to the diagnosis of multiple sclerosis, not only because of the high sensitivity (of the order of 97% using the recommended techniques[24]), but also for the specificity of pathogenesis, which if the patient does not have multiple sclerosis, at least gives a strong indication for an inflammatory disease (this will be discussed in further detail below, box 15.1).

Box 15.1   Antigen-specific IgG studies on CSF

Organism

- Bacteria:
  S pneumoniae
  H influenzae
  N meningitidis
  M tuberculosis
  T pallidum
  B burgdorferi

- Viruses:
  Measles
  Herpes simplex types I, II
  Varicella zoster
  Rubella
  Mumps
  Cytomegalovirus
  JC papova virus
  ECHO virus
  Epstein-Barr virus

- Protozoans:
  Toxoplasma
  Malaria

- Other
  Kveim
  Aspergillus

Qualitative versus quantitative analysis

For many years now IgG, as well as albumin or total protein, have each been determined in CSF and parallel serum with the final evaluation being expressed by various mathematical formulae. These formulations are derived from either presumed simple linear relations or more complex curvolinear relations of IgG to albumin which are then used to quantify amounts of IgG which are ostensibly synthesised within the CNS compartment. It is of some historical note that the first demonstration by Kabat of abnormal CSF immunoglobulins was based on the qualitative method of electrophoresis before he subsequently published his paper on the precipitation of IgG to quantify its amount. The strongest current consensus arrived at by a pan-European committee is that qualitative analysis using isoelectric focusing followed by immunofixation for IgG is a more sensitive and specific test for the diagnosis of multiple sclerosis than the quantitative determination of IgG/albumin in CSF/serum using any of the mathematical formulations, including the various non-linear representations.[24]

Affinity maturation of antibody response

It has been known for many years that patients with multiple sclerosis have locally synthesised antibodies against measles and other neurotropic agents.[25 26] It is not seriously considered, however, that measles or other viral antigens have a primary role in the pathogenesis of multiple sclerosis, merely that these antibodies, which have low affinity, represent a secondary phenomenon. This is by contrast with patients with bona fide viral infections who have antibodies of high affinity.[27] It has also been shown that patients with a viral infection of, for example, measles will have high affinity antibody to the causative virus, but the same patients will also have low affinity antibody against other unrelated viral antigens.[27] Sodium thiocyanate can be used to measure the strength of the antigen-antibody bonds as it dissociates the hydrogen bonds between antigen and antibody. The lower the concentration of thiocyanate required to perform dissociation, the lower the affinity of the antigen/antibody bonding and vice versa.[28] It is our experience that the diagnosis of a viral infection of the nervous system can be improved in some cases by using the combination of thiocyanate with antigen immunoblotting (qualitative) rather than the more traditional ELISA technique (quantitative). It is

453

easy to visualise the qualitative difference between polyclonal, oligoclonal, and monoclonal IgG responses on nitrocellulose blots, whereas given the same IgG clones in solution, there is no discrimination using the ELISA technique between these three different types of antibody response.[29] It is thus important for the determination of local IgG synthesis to compare the clonal pattern in CSF v the corresponding serum, as well as any difference in affinity for the two parallel fluids being analysed. As in other branches of medicine, the diagnosis is often made by pattern recognition, in this case the pattern of the IgG clones. Thus any analysis of CSF should utilise tests for antigen as well as antibody against the specified antigen, as they will often produce complementary results rather than simply suggesting that one test is "better" than the other.

Diseases

Infection: acute; chronic; secondary infections (HIV)

A good indicator of bacterial meningitis is CSF lactate greater than 3·5 mmol/l in combination with a white count of less than 800 cells/μl.[30 31] Concentrations of serum lactate should always be measured in parallel specimens, to prove local synthesis of lactate within the CNS. Another indicator of infection is the serum concentration of C-reactive protein (CRP), which is much more reliable than the CSF concentration of CRP. There are some neurotropic brain pathogens which can be diagnosed using either the ELISA technique followed by affinity titration with thiocyanate, or the preferred additional technique of antigen-specific immunoblotting again followed by thiocyanate titration. Box 15.1 gives a partial list of antibodies which have been detected for specific pathogens.[32]

Inflammation: multiple sclerosis; autoimmune disease

We shall consider in due course the differential diagnosis of a positive oligoclonal response within the CNS. The most common cause is multiple sclerosis; however, other infectious or autoimmune diseases must be excluded. The immunopathological interpretation of an oligoclonal response is that there must be a responsible antigen. In working through the differential diagnosis to try and find infectious antigens, or antibodies against other antigens such as double stranded DNA or cardiolipin antibody which are typical of autoimmune diseases,[33] it is only after exclusion of the entire list of other possible causes of antigenic stimulation, that one can be left with a confident diagnosis of multiple sclerosis.

Neoplasia

Malignant cells can be found in the sediment of CSF and this can be reassuring as a direct demonstration of pathological cells in question. It is important to realise that there must be fluid communication between the tumour and the CSF for the cells to be shed into the CSF. The same is true for the determination of carcinoembryonic antigen (CEA). This is typically expressed as an index—that is, the concentration of CEA in CSF divided by the concentration in serum, which is further normalised by dividing the concentration of CSF albumin by the concentration of serum albumin.[34] This is particularly useful in carcinoma involving the meninges and is generally of more value in secondary (metastatic) than primary CNS tumours. Patients with leukaemic infiltration of the CNS (including myeloma) can have the same index calculation performed in which the CSF concentration of paraprotein divided by its concentration in serum, is again normalised to the CSF albumin divided by the serum albumin. In other cases in which there is no tumour to be found within the CNS, there can be "remote" effects of carcinoma in which there is cross reactivity between various brain antigens and the tumour antigens in, for example, lung or ovarian tumours. These patients can have an oligoclonal pattern or a "mirror" pattern. This is due to the strong systemic response which will be discussed further under the differential diagnosis of the "mirror" pattern.

Injury: CNS trauma

We have previously discussed the use of β_2-transferrin for the detection of CSF rhinorrhoea or otorrhoea. Various brain proteins have been used to diagnose and monitor patients with brain injury (for example, road traffic accidents) using several different brain proteins, mainly myelin basic protein or enolase, and to a lesser degree (although they show the same pattern), proteolipid protein, glial fibrillary acidic protein, ferritin, S-100, N-CAM protein, and myelin associated glycoprotein.[35]

As noted previously, the higher the concentrations or the more persistent the increases of these proteins, the worse is the likely outcome from the injury.

455

Haemorrhage: xanthochromia and ferritin

Although we have previously discussed the use of xanthochromia as an indicator of cerebral haemorrhage, CSF ferritin is a more sensitive marker. Nevertheless, the question of specificity for ferritin must also be considered in the context of possible brain infection.

Destruction: Creutzfeldt-Jakob disease

In Creutzfeldt-Jakob disease the excessive proliferation of prion proteins produces large scale destruction of brain parenchyma due to the accumulation of the amyloid type of cross linked proteins. The extraordinarily high concentrations of normal brain proteins found in the CSF in Creutzfeldt-Jakob disease can also be helpful in its diagnosis, and are presumably related to the massive spongiform destruction of the CNS with the consequence that brain proteins are easily found in CSF and serum.[36]

Brain death: enolase

The concentrations of neuron-specific enolase have been used, but only by some investigators, to confirm the clinical diagnosis of brain death.[37]

Isolated inracranial hypertension: IgG index

Determination of CSF pressure using the manometer at the time of lumbar puncture is important not only for diagnosis but also for monitoring the treatment of isolated inracranial hypertension. An unexpected finding was the increase in the IgG index in this disease.[22] However, the patients had no oligoclonal bands in the CSF. Careful analysis of the serum concentrations of albumin and IgG (with reference to the CSF concentrations of albumin and IgG) showed that imbalance for any of these variables can yield a consequent increase in the IgG index. The primary pathological process is therefore not thought to be related to an intrinsic intrathecal immunological abnormality but is probably related to secondary alterations in the body fluid balance within the compartments of CSF as contrasted with serum, which could thereby alter the relative amounts of CSF IgG when compared with the other three variables of the IgG index.

456

Diagnosis by clinical and paraclinical techniques

Quality assurance for reliable diagnosis

The importance of quality assurance is to give independent objective evidence that the laboratory is sufficiently reliable to be able to support the diagnosis in question, using their chosen technology (which is hopefully up to date), and that their results are being interpreted correctly (as can be seen with the five types of band pattern in isoelectric focusing). Some tests have been subjected to the history of the swinging pendulum—there is an initial burst of enthusiasm, and as soon as people realise the test is not perfect, the pendulum swings back towards doubt. A more appropriate equilibrium is eventually reached. This can be seen not only for tests such as PCR, but also for other paraclinical "tests" such as MRI. It is important to have blind specimens sent to the laboratory in question to ascertain the accuracy of diagnosis, and this also applies to qualitative judgements, not only for the five types of isoelectric focusing patterns but also for the exchange of slides between pathologists and radiographs between radiologists[38] (and chapter 2 of this volume). Clinicians should still request that their colleagues in the pathology and radiology departments provide evidence that results from their techniques have been externally verified.

Oligoclonal bands and MRI are complementary for diagnosis of "early" multiple sclerosis

The relative risk ratio (RR), which is analogous to the predictive value (PV) for a positive result, was essentially the same for MRI and oligoclonal bands in the study of Miller et al.[39] About half the patients who were positive for either MRI or CSF bands went on to develop multiple sclerosis. When both tests were positive, over 80% developed multiple sclerosis, but when both were negative, none developed multiple sclerosis. A subsequent study by Morrissey et al[40] showed a dramatically lower response for CSF, which could either be explained by the few specimens they examined or perhaps more relevant was the fact that the lumbar puncture was often performed early in the disease. By contrast, MRI can more easily be repeated at all stages of progression. Having personally reviewed many of the cases in question, it would seem that the paper of Miller et al[39] is likely to provide the more representative result overall. This continues to be the fruitful subject of ongoing collaborative research. Independent studies of the quality assurance for the different IgG separation techniques[41] have emphasised the idea that each different method for the demonstration of oligoclonal bands can yield dramatic differences, with electrophoresis on agarose with Coomassie staining being much less sensitive than isoelectric focusing followed by immunofixation for IgG.[42] This also reinforces the point that any technique must be regularly assessed using external "blinded" specimens. This will ensure not only reproducibility but also the basic credibility of the laboratory results as well as the underlying methodology.

With the much vaunted recent success attributed to β-interferon trials, more patients are being recruited with "early" multiple sclerosis. It is thus particularly important that the diagnosis of "latent" or possible multiple sclerosis is made as confidently as possible. This means that MRI in itself may not be sufficient and, especially in these early cases, a lumbar puncture should provide the necessary extra degree of confidence to either accept or reject the diagnosis of multiple sclerosis. This has been the conclusion of most investigators in the field.[39 42 43]

Cerebrospinal fluid and MRI are complementary for the diagnosis of "early" multiple sclerosis. When both are positive, there is a very high index of credibility for the disease. Conversely, when both are negative, the obverse is true.

Differential diagnosis of positive oligoclonal bands (local synthesis)

These disorders all have a common pathogenesis—namely, inflammatory disease—with the basic underlying question being what is the antigen? Having ruled out the common antigens, one is left by exclusion with the diagnosis of multiple sclerosis, for which there is as yet no known specific antigen. Box 15.2 gives an illustrative differential diagnosis.

Patients with SSPE will have high affinity antibodies to measles, whereas patients with multiple sclerosis will have low affinity antibodies directed against measles.[27]

There is evidence for intrathecal conversion of complement in Behçet's disease.[44] About half of these patients have CSF polymorphs, which must be giving some clue as to its underlying pathogenesis.

458

Box 15.2   Inflammatory disorders of the CNS associated with oligoclonal IgG bands

Disorder	Approximate incidence of oligoclonal bands (%)	Suggested supplementary investigations
Multiple sclerosis	97	MRI
SSPE	100	Antimeasles antibody
Neurosyphilis	95	Antitreponemal antibody
Neuro-AIDS	80	Anti-HIV antibody
Neuro-Lyme disease	80	Antiborrelia antibody
Neuro-SLE	50	Antinuclear factor
Neuro-Behçet's	20	C'3 and CSF polymorphs
Neuro-sarcoid	40	Kveim test
Ataxia-telangectasia	60	Serum IgA
Adrenoleukodystrophy	100	Long chain fatty acids
Harada's meningitis-uveitis	60	Serum CRP
Acute encephalitis (< 7 days)	< 5	Viral antibody
Acute meningitis (< 7 days)	< 5	CSF lactate, serum CRP
Tumour	< 5	Brain scan

SSPE = subacute sclerosing panencephalitis; SLE = systemic lupus erythematosus; CRP = C reactive protein

In sarcoid just over half have antibodies against the Kveim antigen which is used as a substrate for the immunoblotting after isoelectric focusing.[45]

Because patients with ataxia telangectasia are known to have a low serum IgA, the oligoclonal response may be due to the exogenous immunoglobulins which are given to these patients to help prevent infections. Nevertheless, some still show local synthesis of bands which are not transferred from the serum.[46]

In adrenoleukodystrophy, in which there is no obvious aetiology for the oligoclonal response—the presence of abnormal long chain fatty acids may have a kind of "adjuvant" effect to allow the consequent production of intrathecal immunoglobulins.[47]

459

It may also be worth noting a list of diseases in which we have not found local synthesis of oligoclonal bands as previous techniques may have yielded differing results (box 15.3).[22]

The presence of oligoclonal bands in both serum and CSF, the so-called "mirror" pattern, has different connotations which will be considered under the next section concerning the differential diagnosis of two of the five types of banding patterns seen on isoelectric focusing.

Box 15.3   Disease categories of patients in whom local synthesis of oligoclonal bands is not found

- Bands are not found when infectious disorders are excluded:
  Congenital disorders
  Vascular disorders
  Headache and pain syndromes
  Metabolic disorders
  Paroxysmal disorders
  Toxic disorders
  Traumatic and sequelae
  Skeletal and sequelae including myelopathy
  Systematic disorders
  Psychiatric disorders
  Degenerative
    Parkinson's disease
    Autonomic failure
    Alzheimer's disease and other dementias
    Motor neuron disease
    Spinal muscular atrophy
    Hereditary degenerations
    Idiopathic cerebellar, spinocerebellar degenerations

- Bands are not found when complicating cases are excluded:
  Neuropathies and myopathies
    Peripheral neuropathies (hereditary and acquired)
    Radicular syndromes
    Isolated peripheral nerve lesions
    Metabolic myopathies

- Other groups in which local synthesis of bands is not found:
  Isolated myelopathies
  Guillain-Barré syndrome
  Isolated intracranial hypertension

Differential diagnosis of mirror pattern oligoclonal bands (systemic synthesis)

The "mirror" pattern does not denote local synthesis of IgG within the CNS but rather the preponderance of the systemic oligoclonal response (box 15.4).

The "mirror" pattern typically indicates a systemic type disease[48] whereas the "greater than" pattern is typical of infections (and to a lesser degree autoimmune diseases) and of multiple sclerosis. Given the possibility of infection, the information in box 15.1 should also be considered for specific antigens as well as the infective/autoimmune diseases in box 15.2. The likelihood of a "mirror" pattern is roughly evenly divided between: infection, autoimmune diseases, neoplastic disease (paraneoplastic to a lesser degree), Guillain-Barré syndrome, and other peripheral neuropathies, but occasionally vascular (autoimmune) or degenerative disease.

Either pattern basically reflects systemic synthesis of antibody which could bind to infectious antigens and we therefore require the additional technique of impregnating the nitrocellulose with

---

Box 15.4 Differential diagnosis for the "mirror" and "greater than" patterns of oligoclonal response with % given for each pattern (number of cases)

Mirror	Diagnosis	Greater than
14 (8)	Infection	29 (13)
18 (10)	Autoimmune	9 (4)
16 (9)	Neoplastic	2 (1)
5 (3)	Paraneoplastic	1 (2)
16 (9)	Guillain-Barré syndrome	0 (0)
18 (10)	Peripheral neuropathy	0 (0)
2 (1)	Multiple sclerosis	57 (26)
5 (3)	Vascular	0 (0)
5 (3)	Degenerative	0 (0)
(56)	Total	(46)

---

the antigen in question so that only the stereospecific antibodies will bind. With the more general technique applied to the diagnosis of multiple sclerosis, the total IgG population is bound to nitrocellulose regardless of antigenic specificity. Some patients with multiple sclerosis have systemic bands, which must be giving us some clue concerning the pathogenesis of this disease. Further work is thus indicated.

Prognosis and "predicting" response to treatment

Although some brain specific proteins (including the best studied case of myelin basic protein), have been found in CSF, blood, and urine, the main use of these proteins has been in sequential studies of their serum concentrations as an aid to prognosis in brain trauma. The higher the concentrations, as well as the longer their persistence at high concentrations, the worse the prognosis.[49]

Most predictive studies have been applied to the question of isolated syndromes such as optic neuritis—that is, will they progress to multiple sclerosis? Many investigators agree that the presence of oligoclonal bands makes it more likely that the patient will develop full blown multiple sclerosis, but the difference is not sufficiently great to be of help in giving advice to individual patients.[50] Nevertheless, because of the statistically significant findings, it does reinforce the idea that oligoclonal bands play some part in the pathogenesis, although their precise role remains uncertain. The amount of IgG in the CSF correlates with the Kurtzke disability scale, but not with the duration of the disease.[51] Patients with recent exacerbations have increased numbers of bands of free light chains, as determined by electrophoretic separation followed by immunofixation.[52 53] Conversely, in patients with a long duration (typically more than seven years), free light chains tend to disappear.

Clinical correlations can be found with raised CSF IgG and whether multiple sclerosis pursues a "benign" or "malignant" course—namely, the Kurtzke score divided by the duration as defined by Poser.[51 54]

There is a separate aspect to prognosis— namely, its broad use in terms of prediction of response to treatment. Myelin basic protein constitutes a major marker for destruction and possible remyelination of white matter.[55] Whitaker et al were able to show

462

statistically significant differences in the positive response to steroids over five to 40 days when they separated patients into two groups using the cut off value of 0·1 ng/ml CSF myelin basic protein, whereas there was no significant difference in the first five days.[56] Thus patients with increased concentrations were more likely to show a response to steroids over two to five weeks than those with no increase in CSF myelin basic protein.

Treatment and the search for surrogate markers

Re-examination of CSF is helpful in monitoring the expected response to drug treatment in diseases such as tuberculous meningitis and syphilis.

The more fundamental question relates to what markers can be used (either molecular, functional, or anatomical) for response to therapy—namely, the quest for surrogate markers which can supply additional information to clinical signs and symptoms. This is a slightly different question from trying to distinguish responders from non-responders—that is, how great is the response of the surrogate marker, and does it parallel the clinical response? In comparing the clinical with the anatomical (MRI) and the molecular (immunology), these can be thought of as successively lower layers of the "iceberg" in which we normally only see the clinical "tip". Just as MRI shows additional (non-clinical) activity, so also the immunological studies show additional (non-MRI!) activity.[19] Longitudinal studies of CSF light chain bands have shown that treatment of patients with multiple sclerosis with cyclosporin A showed a significant decrease in their production compared with placebo controls.[57]

Myelin basic protein is also being revisited because of the search for potential surrogate markers in response to β-interferon and other therapies. The studies of Whitaker et al on urinary myelin basic protein were less rewarding in predicting who might respond to β-interferon than the statistically significant difference which they found for CSF myelin basic protein in predicting response to steroids which was described in the previous section.[58] Nevertheless, large amounts of urinary myelin basic protein were found in patients with the progressive form of multiple sclerosis. It is especially important to look for surrogate markers in the patients with the progressive form of the disease, as their MRIs do not usually show gadolinium enhancement, unlike the scans in the relapsing and remitting forms.

Summary

Cerebrospinal fluid has been used in the main to support the diagnosis of multiple sclerosis, in which more than 95% of specimens show oligoclonal bands. This finding has become even more relevant for various treatment of "early" multiple sclerosis, in which the diagnosis should not rest on MRI grounds alone. In addition, some other immunological variables can be studied as potential surrogate markers to help predict which particular subgroup of patients will respond to treatment and which will not.

Diagnostic information can be provided for a number of inflammatory or infective brain diseases. It is also relevant to study brain specific proteins in CSF as an indicator of prognosis in a number of conditions, whether degenerative or traumatic in origin. In addition to studies of antibodies, some antigens (for example, herpes simplex virus) can now be amplified with (PCR).

Recent advances in methodology, which emphasise the qualitative analysis of the antibody response (for example, its clonality and affinity), are supplying new and valuable information beyond that provided by the traditional quantitative analysis of proteins in CSF and serum.

1 Streilein JW. Immunology, regional. In: Streilein JW, ed. *Encyclopedia of human biology*. New York: Academic Press, 1991:391–400.
2 Cserr HF, Knopf PM. Cervical lymphatics, the blood-brain barrier and the immunoreactivity of the brain: a new view. *Immunology Today* 1992;**13**:507–12.
3 Felgenhauer K. Protein size and cerebrospinal fluid composition. *Klinische Wochenschrift* 1974;**52**:1158–64.
4 Norman PM. Cerebrospinal fluids. In: Coleman DV, Chapman PA, eds. *Clinical cytotechnology*. London: Butterworths, 1989:293–301.
5 Schädlich HJ, Felgenhauer K. Diagnostic significance of IgG-synthesizing activated B cells in acute inflammatory diseases of the central nervous system. *Klinische Wochenschrift* 1985;**63**:505–10.
6 Thompson EJ, Norman P, MacDermot J. The analysis of cerebrospinal fluid. *Br J Hosp Med* 1975;**14**:645–52.
7 McLean BN. *The detection of viral antigen in the cerebrospinal fluid of patients with herpes simplex virus encephalitis*. MD thesis, University of Edinburgh, 1990:1–267.
8 Boerman RH, Arnoldus EPJ, Bloem BR, Raap AK, Peters ACB. PCR in herpes simplex virus infections of the central nervous system. *Serodiagnosis and Immunotherapy in Infectious Disease* 1994;**6**:179–84.
9 Tyler KL. Polymerase chain reaction and the diagnosis of viral central nervous system diseases. *Ann Neurol* 1994; **36**:809–11.
10 Noordhoek GT, Kolk AHJ, Bjune G, *et al*. Sensitivity and specificity of PCR for detection of *Mycobacterium tuberculosis*: a blind comparison study among seven laboratories. *J Clin Microbiol* 1994;**32**:277–84.
11 Baringer JR, Pisani P. Herpes simplex virus genomes in human nervous system tissue analyzed by polymerase chain reaction. *Ann Neurol* 1994;**36**:823–9.
12 Kamei S, Tetsuka T, Takasu T, Shimizu K. New noninvasive rapid diagnosis of herpes-simplex virus encephalitis by quantitative detection of intrathecal antigen with a chemiluminescence assay. *J Neurol Neurosurg Psychiatry* 1994;**57**:1112–4.

13 Wahlgren NG, Lindquist C. Haem derivatives in the cerebrospinal fluid after intracranial haemorrhage. *Eur Neurol* 1987;**26**:216–21.

14 Keir G, Tasdemir N, Thompson EJ. Cerebrospinal fluid ferritin in brain necrosis: evidence for local synthesis. *Clin Chim Acta* 1993;**216**:153–66.

15 Keir G, Zeman A, Brookes G, Porter M, Thompson EJ. Immunoblotting of transferrin in the identification of cerebrospinal fluid otorrhoea and rhinorrhoea. *Ann Clin Biochem* 1992;**29**:210–3.

16 McLean BM, Zeman A, Barnes D, Thompson EJ. Patterns of blood brain barrier impairment and clinical features in multiple sclerosis. *J Neurol Neurosurg Psychiatry* 1993; **56**:356–60.

17 Hans P, Albert A, Franssen C, Born J. Improved outcome prediction based on CSF extrapolated creatine kinase BB isoenzyme activity and other risk factors in severe head injury. *J Neurosurg* 1989;**71**:54–8.

18 Sindic CJM, Collet-Cassart D, Depré A, Laterre EC, Masson PL. C-reactive protein in serum and cerebrospinal fluid in various neurological disorders. *J Neurol Sci* 1984;**63**:339–44.

19 Dowling PC, Cook SD. Disease markers in acute multiple sclerosis. *Arch Neurol* 1976;**33**:668–70.

20 Fredrikson S, Link H, Eneroth P. CSF neopterin as marker of disease activity in multiple sclerosis. *Acta Neurol Scand* 1987;**75**:352–5.

21 Giovannoni G, Thorpe JW, Kidd D, *et al*. Soluble E-selectin in multiple sclerosis: clinical and MRI correlation. *J Neuroimmunol* 1994;**54**:164.

22 McLean BN, Luxton RW, Thompson EJ. A study of immunoglobulin G in the cerebrospinal fluid of 1007 patients with suspected neurological disease using isoelectric focusing and the log IgG index. *Brain* 1990;**113**:1269–89.

23 Luxton RW, McLean BN, Thompson EJ. Isoelectric focusing versus quantitative measurements in the detection of intrathecal local synthesis of IgG. *Clin Chim Acta* 1990; **187**:297–308.

24 Andersson A, Alvarez-Cermeño J, Bernardi G, *et al*. The role of cerebrospinal fluid analysis in the diagnosis of multiple sclerosis: a consensus report. *J Neurol Neurosurg Psychiatry* 1994;**7**:897–903.

25 Felgenhauer K, Schädlich H-J, Nekic M, Ackermann R. Cerebrospinal fluid virus antibodies. A diagnostic indicator for multiple sclerosis? *J Neurol Sci* 1985;**71**: 291–9.

26 Reiber H, Lange P. Quantification of virus-specific antibodies in cerebrospinal fluid and serum: sensitive and specific detection of antibody synthesis in brain. *Clin Chem* 1991; **37**:1153–60.

27 Luxton RW, Zeman A, Holzel H, *et al*. Affinity of antigen specific-IgG distinguishes multiple sclerosis from encephalitis. *J Neurol Sci* 1995;**132**:11–9.

28 Luxton RW, Thompson EJ. Affinity distribution of antigen-specific IgG in patients with multiple sclerosis and in patients with viral encephalitis. *J Immunol methods* 1990; **131**:277–82.

29 Luxton RW, Thompson EJ. Differential oligoclonal band patterns on polyvinyldifluoride membranes. *J Immunol Meth* 1989;**121**:269–74.

30 Lindquist L, Linné T, Hansson L-O, Kalin M, Axelsson G. Value of cerebrospinal fluid analysis in the differential diagnosis of meningitis: a study in 710 patients with suspected central nervous system infection. *Eur J Clin Microbiol Infect Dis* 1988;**7**:374–380.

31 Kleine TO, Baerlocher K, Niederer V, *et al*. Diagnostiche Bedeutung der lactat bestimmung im liquor bei meningitis. *Dtsch Med Wochenschr* 1979;**104**:553–7.

32 Thompson EJ. Nervous system. In: Noe DA, Rock RC, eds. *Laboratory medicine:* New York: Williams and Wilkins, 1994:462–75.

33 Hughes GRV. The antiphospholipid syndrome: ten years on. *Lancet* 1993;**342**:341–4.

34 Jacobi C, Reiber J, Felgenhauer K. The clinical relevance of locally produced carcinoembryonic antigen in cerebrospinal fluid. *J Neurol* 1986;**233**:358–61.

35 Thompson EJ. *CSF Proteins: a biochemical approach*. Amsterdam: Elsevier, 1988:117–20.

36 Jimi T, Wakayama Y, Shibuya S, *et al*. High levels of nervous system-specific proteins in cerebrospinal fluid in patients with early stage Creutzfeldt-Jakob disease. *Clin Chim Acta* 1992;**211**: 37–46.

37 Schaarschmidt H, Prange HW, Reiber H. Neurone-specific enolase concentrations in blood as a prognostic parameter in cerebrovascular diseases. *Stroke* 1994;**25**:558–65.

38 Moseley I. Imaging the adult brain. *J Neurol Neurosurg Psychiatry* 1995;**58**:7–21.

39 Miller DH, Ormerod IEC, Rudge P, Kendall BE, Moseley IF, McDonald WI. The early

risk of multiple sclerosis following isolated acute syndromes of the brainstem and spinal cord. *Ann Neurol* 1989;26:635–9.

40 Morrissey SP, Miller DH, Kendall BE, *et al.* The significance of brain magnetic resonance imaging abnormalities at presentation with clinically isolated syndromes suggestive of multiple sclerosis. *Brain* 1993;116: 135–46.

41 Reiber H. External quality assessment in clinical neurochemistry—survey of analysis for cerebrospinal fluid (CSF) proteins based on CSF serum quotients. *Clin Chem* 1995; 41:256–63.

42 Paty DW, Oger JJF, Kastrukoff LF, *et al.* MRI in the diagnosis of MS: a prospective study with comparison of clinical evaluation, evoked potentials, oligoclonal banding, and CT. *Neurology* 1988;38:180–3.

43 Filippini G, Comi GC, Cosi V, *et al.* Sensitivities and predictive values of paraclinical tests for diagnosing multiple sclerosis. *J Neurol* 1994;241:132–7.

44 Aoyama J, Inaba G, Shimizu T. Third complement in cerebrospinal fluid in neuro-Behçets syndrome. *J Neurol Sci* 1979;41:183–90

45 McLean BN, Mitchell DN, Thompson EJ. Local synthesis of specific IgG in the cerebrospinal fluid of patients with neurosarcoidosis detected by antigen immunoblotting using Kveim material. *J Neurol Sci* 1990;99:165–75.

46 Lowenthal A, Adriaenssens K, Colfs B, Karcher D, Van Heule R. Oligoclonal gammopathy in ataxia-telangiectasia. *Zeitschrift für Neurologie* 1972;202:58–63.

47 Bernheimer H, Budka H, Müller P. Brain tissue immunoglobulins in adrenoleukodystrophy: a comparison with multiple sclerosis and systemic lupus erythematosus. *Neuropathology* 1983;59:95–102.

48 Zeman A, McLean BN, Keir G, Luxton RW, Sharief MK, Thompson EJ. The significance of serum oligoclonal bands in neurological diseases. *J Neurol Neurosurg Psychiatry* 1993; 56:32–5.

49 Thomas DGT, Palfreyman JW, Radcliffe DIG. Serum myelin basic protein assay in diagnosis and prognosis of patients with head injury. *Lancet* 1978;i:113–5.

50 Moulin D, Paty DW, Ebers GC. The predictive value of cerebrospinal fluid electrophoresis in "possible" multiple sclerosis. *Brain* 1983;106:809–16.

51 Walker RWH, Thompson EJ, McDonald WI. Cerebrospinal fluid in multiple sclerosis: relationships between immunoglobulins, leucocytes and clinical features. *J Neurol* 1985;232:250–9.

52 Vakaet A, Thompson EJ. Free light chains in the cerebrospinal fluid: an indicator of recent immunological stimulation. *J Neurol Neurosurg Psychiatry* 1985;48:995–8.

53 Lolli F, Siracusa G, Amato MP, *et al.* Intrathecal synthesis of free immunoglobulin light chains and IgM in initial multiple sclerosis. *Acta Neurol Scand* 1991;83:239–43.

54 Stendahl-Brodin L, Link H. Relation between benign course of multiple sclerosis and low-grade humoral immune response in cerebrospinal fluid. *J Neurol Neurosurg Psychiatry* 1980;43:102–5.

55 Cohen SR, Brooks BR, Herndon RM, Jubelt B, McKhann GM. A diagnostic index of active demyelination: myelin basic protein in cerebrospinal fluid. *Ann Neurol* 1980; 8:25–31.

56 Whitaker JN, Layton BA, Herman PK, Kachelhofer RD, Burgard S, Bartolucci AA. Correlation of myelin basic protein-like material in cerebrospinal fluid of multiple sclerosis patients with their response to glucocorticoid treatment. *Ann Neurol* 1993;33:10–7.

57 McLean BN, Rudge P, Thompson EJ. Cyclosporin A curtails the progression of free light chain synthesis in the CSF of patients with multiple sclerosis. *J Neurol Neurosurg Psychiatry* 1989;52:529–31.

58 Whitaker JN, Williams PH, Layton BA, *et al.* Correlation of clinical features and findings on cranial magnetic resonance imaging with urinary myelin basic protein-like material in patients with multiple sclerosis. *Ann Neurol* 1994;35:577–85.

16 Multimodal monitoring in neurointensive care

P J KIRKPATRICK, M CZOSNYKA, J D PICKARD

The pathophysiological mechanisms occurring in cerebral ischaemia are multiple, complex, and incompletely understood.[1] However, despite the diverse aetiology for brain injury, different processes operate to cause common manifestations such as raised intracranial pressure (ICP), derangements in cerebral blood flow (CBF), and brain hypoxia.[1 2] Such changes in the pathophysiological state of the cerebral tissues may be transient and last only a few minutes. Although intermittent monitoring with serial cranial imaging methods (such as enhanced computerised and emission tomography) in specialised institutions[3-5] provide good spatial information, they are likely to miss transient events. Also, the necessary intensive support for these precarious patients is difficult to maintain within such imaging facilities. Thus methods for assessing brain function in an uninterrupted fashion have attracted increased clinical attention,[6-11] particularly those that can be adapted for bedside monitoring, which reduces the need for patients' transfer.

A single monitored cerebral event, such as a period of raised ICP, may be a manifestation of various different pathophysiological changes. Cerebral swelling from ischaemia (oligaemia), and increased cerebral blood volume from hyperaemia are examples in which the contrast in pathology is extreme. Blind ICP treatment in both instances using agents such as mannitol may be beneficial in the first case, but potentially aggravate the raised ICP in the second.[12 13] Thus directing treatment according to one measured variable may be inappropriate. Similarly, whereas controlled hyperventilation has traditionally been used to treat raised ICP by encouraging reactive vasoconstriction, recent evidence suggests that in situations of cerebral oligaemia these manoeuvres can increase cerebral ischaemia and lactic acid production.[14] By monitoring several different variables, each providing relevant information on different aspects of brain physiology, a greater understanding of the individual situation can be gathered. The aim would be a more accurate targeting and policing of treatment. Computer support of multimodality monitoring[15] helps the observer to identify important cerebral events among the background noise and artefacts (often induced within the hostile environment of an intensive care unit), and helps in the interpretion of complex information.

The purpose of this chapter is to provide an introduction to the novel methods that are available for the real time assessment of cerebral perfusion, haemodynamics, and oxygenation. Continuous monitoring techniques for different variables concerning the health of the brain are now available, and these include measurements of ICP, cerebral perfusion pressure (CPP), jugular venous oxygen saturation (SjO_2), and cortical electrical activity.[6-11 16-18] General systems monitors, such as pulse oximetry, end tidal CO_2, and temperature are clearly of importance but will not be discussed here. More recently additional methods have been introduced such as transcranial Doppler,[6 8] laser Doppler flowmetry,[9 10] and near infrared spectroscopy.[11]

Computing support of data analysis

In an established neurointensive care facility enormous quantities of data can be captured from each patient from which information on cerebral autoregulation, oxygenation, metabolite production, and function can be obtained. Recognition of changing cerebrovascular haemodynamics and oxygenation demands not only reliable monitoring techniques, but also complex and time consuming signal analysis. This can only be provided by dedicated computer support.

The first specialised computer based systems for neurointensive care were introduced at the beginning of the 1970s. Initially, these systems were oriented to the monitoring of ICP and arterial blood pressure (ABP), allowing calculation of CPP and a basic analysis of the pulsatile ICP waveform.[19 20] By contrast, contemporary systems are highly complex multichannel digital trend recorders with built in options for complex signal processing. The considerable flexibility of such systems[15 20 21] permits almost unlimited signal analysis which in itself can generate a state of data chaos. Thus the modern user is faced with the problem of which variables should be considered, and how the data should be interpreted. This information should then be presented in a manner comprehensible to medical and nursing staff. The mechanism of presentation is also important. Although personal computers with designated software are portable, they have yet to gain widespread clinical acceptance as an intensive care tool. They are seen as stand alone instruments requiring specialised skills for their operation, and occupying precious space. By contrast, commercial hardware systems with a customised console are more user friendly, but are far more expensive and less flexible.

The intensive multimodality monitoring system adopted in the Cambridge Neurosurgical Intensive Care Unit is based on software for the standard IBM compatible personal computer, equipped with a digital to analogue converter and RS232 serial interface. It was introduced into clinical practice in Poland, Denmark, and the United Kingdom in the late 1980s and has recently been extended into a system for multimodal neurointensive care monitoring and waveform analysis.[15] Most data have been derived from patients with head injuries, common occupants of the neurointensive care unit. However, the same techniques are being increasingly applied to those with severe stroke, subarachnoid haemorrhage, cerebral infections, and encephalopathies.[22]

Intracranial pressure and cerebral perfusion pressure

Pathophysiological mechanisms responsible for stabilisation of ICP within a rigid skull vault are complex.[6] Changes in the CSF and cerebral blood volume may compensate for longstanding volumetric changes of cerebral tissue. However, in acute injury small changes in cerebral parenchymal volume can cause gross changes in ICP and CPP. Accompanying cerebral haemodynamic deterioration may occur with the possible sequel of secondary ischaemic brain damage. Thus the continuous assessment of ICP is a key component of any cerebral multimodality monitoring system.

Reliable measurement of ICP still depends on invasive systems. Non-invasive methods, such as transfontanometry,[23] tympanic

469

membrane displacement,[24] and assessment of transcranial Doppler flow velocity pulse waveform,[25] are difficult to calibrate and have not achieved suitable accuracy. The least invasive systems available use epidural probes, but there is still uncertainty regarding the precise relation between ICP and pressure in the extradural space. Intraventricular or subdural fluid filled catheters with external pressure sensitive elements can measure ICP directly but display signal drift, have limited frequency response,[26] and present a risk of infection. By contrast, ICP microtransducers measure CSF or intraparenchymal pressures with high accuracy, minimum signal drift, and a good frequency response,[27-30] and as their support bolt provides an airtight seal with the skull bone they can be safely used for long term monitoring without concern for infection.

Intracranial pressure measurements are used to estimate CPP; providing that ICP estimates intracerebral venous pressure:

$$\text{mean CPP} = \text{mean ABP} - \text{mean ICP}$$

Sufficient CPP is required to maintain a stable CBF with an autoregulatory reserve. A CPP below 60–70 mm Hg may result in a compromise in various haemodynamic modalities.[3 8 31 32] There is also an increased chance of a poor outcome if CPP falls below these thresholds in patients with head injury.[33-35] However, policies to therapeutically maintain a high CPP are controversial. Non-reactive vessels may result in hyperaemia, increasing vasogenic oedema, and secondary increase in ICP. It is also probable that there are considerable patient dependent differences in the optimal level of CPP. Thus although many authors evaluate such thresholds in their group analysis[31 32 35 36] and demonstrate critical values ranging from 55 to 80 mm Hg, a general threshold between adequate and non-adequate CPP for each patient is difficult to define. The threshold of CPP causing haemodynamic deficit should be considered as a time dependent factor,[37 38] hence the real time assessment of the relation between haemodynamic modalities and CPP is essential.

One approach to identifying a "safe pressure" zone in the individual patient is to use information derived from the ICP and CPP waveforms. For example, the analysis of the relation between the mean ICP and the amplitude of its waveform,[39 40] the analysis of the shape of pulse wave[39] and its relation to respiratory oscillations,[41] the transmission of the arterial blood pressure wave into the intracranial compartment,[42 43] and the spectral analysis of the fundamental[44][45] and subsequent ICP waveform harmonics[46] have all been considered. The basic phenomenon of an increase in ICP amplitude with rising mean ICP was seen in the early recordings made by Ryder *et al* in 1953.[47] Using a monoexponential model of cerebrospinal pressure-volume relation Langfitt *et al*[48] later postulated that if an increase in cerebral blood volume during one heart contraction was constant, it would produce a higher pressure response when the ICP level was raised. However, when the ICP becomes very high with a compensatory maximal vasodilatation a secondary decrease in the ICP pulse amplitude is seen (figure 16.1). The linear correlation coefficient between mean ICP and ICP pulse amplitude values can be calculated and has been

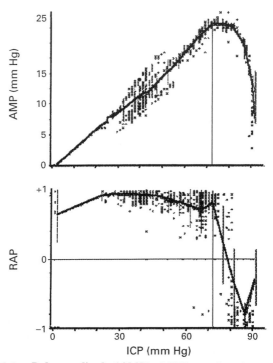

Figure 16.1 *Pulse amplitude (AMP) of ICP waveform increases with mean ICP until a critical threshold is reached above which a decrease occurs (upper graph). The correlation coefficient between AMP and mean ICP (RAP— bottom graph) marks this threshold by switching from positive to negative values. Redrawn from Pickard and Czosnyka*[6]

471

termed RAP (R = symbol of correlation, A = amplitude, P = pressure).[44 49] This index describes time dependent changes in the relation between mean ICP and the pulse amplitude. The advantage is that the coefficient has a normalised value from − 1 to +1 (figure 16.1), allowing comparison between patients. The relation of RAP and ICP or CPP in pooled analysis of patients with head injury shows that a positive index close to +1 is expected in such patients with moderately raised ICP (>15 mm Hg) and CPP above 50 mm Hg. A decrease in RAP to 0 is found with very high ICP and very low CPP (figure 16.2), which are predictive of a

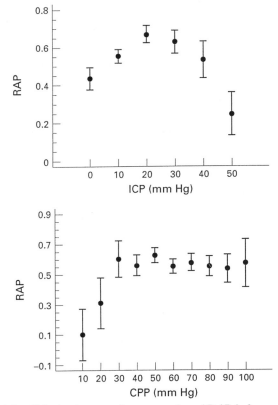

Figure 16.2 *Relation between the mean value of RAP index and the day average ICP (upper graph) and CPP (bottom graph) in a group of 56 patients after head injury (bars denote 95% confidence intervals for mean value). Redrawn from Czosnyka et al*[50]

poor outcome (figure 16.3).[50] The RAP index as a time related factor often anticipates brainstem herniation due to an excessive rise in ICP (figure 16.4). Because the RAP coefficient is calculated using the fundamental harmonic of the ICP pulse wave, the practical advantage of this index is that there is no need to use a pressure transducer with a wide bandwidth; a simple subdural catheter connected to an external membrane transducer will suffice.

Transcranial Doppler ultrasonography

Transcranial Doppler ultrasonography[51] allows non-invasive measurement of blood flow velocity in basal cerebral arteries. Most data have been derived from the middle cerebral artery as this vessel is technically the simplest to insonate, and is the most significant as 80% of supratentorial cerebral blood flow passes through it. Although blood flow velocity cannot express volume flow,[52] the dynamic changes of CBF are almost always reflected in transcranial Doppler readings. Experience with TCD in neurointensive care monitoring is still limited because of problems of long term fixation of the ultrasound probe and of interfacing with a computerised system.[15] However, the high dynamic resolution provided, and con-

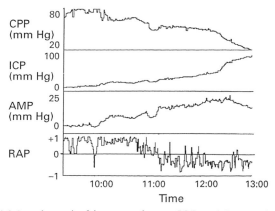

Figure 16.3   *A terminal increase of mean ICP and decrease in CPP leading to brain stem herniation at 12:30 (x axis: time in hours). RAP coefficient decreased from positive to negative values 1·5 hours earlier showing generalised deterioration of cerebrovascular reactivity reserve. AMP-pulse amplitude of ICP waveform. Redrawn from Czosnyka et al[15]*

473

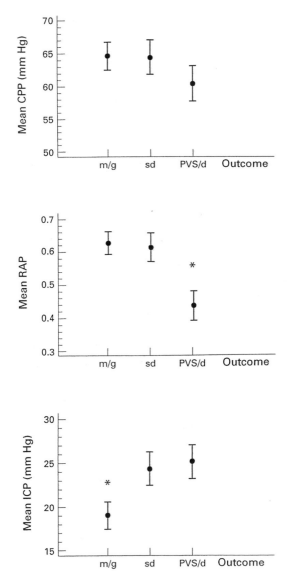

Figure 16.4   *Mean values of CPP, RAP, and ICP over a 24 hour period in 42 patients with head injury in different outcome groups. ICP is significantly lower for moderate/good (m/g) patients. RAP is significantly lower for dead or persistent vegetative (PVS/d) patients. RAP = correlation coefficient between pulse amplitude (first harmonic) and mean intracranial pressure; sd = severely disabled patients. Redrawn from Czosnyka et al[37]*

474

firmed correlation with other haemodynamic modalities is encouraging increasing numbers of neurointensivists to adopt the technique.[31 32 38 53-55] In addition to calculating the time averaged mean FV, recent TCD machines provide information on the flow waveform, which is affected by pulsations of CPP and by the resistance and compliance (mechanoelastic properties) of the cerebrovascular bed.[56] Thus transcranial Doppler provides great potential in cerebrovascular investigations[32 37 38] for assessment of cerebrovascular autoregulatory reserve, reactivity, cerebral perfusion pressure, cerebral hyperaemia, post-traumatic spasm, and in the estimation of cerebral tamponade.[57]

Cerebral autoregulation

With continuous transcranial Doppler, autoregulation can be assessed by observing the responses to spontaneous changes in ABP, transient changes in CPP induced by a three second carotid compression, or longer periods (20–40 s) of reduced CPP induced by inflating and releasing large blood pressure cuffs applied to the legs.[58-61] Continuous assessment of TCD pulsatility indices which vary according to the state of autoregulation[31 32 37 38] can be useful for the on line monitoring of critical thresholds in CPP (see later). More recently an evaluation of the gradient of linear regression between the different components of the flow velocity waveform (systolic, mean, and diastolic) and the CPP (figure 16.5)[37] show that these gradients are dependent on mean CPP and correlate with outcome after head injury (figure 16.6).

Cerebrovascular reactivity

The response of flow velocity to changes in CO_2 concentration characterises vascular reactivity. Decreased reactivity is reported with decreasing CPP[62] and in patients with poor outcome after head injury.[63]

Spasm and hyperaemia

Flow velocity in excess of 100 cm/s occurs in 10% to 20% of patients after head injury,[64 65] but the differentiation between hyperaemia and vasospasm can be difficult and often requires measurement of a further variable such as jugular venous oximetry.[48] If the ratio of middle cerebral artery flow velocity to the internal carotid artery flow velocity exceeds 3 then vasospasm is likely.[66]

475

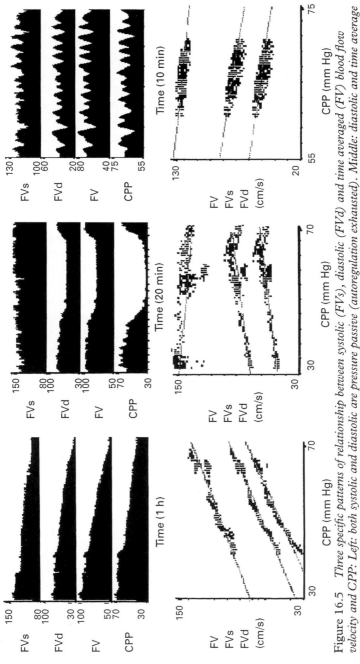

Figure 16.5 *Three specific patterns of relationship between systolic (FVs), diastolic (FVd) and time averaged (FV) blood flow velocity and CPP: Left: both systolic and diastolic are pressure passive (autoregulation exhausted). Middle: diastolic and time average FV pressure passive but systolic FV not pressure passive (autoregulatory reserve compromised). Right: systolic and diastolic FV are not pressure passive (good autoregulatory reserve). Figure redrawn from poster presented at the 3rd International Neurotrauma Symposium, Toronto, 1995*

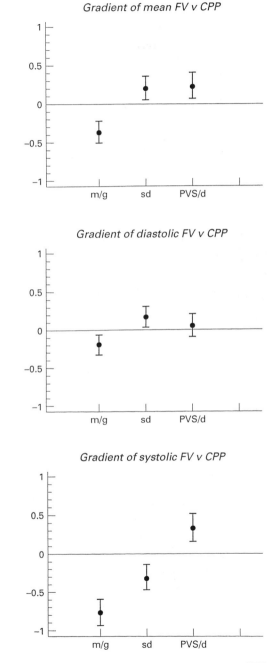

Figure 16.6 *Analysis of the gradient of average, systolic, and diastolic flow velocity time versus CPP in different outcome groups (62 patients with head injury; transcranial Doppler examinations done daily). Black bars show 95% confidence intervals for mean. m/g = moderate/good outcome; sd = severe disability; PVS/d = persistant vegetative or dead patients. syst FV = systolic flow velocity*

Detailed flow velocity waveform analysis and detection of a dicrotic notch in the pulse pattern[67] are not very helpful.

Non-invasive assessment of cerebral perfusion pressure

The pulsatility index (PI = flow velocity amplitude/flow velocity mean) is a dimensionless index that is independent of sampling variation provided the signal to noise ratio is good and the gain setting of the instrument is constant. Most modern software packages provided with transcranial Doppler automatically calculate the pulsatility index which is averaged from several cardiac cycles. The potential importance of the pulsatility index in brain injury is that increases in the index provide a non-invasive artefact free measure of failing autoregulation.[8 21 25] Clinical experience has shown a closer correlation between CPP and pulsatility index than between mean flow velocity and CPP which has facilitated the use of this parameter for the non-invasive estimation of CPP in patients with head injury (figure 16.7).

Detection of cerebral tamponade

Transcranial Doppler has been used to assist in the diagnosis of brain death. At very low levels of CPP the critical closing pressure for cerebral arterioles is reached resulting in the collapse of the microcirculation and vascular infarction. Net forward blood flow

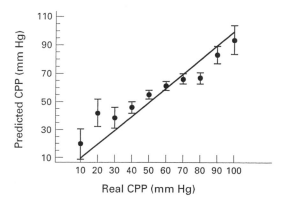

Figure 16.7   *Relation between real CPP (x axis) and estimated CPP (y axis) in 42 patients with head injury. The method overestimates real CPP for pressure under 60 mm Hg. From Czosnyka et al*[25]

diminishes and the transcranial Doppler pattern shows reversal of flow during diastole.[57]

Laser Doppler flowmetry

Laser Doppler flowmetry is a technique which provides a continuous measure of relative microcirculatory flow.[68-70] The final signal generated is a measure of microcirculatory red cell flux (the product of red cell concentration and the red cell velocity). Experimental use of laser Doppler flowmetry in vitro and in vivo has consistently shown a close linear correlation between laser Doppler flowmetry flux and CBF measured with various standard methods, and the laser light used does not seem to alter the morphological and physiological characteristics of the vascular bed examined.[71-73] The method has shown particular use in the observation of changes in microcirculatory flow induced by physiological and pharmacological stimuli.[74] However, laser Doppler flowmetry is not quantitative, records from a small tissue volume, and provides no information on the direction of blood flow. Further, experience has shown that the flux signal is very sensitive to the artefacts of local tissue pressure and movement, so that the reliability of the technique is critically dependent on the method of application.[55] Despite these drawbacks, laser Doppler flowmetry has already shown potential for blood flow measurements in several clinical disciplines including neurosurgery.[10 75-77]

Using rigid support bolts which are fixed into the skull, reliable long term recordings from ventilated patients with head injury has been achieved.[10] Figure 16.8A gives an example of a recording captured from one patient with a severe diffuse head injury during spontaneous changes in CPP. Fluctuations in ICP resulted in variations in CPP which were accompanied by changes in the laser Doppler flowmetry signal. Although cerebral events resulting in changes of CPP usually cause very similar trends in middle cerebral artery flow velocity and laser Doppler flowmetry, uncoupling between flow velocity and laser Doppler flowmetry can occur (figure 16.8B).

The advantage of laser Doppler flometry is that the technique provides a real time measure of relative changes in capillary perfusion which is particularly suitable for assessing the microcirculatory response to a therapeutic challenge. Figure 16.9 shows the effect of mannitol infusion on cerebral microcirculatory flow in

479

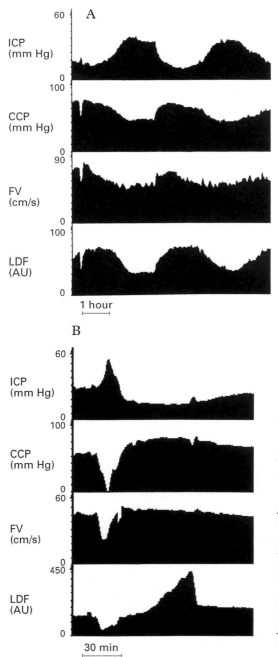

Figure 16.8 *Laser Doppler flowmetry in patients with head injury: A: closely correlated changes in middle cerebral artery flow velocity and cortical laser Doppler capillary flow during plateau wave activity. From Kirkpatrick et al.[11] B: uncoupled "big" and "small tube" flow in head injury. FV = blood flow velocity in MCA; LDF = cortical laser Doppler flux*

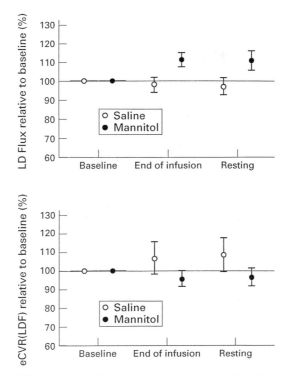

Figure 16.9   *Effect of mannitol infusion on laser Doppler flux (upper) and estimated cerebrovascular resistance (eCVR calculated using relative changes in cortical laser Doppler signal: lower graph) after a 200 ml bolus of 20% mannitol compared with a 200 ml bolus of normal saline*

patients with head injury indicating a fall in cerebrovascular resistance with increased red cell flow independent of any significant change in CPP.

Jugular venous oximetry

Cerebral tissues can tolerate limited changes in CPP without compromising neuronal function. A fall in CPP to below certain thresholds results in loss of neuronal electrical activity and, on further reduction, loss of membrane stability resulting in cell death.[1] The critical thresholds at which damage ensues is difficult to ascertain in a patient, and may be different with differing pathological states. A measure of the metabolic response to cerebral

481

hypoperfusion can be obtained by measuring the oxygen and metabolite concentrations in the venous effluent from the brain.[15] [16] This is usually achieved by passing a cannula or optic fibre into the jugular vein and subsequently into the jugular bulb.[15 16 78] The second allows continuous measurement of jugular venous saturation (SjO_2). Intermittent measures of arteriovenous oxygen and lactate difference provides additional measures of the cerebral oxygenation and metabolic state.[78] However, the technique is notoriously difficult and a high percentage of SjO_2 readings are erroneous due to complications of catheter position, impaction, or thrombus formation.[78-81] Further, it is still unclear as to which side should be cannulated.[82] Consequently, other cerebral variables need to be monitored to assist in the interpretation of changes in SjO_2. Despite these difficulties the method has added support to the notion that thresholds of CPP exist below which the cerebral oxygenation and metabolic state deteriorates, and that such states are associated with a poor outcome.[31]

Near infrared spectroscopy

Near infrared spectroscopy is a non-invasive method which attempts to measure cerebral levels of oxyhaemoglobin and deoxy-haemoglobin by observing the absorption of near infrared light. The method has been used most extensively in the neonate where interperional transmission of light (transmission spectroscopy) can occur.[83 84] An absolute measure of changing brain haemoglobin saturation and blood volume is possible, and has provided a means of monitoring the cerebrovascular response to certain therapeutic manipulations in critically ill infants.[85]

In adults, scattering of light during passage through a greater thickness of tissue prevents adequate transmission of light to the opposite side of the skull.[86-88] Thus scattered light has to be sampled by a receiving probe placed ipsilateral to the source probe (reflectance spectroscopy). This results in limited topographical resolution, as it is not clear to what depth near infrared light penetrates the adult brain. Further, the thicker extracranial tissue will influence the sampled signal to a greater proportion when the technique is used in adults, and the significance of this remains unresolved.[89] Hence, although an estimate of the light path length transgressed is possible, the use of near infrared spectroscopy in the adult brain is presently considered non-quantitative. Despite these concerns, the technique has been used to demonstrate predictable physiological changes in cerebral oxyhaemoglobin and deoxyhaemoglobin content during respiration,[90] in response to various manoeuvres such as a CO_2 stress test,[91] and in response to internal carotid artery cross clamping during carotid endarterectomy.[92]

Experience using near infrared spectroscopy in the neurointensive care setting is limited due in part to the practical difficulties of maintaining probe positioning long term. However, our own experience indicates that it can provide warning of a fall in cerebral oxygenation with greater sensitivity than jugular venous oximetry (figure 16.10).[11] In addition, calculations of total haemoglobin allow characterisation of different events causing a fall in CPP (hyperaemia versus primary increases in ICP (figure 16.11)). The advantage of a non-invasive technique which provides estimates of cerebral oxygenation with high temporal resolution[11 93] is clear to all those interested in monitoring cerebrovasular status, but the use of near infrared spectroscopy in adults is in a state of evolution requiring considerable efforts with future clinical validation studies.

Intraparenchymal probes

Direct measurement of substances in brain tissue has been slow to evolve in the clinical setting for practical and ethical reasons. However, modern probes can now be placed with minimal risks of added morbidity, and experience is accumulating. The measurement of relevant chemicals (such as excitatory amino acids) in traumatised adult brain using microphoresis techniques indicates similar chemical profiles to those seen in experimental animals.[94] Similarly, oxygen measuring electrodes can be employed for direct measurement of parenchymal oxygen concentration and are beginning to provide novel information regarding the response of the cerebral tissues to specific manoeuvres such as hyperventilation.[95 96] However, whether such focal measures will provide a sufficiently accurate estimation of the condition of the brain for targeted treatment remains to be seen.

The future for multimodality monitoring

All the aforementioned techniques have largely evolved independently of each other and have all identified their own limita-

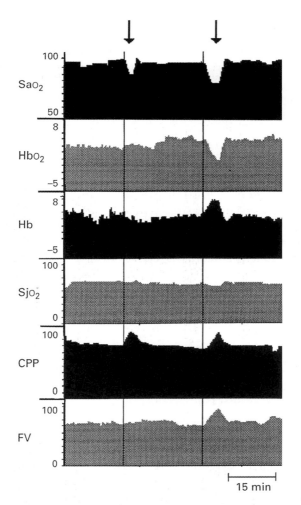

Figure 16.10   *Two successive episodes of peripheral desaturation occur in this head injured patient as recorded with peripheral pulse oximetry. The second event arrowed shows the Sao_2 falling to below 80% and is accompanied by a fall in oxyhaemoglobin and reciprocal rise in deoxyhaemoglobin. The Sjo_2 monitor failed to register this event. From Kirkpatrick et al.[11] ICP = intracranial pressure (mm Hg); CPP = cerebral perfusion pressure (mm Hg), FV = right middle cerebral artery flow velocity (cm/s); LDF = laser Doppler flux from the right frontal region (AU). NIRS = near infrared spectroscopy (recording from the right frontal region); HbO_2 = oxyhaemoglobin (μmol/l); Hb = deoxyhaemoglobin (mmol/l), tHb = total haemoglobin (mmol/l), (Sjo_2 = right jugular venous oxygen saturation (%). Sao_2 = peripheral oxygen saturation (%)*

Figure 16.11 Examples of different types of ICP waveform detected using multimodality monitoring methods. From Kirkpatrick et al.[11] Left: NIRS signals register a fall in HbO_2 (arrowed) and rise in Hb indicating cerebral oxygen desaturation confirmed by the fall in SjO_2. The CPP, FV and LDF also fall indicating primary intracerebral hypertension with a secondary fall in cerebral blood flow. Right: In this event (arrowed) increases in tHb, FV, and LDF all indicate that the rise in ICP was due to cerebral hyperaemia. Abbreviations as in fig 16.10

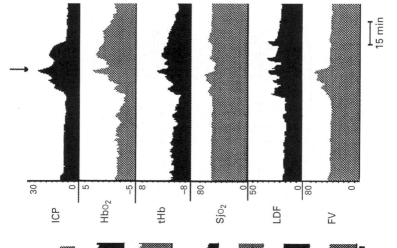

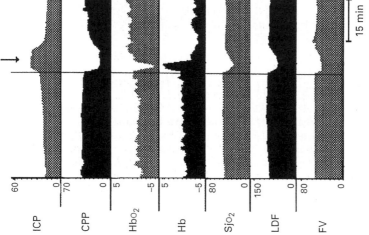

485

tions and artefacts. However, the disadvantages of one modality does not necessarily overlap with those of another. As a result there has been a growing tendency to adopt a multimodality approach to patients in neurointensive care which allows a more informed interpretation of an individual patient's cerebral state and helps to identify artefacts. Thus an event characterised by changes in several monitored variables (figure 16.11) provides credence to the finding. As experience gathers we anticipate that certain modalities will eventually evolve as those providing the essential key information. If the errors provided by these selected modalities are acceptable, the system can be trimmed for simplicity and reliability, features which are clearly necessary before these systems gain a wider clinical acceptance.

The advantage of multimodality monitoring is the increased power of interpretation. Most patients with brain injury are treated according to general principles maintaining low ICP and adequate CPP. With increasing experience we are learning to recognise situations in which general principles of treatment may at best be inappropriate, at worst detrimental. We envisage that the future management for brain injury will become more precise and increasingly dependent on monitored information gathered real time.

Summary

After cerebral injury secondary damaging events may occur which can be short lived and frequent. Their detection depends on real time monitoring as standard imaging techniques are likely to miss these episodes. Techniques for measurement of intracranial pressure and arterial blood pressure are now established in many neurointensive care facilities allowing the estimation of CPP. Although long periods of significantly reduced CPP are now known to be associated with a bad outcome, the precise relation between cerebral perfusion and brain function or injury for each person are not clearly understood. Other monitored modalities measured real time may help to provide more detailed information on the condition of the cerebral tissue. These include monitoring of venous oxygen saturation by jugular oximetry, measurement of relative cortical oxygenation using near infrared spectroscopy, and relative measures of cerebral blood flow including transcranial

Doppler ultrasonography and laser Doppler flowmetry. In addition, invasive real time monitors of brain tissue oxygenation and biochemical state using direct oximetry and microdialysis respectively have been recently introduced.

Although a complex computer system is needed to collate large volumes of data, the advantage of multimodality monitoring is that it allows for improved interpretation of each cerebral episode. Artifacts are more readily identified, and delays in implementing treatment are potentially reduced. If the pathophysiological mechanisms are more accurately identified, treatment can be specifically targeted, hence avoiding inappropriate (and possibly dangerous) intervention. The implementation of these techniques into standard intensive care units awaits improved reliability and selection of key modalities.

1 Sjeso BK. Pathophysiology and treatment of focal cerebral ischaemia. Parts I and II. *J Neurosurg* 1992;77:169–84; 337–54.
2 Macpherson P, Graham DI. Arterial spasm and slowing of the cerebral circulation in the ischaemia of head injury. *J Neurol Neurosurg Psychiatry* 1973;48:560–4.
3 Marion DW, Darby J, Yonas H. Acute regional cerebral blood flow changes caused by severe head injuries. *J Neurosurg* 1991;74:407–14.
4 Goncalves JM, Vaz R, Cereo A, *et al*. HM-PAO SPECT in head trauma. *Acta Neurochir suppl (Wien)* 1994;55:11–13.
5 Obrist WD, Wilkinson WE. Regional cerebral blood flow measurement in humans by xenon-133 clearance. *Cerebrovasc Brain Metab Rev* 1990;2:283–327.
6 Pickard JD, Czosnyka M. Management of raised intracranial pressure. *J Neurol Neurosurg Psychiatry* 1993;56:845–58.
7 Cruz J. On-line monitoring of global cerebral hypoxia in acute brain injury. Relationship to intracranial hypertension. *J Neurosurg* 1993;79:228–33.
8 Chan KH, Dearden NM, Miller JD, *et al*. Multimodality monitoring as a guide to treatment of intracranial hypertension after severe brain injury. *Neurosurgery* 1993;32:547–52.
9 Muir JK, Boerschel M, Ellis EF. Continuous monitoring of posttraumatic cerebral blood flow using laser-Doppler flowmetry. *J Neurotrauma* 1992;9:355–62.
10 Kirkpatrick PJ, M Czosnyka, P Smielewski, *et al*. Continuous monitoring of cortical perfusion using Laser Doppler flowmetry in ventilated head injured patients. *J Neurol Neurosurg Psychiatry* 1994;57:1382–8.
11 Kirkpatrick PJ, Smielewski P, Czosnyka M, *et al*. Provisional observations with near infrared spectroscopy in head injured patients. *J Neurosurg* 1995;83:963–70.
12 Marmarou A, Anderson RL, Ward JD, *et al*. Impact of ICP instability and hypotension in patients with severe head trauma. *J Neurosurg* 1991;75:859–66.
13 Miller JD. Head injury. *J Neurol Neurosurg Psychiatry* 1993;56:440–7.
14 Gold GE. Does acute hyperventilation provoke cerebral oligoemia in comatose patients after acute head injury? *Acta Neurochir (Wien)* 1989;96:100–6.
15 Czosnyka M, Whitehouse H, Smielewski P, *et al*. Computer supported multimodal monitoring in neuro intensive care. *International Journal of Clinical Monitoring and Computing* 1994;11:223–32.
16 Lewis SB, Miner ME, Allen SJ, *et al*. Continuous monitoring of cerebral oxygenation in acute brain injury: assessment of cerebral hemodynamic reserve. *Neurosurgery* 1991;29:743–49.
17 Gopinath PS, Robertson CS, Contant CF, *et al*. Jugular venous desaturation and outcome after head injury. *J Neurol Neurosurg Psychiatry* 1994;57:717–23.
18 Robertson CS, Simpson RK Jr. Neurophysiologic monitoring of patients with head injuries. *Neurosurg Clin N Am* 1991;2;285–99.

19 Szewczykowski J, Dytko P, Kunicki A, *et al.* Method of estimating intracranial decompensation in man. *J Neurosurg* 1976;45:155.

20 Gaab M, Ottens M, Busche F, *et al.* Routine computerized neuromonitoring. In: Miller JD, Teasdale GM, *et al,* eds. *ICP VI.* Berlin: Springer Verlag, 1986:240–7 .

21 Newell DW, Aaslid R, Stooss R, Reulen HJ. The relationship of blood flow velocity fluctuations to intracranial pressure B waves. *J Neurosurg* 1992;76:415–21.

22 Lee WM. Acute liver failure. *Am J Med* 1994;96(1A):3S-9S.

23 Plandsoen WCG, Jong DA de, Maas AIR, *et al.* Fontanelle pressure monitoring in infants with the Rotterdam teletransducer: a reliable technique. *Med Prog Technol* 1987;13:261–71.

24 Reid A, Marchbanks RJ, Martin R, *et al.* Mean intracranial pressure monitoring by an audiological technique—a pilot study. *J Neurol Neurosurg Psychiatry* 1989;52:610–2.

25 Czosnyka M, Kirkpatrick P, Guazzo E, *et al.* Can TCD pulsatility indices be used for a non-invasive assessment of cerebral perfusion pressure in head injured patients ? In: Nagai H, Kamiya K, Ishii S, eds. *Intracranial pressure IX.* Berlin: Springer Verlag, 1994:146–9.

26 Gaab MR, Heissler HE, Ehrhardt K: Physical characteristics of various methods for measuring ICP, In: Hoff JT, Betz AL, eds. *Intracranial pressure VII.* Berlin: Springer Verlag, 1989:16–21.

27 Gopinath SP, Robertson CS, Narayan RG, *et al.* Evaluation of a microsensor intracranial pressure transducer. In: Nagai H, Kamiya K, Ishii S, eds. *Intracranial pressure IX.* Berlin: Springer Verlag, 1994:2–5.

28 Luerssen TG, Shields PF, Vos HR, *et al.* Clinical experience with fiber optic brain parenchymal pressure monitor, in: Hoff JT, Betz AL, eds. *Intracranial pressure VII.* Berlin: Springer Verlag, 1989:35–7.

29 Marmarou A, Tsuji O, Dunbar JG. Experimental evaluation of a new solid state ICP monitor, in: Nagai H, Kamiya K, Ishii S, eds. *Intracranial pressure IX.* Berlin: Springer Verlag, 1994:15–19.

30 Czosnyka M, Czosnyka Z, Pickard JD: Laboratory testing of three intracranial pressure microtransducers—a technical report. *Neurosurgery* 1996;38:216–24.

31 Chan KH, Miller DJ, Dearden M, *et al.* The effect of changes in cerebral perfusion pressure upon middle cerebral artery blood flow velocity and jugular bulb venous oxygen saturation after severe brain trauma. *J Neurosurg* 1992;77:55–61.

32 Czosnyka M, Guazzo E, Iyer V, *et al.* Testing of cerebral autoregulation by waveform analysis of blood flow velocity and cerebral perfusion pressure. *Acta Neurochir suppl (Wien)* 1994;60:468–71.

33 Contant CF, Robertson CS, Gopinath SP, *et al.* Determination of clinically important thresholds in continuous monitored patients with head injury. *J Neurotrauma* 1992;10 (suppl 1):S57.

34 Jones PA, Andrews PJD, Midgley S, *et al.* Assessing the burden of secondary insults in head injured patients during intensive care. *J Neurol Neurosurg Psychiatry* 1993;56:571–2.

35 Chambers IR, Mendelow AD. Receiver operator characteristic (ROC) curve analysis applied to CPP, ICP and outcome in severely head injured patients. In: Nagai H, Kamiya K, Ishii S, eds. *Intracranial pressure IX.* Berlin: Springer Verlag, 1994:64–7.

36 McGraw P. A cerebral perfusion pressure greater than 80 mm Hg is more beneficial. In: Hoff JT, Betz AL, eds. *Intracranial pressure VII.* Berlin: Springer Verlag, 1989:839–41.

37 Czosnyka M, Kirkpatrick P, Guazzo E, *et al.* Assessment of the autoregulatory reserve using continuous CPP and TCD blood flow velocity measurement in head injury. In: Nagai H, Kamiya K, Ishii S, eds. *Intracranial pressure IX.* Berlin: Springer Verlag, 1994:593–4.

38 Wong FC, Piper IR, Miller JD. Waveform analysis of blood pressure, intracranial pressure and transcranial Doppler signals and their relationship to cerebral perfusion pressure in head injured patients. In: Nagai H, Kamiya K, Ishii S, eds. *Intracranial pressure IX.* Berlin: Springer Verlag, 1994:144–5.

39 Avezaat CJJ, van Eijndhoven JHM. Thesis. The Hague: A Jongbloed and Zoon Publishers, 1984.

40 Price JD, Czosnyka M, Williamson M. Attempts to continuously monitor autoregulation and compensatory reserve in severe head injuries. In: Avezaat CJJ, van Eijndhoven JHM, Maas AIR ,Tans JTJ, eds. *Intracranial pressure VIII.* Berlin: Springer Verlag, 1993:61–6

41 Dearden NM, Miller JD. Paired comparison of hypnotic and osmotic therapy in the reduction of raised intracranial pressure after severe head injury. In: Hoff JT, Betz AL, eds. *Intracranial pressure VII.* Berlin: Springer Verlag, 1989:474–81.

42 Piper I, Miller JD, Dearden M, et al. System analysis of cerebrovascular pressure transmission: an observational study in head injured patients. *J Neurosurg* 1990;**73**:871–80.

43 Portnoy HD, Chopp M, Branch C, et al. Cerebrospinal fluid pulse pressure waveform as an indicator of cerebral autoregulation. *J Neurosurg* 1982;**56**:666–78.

44 Czosnyka M, Wollk-Laniewski P, Batorski L. Analysis of intracranial pressure waveform during infusion test. *Acta Neurochir (Wien)* 1989;**93**:140–5,

45 Czosnyka M, Price JD, Williamson M. Monitoring of cerebrospinal dynamics using continuous analysis of intracranial pressure and cerebral perfusion pressure in head injury. *Acta Neurochir (Wien)* 1994;**126**:113–9.

46 Robertson CS, Narayan RK, Contant CF, et al. Clinical experience with a continuous monitor of intracranial compliance. *J Neurosurg* 1989;**71**:673–80.

47 Ryder HW, Epsey FP, Kimbell FD. The mechanism of the change in cerebrospinal fluid pressure following an induced change in the volume of the fluid space. *J Lab Clin Med* 1953;**41**:428–35.

48 Langfitt TW, Weinstein JD, Kassell NF. Cerebral vasomotor paralysis produced by intracranial pressure. *Neurology* 1965;**15**:622–41.

49 Czosnyka M, Laniewski P, Batorski L, et al. Remarks on amplitude-pressure characteristic phenomenon, In: Hoff JT, Betz AL, eds. *Intracranial pressure VII*. Springer Verlag, 1989:255–9.

50 Czosnyka M, Guazzo E, Kirkpatrick P, et al. Prognostic value of the ICP pulse waveform analysis after severe head injury. In: Nagai H, Kamiya K, Ishii S, eds. *Intracranial pressure IX*. Berlin: Springer Verlag, 1994:200–3.

51 Aaslid R. Cerebral hemodynamics. In: Newell DW, Aaslid R, eds. *Transcranial Doppler*. New York: Raven Press, 1992:49–58.

52 Kontos HA. Validity of cerebral arterial blood calculations from velocity measurements. *Stroke* 1989;**20**:1–3.

53 Nelson RJ, Czosnyka M, Pickard JD, et al. Experimental aspects of cerebrospinal haemodynamics: the relationship between blood flow velocity waveform and cerebral autoregulation. *Neurosurgery* 1992;**31**:705–10.

54 Czosnyka M, Richards H, Kirkpatrick P, Pickard J. Assessment of cerebral autoregulation using ultrasound and laser doppler waveforms—an experimental study in anaesthetized rabbits. *Neurosurgery* 1994;**35**:287–93.

55 Richards HK, Czosnyka M, Kirkpatrick P, Pickard JD. Estimation of laser doppler flux biological zero using basilar artery flow velocity in the rabbit. *Am J Physiol* 1995;**268**:H213–17.

56 Czosnyka M, Richards H, Pickard JD, Iyer V. Frequency-dependent properties of cerebral blood transport—An experimental study in rabbits. *Ultrasound Med Biol* 1994;**20**:391–9.

57 Hassler W, Steinmets H, Gawlowski J. Transcranial Doppler ultrasonography in raised intracranial pressure and intracranial circulatory arrest. *J Neurosurg* 1988;**68**:745–51.

58 Aaslid R, Lindegaard KF, Sorteberg W, Helge N. Cerebral autoregulation dynamics in human. *Stroke* 1989;**20**:45–52.

59 Giller CA. A bedside test for cerebral autoregulation using transcranial Doppler ultrasound. *Acta Neurochir (Wien)* 1991;**108**:7–14,.

60 Czosnyka M, Pickard J, Whitehouse HS. The hypearemic response to a transient reduction in cerebral perfusion pressure—a modelling study. *Acta Neurochir (Wien)* 1992;**115**:90–7.

61 P Smielewski, M Czosnyka, V Iyer, et al. Computerised transient hyperaemic response test—a method for the assessment of cerebral autoregulation. *Ultrasound in Medical Biology* 1995;**21**:599–611.

62 Newell DW, Aaslid R, Stooss R, Reulen HJ. Evaluation of closed head injury patients using transcranial Doppler monitoring. In: Avezaat CJJ, van Eijndhoven JHM, Maas AIR, Tans JTJ, eds. *Intracranial pressure VIII*. Berlin: Springer Verlag, 1993:309–12.

63 Grosset DG, Strebel S, Straiton J, et al. Impaired carbon dioxide reactivity predicts poor outcome in severe head injury: a transcranial Doppler study . In: Avezaat CJJ, van Eijndhoven JHM, Maas AIR, Tans JTJ, eds. *Intracranial pressure VIII*. Berlin: Springer Verlag, 1993:322–6.

64 Chan KH, Dearden M, Miller JD. The significance of postraumatic increase in cerebral blood flow velocity: a transcranial Doppler ultrasound study. *Neurosurgery* 1992;**30**:697–700.

65 Compton JS, Teddy PJ. Cerebral arterial vasospasm following severe head injury—a transcranial Doppler study. *Br J Neurosurg* 1987;**1**:435–9.

66 Weber M, Grolimund P, Seiler RW. Evaluation of post-traumatic cerebral blood flow velocity by transcranial Doppler ultrasonography. *Neurosurgery* 1990;**27**:106–12.

67 Chan KH, Dearden M, Miller JD, et al. Transcranial Doppler waveform differences in hyperemic and nonhyperemic patients after severe head injury. Surg Neurol 1992;32:433–6.

68 Haberl RL, Heizer ML, Ellis EF. Laser-Doppler assessment of brain microcirculation: effect of systemic alterations. Am J Physiol 1989;256:H1247–54.

69 Haberl RL, Heizer ML, Ellis EF. Laser-Doppler assessment of brain microcirculation: effect of local alterations. Am J Physiol 1989;256:H1255–60.

70 Shepherd AP, Riedel GL, Kiel JW, et al. Evaluation of an infrared laser Doppler blood flowmeter. Am J Physiol 1987;252:G832–9.

71 Skarphedinsson JO, Harding H, Thoren P. Repeated measurements of cerebral blood flow in rats. Comparisons between the hydrogen clearance method and laser Doppler flowmetry. Acta Physiol Scand 1988;134:133–42.

72 Eyre JA, Essex JTH, Flecknell PA, et al. A comparison of measurements of cerebral blood flow in the rabbit using laser Doppler spectroscopy and radionuclide labelled microspheres. Clin Phys Physiol Meas 1988;9:65–74.

73 Florence G, Seylaz J. Rapid autoregulation of cerebral blood flow: a laser-doppler flowmetry study. J Cereb Blood Flow Metab 1992;12:674–80.

74 Skarphedinsson JO, Delle M, Hoffman P, Thoren P. The effects of naloxone on cerebral blood flow and cerebral function during relative cerebral ichemia. J Cereb Blood flow Metab 1989;9:515–22.

75 Fasano VA, Urciuoli R, Bolognese P, Mostert M. Intraoperative use of laser Doppler in the study of cerebral microvascular circulation. Acta Neurochir (Wien) 1988;95:40–8.

76 Meyerson BA, Gunasekera L, Linderoth B, Gazeliu B. Bedside monitoring of regional cortical blood flow in comatose patients using laser Doppler flowmetry. Neurosurgery 1991;297:50–5.

77 Rosenblum BR, Bonner RF, Oyield EH. Intraoperative measurement of cortical blood flow adjacent to cerebral AVM using laser Doppler velocimetry. J Neurosurg 1987;66:396–9.

78 Andrews PJD, Dearden NM, Miller JD. Jugular bulb cannulation: description of a cannulation technique and validation of a new continuous monitor. Br J Anaesthesiol 1991;67:553–8.

79 Cruz J. Contamination of jugular bulb venous oxygen measurements. J Neurosurg 1992;77:975–6.

80 Sheinberg M, Kanter MJ, Robertson CS, et al. Continuous monitoring of jugular venous oxygen saturation in head-injured patients. J Neurosurg 1992;76:212–7.

81 Dearden NM, Midgley S. Technical considerations in continuous jugular venous oxygen saturation measurement. Acta Neurochir suppl (Wien)1993;59:91–7.

82 Stocchetti N, Paparella A, Bridelli F, et al. Cerebral venous oxygen saturation studied with bilateral samples in the internal jugular veins. Neurosurgery 1994;34:38–44.

83 Cope M, Delpy DT. A system for long term measurement of cerebral blood and tissue oxygenation in newborn infants by near infrared transillumination. Med Biol Eng Comput 1988;26:289–94.

84 Wyatt JS, Cope M, Delpy DT, et al. Quantification of cerebral oxygenation and haemodynamics in sick newborn infants by near infrared spectrophotometry. Lancet 1986;ii:1063–6.

85 Edwards AD, McCormick DC, Roth SC, et al. Cerebral hemodynamic effects of treatment with modified natural surfactant investigated by near infrared spectroscopy. Pediatr Res 1992;32:532–6.

86 Delpy DT, Cope M, van der Zee P, et al. Estimation of optical pathlength through tissues by direct time of flight measurement. Phys Med Biol 1988;33:1433–42.

87 Elwell CE, Cope M, Edwards AD, et al. Measurement of cerebral blood flow in adult humans using near infrared spectroscopy—methodology and possible errors. Adv Exp Med Biol 1992;317:235–4.

88 Hampson NB, Camporesi EM, Stolp BW, et al. Cerebral oxygen availability by NIRS spectroscopy during transient hypoxia in humans. J Appl Physiol 1990;69:907–13.

89 Germon TJ, Kane NM, Manara AR, et al. Near infrared spectroscopy in adults: effects of extracranial ischaemia and intracranial hypoxia on estimation of cerebral oxygenation. J Anaesthesiol 1994;73:503–6.

90 Elwell CE, Owen-Reece H, Cope M, et al. Measurement of changes in cerebral haemodynamics during inspiration and expiration using near infrared spectroscopy. Adv Exp Med Biol 1993;345:619–26.

91 Smielewski P, Minhas P, El Zayat S, et al. Cerebral CO_2 reactivity testing using TCD ultrasound and near-infrared spectroscopy—study in normal volunteers. Cerebrovascular Diseases 1994;4(suppl 3):23.

92 Kirkpatrick PJ, Smielewski P, Whitfield P, et al. An observational study of near infrared spec-

troscopy during carotid endarterectomy. *J Neurosurg* 1995;**82**:756–63.

93 Kato T, Kamei A, Takashima S, Ozaki T. Human visual cortical function during photic stimulation monitoring by means of near infrared spectroscopy. *J Cereb Blood Flow Metab* 1993;**13**:516–20.

94 Bullock R, Zauner A, Tsuji O, *et al*. Excitatory amino acid release after severe human head trauma: effect of intracranial pressure and cerebral perfusion pressure changes. In: Nagai H, Kamiya K, Ishii S, eds. *Intracranial pressure IX*. Berlin: Springer Verlag, 1994:264–7.

95 Mass AIR, Fleckenstein W, De Jong DA, *et al*. Monitoring cerebral oxygenation: experimental studies and preliminary clinical results of continuous monitoring of cerebrospinal fluid and brain tissue oxygen tension. *Acta Neurochir Suppl (Wien)* 1993;**59**:50–7.

96 Von Santbrink H, Maas AIR, Avezaat CJJ. Continuous monitoring of brain tissue po_2 after severe head injury. In: Nagai H, Kamig K, Ishii, eds. *Intracranial pressure IX*. Berlin, Springer Verlag, 1994:582–4.

Index

493